TCH CARDIOLOGY

Noninvasive Cardiology

CLINICAL CARDIOLOGY MONOGRAPHS

SERIES CONSULTANTS

J. Willis Hurst, M.D.
Professor and Chairman, Department of Medicine,
Emory University School of Medicine, Atlanta, Georgia

and

Dean T. Mason, M.D.
Professor, Department of Medicine and Physiology,
and Chief, Section of Cardiovascular Medicine,
University of California School of Medicine, Davis, California

Noninvasive Cardiology

Edited by

Arnold M. Weissler, M. D.

Professor and Chairman
Wayne State University School of Medicine
Detroit, Michigan

GRUNE & STRATTON
A Subsidiary of Harcourt Brace Jovanovich, Publishers
New York   San Francisco   London

Library of Congress Cataloging in Publication Data
Weissler, Arnold M
    Noninvasive cardiology.
    (Clinical cardiology monographs)
    Includes bibliographical references.
    1. Heart function tests. 2. Heart—Diseases—
Diagnosis. I. Title. [DNLM: 1. Heart diseases—
Diagnosis. WG141 N813 1973]
RC683.W395   616.1′2′075   73-12152
ISBN 0-8089-0815-4

Grune & Stratton, Inc.
111 Fifth Avenue
New York, New York 10003

Library of Congress Catalog Card Number 73-12152
International Standard Book Number 0-8089-0815-4
Printed in the United States of America

Contents

Contributors

NAYAD ALI, M.D., Cardiologist, District of Columbia General Hospital, Washington, D.C.

EZRA A. AMSTERDAM, M.D., Assistant Professor of Medicine, Assistant Professor of Pharmacology, and Director, Coronary Care Unit, Section of Cardiovascular Medicine, University of California School of Medicine, Davis, California

JOSEPH A. BONANNO, M.D., Assistant Professor of Medicine, Director, Cardiovascular Rehabilitation, and Co-Director, Echocardiography, Section of Cardiovascular Medicine, University of California School of Medicine, Davis, California

ERNEST CRAIGE, M.D., Henry A. Foscue Distinguished Professor of Cardiology, University of North Carolina School of Medicine, Chapel Hill, North Carolina

ANTHONY N. DEMARIA, M.D., Assistant Professor of Medicine, Director, Exercise Physiology Laboratory, and Co-Director, Echocardiography, Section of Cardiovascular Medicine, University of California School of Medicine, Davis, California

E. E. EDDLEMAN, M.D., Professor of Medicine, University of Alabama School of Medicine; Associate Chief of Staff, Veterans Administration Hospital, Birmingham, Alabama

WILBUR F. FORESTER, M.S., Research Associate, Division of Cardiology, The Ohio State University College of Medicine. Columbus, Ohio

DONALD C. HARRISON, M.D., Chief, Cardiology Division, and William G. Irwin Professor of Cardiology, Stanford University School of Medicine, Stanford, California

RICHARD F. LEIGHTON, M.D., Associate Professor of Medicine and Director, Cardiovascular Catherization Laboratories, Division of Cardiology, The Ohio State University College of Medicine, Columbus, Ohio

RICHARD P. LEWIS, M.D., Associate Professor of Medicine and Director, Division of Cardiology, The Ohio State University College of Medicine, Columbus, Ohio

DEAN T. MASON, M.D., Professor of Medicine, Professor of Physiology, and Chief, Cardiovascular Medicine, University of California School of Medicine, Davis, California

RASHID A. MASSUMI, M.D., Professor of Medicine and Director, Electrocardiography, University of California School of Medicine, Davis, California

BERTRAM PITT, M.D., Associate Professor of Medicine, Division of Cardiology, The Johns Hopkins Hospital, Baltimore, Maryland

RICHARD L. POPP, M.D., Director, Cardiac Noninvasive Laboratory, and Assistant Professor of Medicine, Stanford University School of Medicine, Stanford, California

N. TY SMITH, M.D., Associate Professor of Anesthesia and Vice Chairman, Department of Anesthesia, University of California, San Diego, Veterans Administration Hospital, La Jolla, California

H. WILLIAM STRAUSS, M.D., Associate Professor of Radiology, Medicine and Environmental Health, The Johns Hopkins Medical Institutions, Baltimore, Maryland

ARNOLD M. WEISSLER, M.D., Professor and Chairman, Department of Medicine, Wayne State University School of Medicine, Detroit, Michigan

ROBERT ZELIS, M.D., Associate Professor of Medicine, Associate Professor Physiology, and Chief, Laboratory of Clinical Physiology, University of California School of Medicine, Davis, California

Preface

The study of the details of the pulsatile phenomena appearing at the body's surface with each cardiac beat has attracted physicians from the very beginnings of medicine. Indeed, until recently the history of the clinical discipline of cardiology was strongly influenced by the insights provided by the recording of such surface potentials and pulsations. A major limitation of these methods in the past was their failure to yield sufficient quantitation to permit critical analysis of the state of left ventricular performance in patients with cardiac disease. It is understandable, therefore, that the availability of new methods for characterizing the physiologic events of the human heart through modification of the techniques of cardiac catheterization and contrast angiography has divert interest from surface recording techniques. The newer approaches to assessing cardiac function have permitted a degree of physiologic quantitation of the function of the human heart heretofore available only in the experimental laboratory. These direct approaches to the assessment of cardiac performance in man, however, have their own limitations, notably that they are time-consuming and often arduous procedures which do not lend themselves to frequent repetition at the bedside or in the physician's office. Furthermore, the techniques of cardiac catheterization and contrast angiography have a finite morbidity and are performed only in centers in which expertise in techniques and interpretation can be concentrated. These limitations have once again directed investigative interest toward the newer non-invasive measures of cardiac performance. This renewed interest derives not only from a desire to simplify quantitative cardiac diagnosis, but also from the knowledge that newly developed noninvasive measures can now be subjected to a more objective and scientific scrutiny. Consequently a vast contemporary literature on noninvasive methods of cardiovascular evaluation has evolved in recent years. This volume provides a critical review of recent research into the physiologic basis and clinical application of these methods. In selecting areas for presentation, primary attention has been focused on the procedures that lend themselves to the assessment of the contractile performance of the heart. This compendium cannot include all techniques currently under investigation. As an arbitrary approach, I have selected those newer methods that have had extensive and critical laboratory investigation as well as more conventional approaches which have been popularized by new conceptual or technical advances.

I would like to express my gratitude to the authors of the chapters, all experts in their field, who have given willingly of their talent and efforts so that this needed critique could be compiled. In addition my deep appreciation goes to my editorial assistant, Mrs. Lois Scoles, for her invaluable support and her able and efficient handling of the manuscript material.

Arnold M. Weissler, M.D.

Ernest Craige

1
Apexcardiography

INTRODUCTION

The term *apexcardiography* is widely used to describe a method for the graphic recording of precordial movements. This appellation, although in general use and therefore selected for the title of this chapter, is not ideal for two reasons: (1) it implies a restriction of observations to the cardiac apex, and (2) it de-emphasizes the importance of simultaneous registration of various other auscultatory and pulsatile events. European[1] and Mexican[2] cardiologists have for a long time used the more general term *mechanocardiography* to designate the use of multi-channel recordings of various combinations of carotid and venous pulsations, precordial movements, and phonocardiograms to provide more comprehensive diagnostic information.

At the present time, with the help of suitable electronic techniques, the echocardiogram can also be obtained in conjunction with the other previously available phenomena.[3] This technique permits observation of valve movements and chamber dimensions in association with heart sounds, murmurs and the apexcardiogram, and provides exciting information regarding the pathogenesis of auscultatory and palpable phenomena.[3] Thus, a modern approach to the diagnosis of heart disease by noninvasive techniques should include a carefully selected battery of graphic records appropriate to the particular clinical situation. In such a context the apexcardiogram can make a significant contribution.

HISTORICAL REVIEW

Clinicians have been interested in palpation of the precordium in the diagnosis of heart disease for many years. The classic textbook of James Hope in 1842, for instance, contains excellent descriptions of precordial movements in the presence of aortic aneurysm and a variety of other cardiac abnormalities.[4] Interest in graphic recordings of precordial movement led Marey, in France, to devise a capsule for sensing pulsations and transcribing them onto a smoked drum. His studies were published over 100 years ago.[5] Another great French clinician, Potain, realized the value of simultaneous recordings of various pulsatile phenomena and provided tracings of apex movements with accompanying venous and arterial curves.[6] Despite the pioneer efforts of these investigators, however, the graphic representation of precordial movements has enjoyed only a fitful popularity until recently.[7] Often, palpation (as well as the graphic registration of pulsatile phenomena) has been accorded only passing attention compared to that devoted to the more glamorous art of auscultation, supported by phonocardiography.

LIMITATIONS OF THE METHOD

Several reasons exist for the delay in general interest in recordings of precordial movement.[8] These include (1) the empirical nature of interpretation of movements recorded over the chest wall until the comparatively recent availability of cardiac catheterization and angiocardiography, (2) a confusing multiplicity of published records from different laboratories using various types of apparatus and methodology, (3) widespread use of equipment that is inadequate for the purpose, with resulting distortion of temporal and morphological landmarks, and (4) lack of methods for quantifying *amplitude* of movement and thus for making comparisons between excursions of normal and of exaggerated dimensions. Now, fortunately, many of these problems are under study and solutions are being found. For example, carefully controlled investigations using catheter-tipped manometers in the left ventricle in dogs have yielded information regarding the physiologic relationships of the left apexcardiogram,[9] thus making interpretation less empirical. In addition, there is a better understanding in many laboratories of the characteristics of the transducer-recorder system necessary for adequate recordings.[1,8,10–12] Angiographic studies in man have been used to explain external pulsations from the chest wall.[13] Finally, methods of quantitating apex movements have been devised which may make it possible to separate normal from hyperdynamic movements.[14–16]

PHYSIOLOGIC CORRELATIONS

In the studies of Willems et al cited above,[9] the temporal relationships between the left ventricular apexcardiogram and simultaneous intraventricular pressures were painstakingly established by experiments in dogs. Catheter-tipped micromanometers were placed in the left ventricle to obtain pressure curves free from catheter delay or artifact. These studies showed a very precise synchronism in the upstroke of the systolic wave of the left apexcardiogram and the rise in left ventricular pressure (Fig. 1–1). A similar relationship in human subjects has been reported

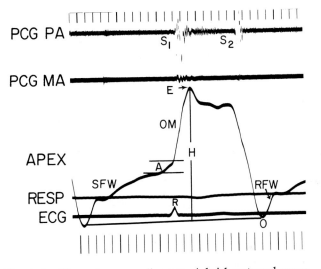

Fig. 1–1. Normal apexcardiogram. A brisk outward movement (OM) occurs during the isovolumic portion of systole, culminating in a peak (E) at approximately the time of onset of ejection. There is an inward movement manifested by a decline of the curve during systole with a more rapid fall beginning just prior to the aortic component of the second sound (S_2). A nadir (O) is reached at approximately the time of opening of the mitral valve. This is followed by a rapid-filling wave (RFW) and slow-filling wave (SFW). The A wave (A) is small in comparison to the total amplitude of the apexcardiogram (H). Other abbreviations include PCG-PA and PCG-MA, phonocardiograms in pulmonary and mitral areas; S_1, first heart sound; R, R wave of the electrocardiogram (ECG); times lines, 0.04 sec. (From Parker E, Craige E, and Hood, WP Jr: The Austin Flint murmur and the A wave of the apexcardiogram in aortic regurgitation. Circulation 43: 349–359, 1971, with permission.)

by Bush et al.[17] The early diastolic nadir in the apexcardiogram and that in the left ventricular pressure curve were also simultaneous. These relationships obtained during a wide variety of physical and pharmacologic interventions. The rapid upstroke of the apexcardiogram therefore initiates and occurs during the isovolumic phase of systole (Fig. 1–1). During this phase the external circumference of the heart is known to increase in proportion to the increase in intraventricular pressure.[18] The upstroke terminates in normal subjects with the E point, which occurs at approximately the onset of ejection.[19] The E point, however, becomes obliterated either with a pressure overload on the heart[15] or with myocardial disease resulting in dilatation of the ventricle,[16] and under these circumstances loses its value as a temporal landmark.

During the remainder of systole in normal subjects, the apexcardiogram describes a declining plateau as the volume of the heart diminishes. A more abrupt decline occurs beginning just before the second heart sound, and a nadir, or *o* point, is reached in early diastole. The *o* point is reached approximately at the time of opening of the mitral valve, and this relationship is useful in clinical situations to help in the identification of sounds in early diastole.[19] The remaining events in diastole, the rapid-filling and slow-filling waves in the left ventricular pressure pulse, are clearly reflected in similar curves obtained externally as shown in the animal studies of Willems et al. In these studies, the A wave, which is the result of left atrial systole, was less clearly seen in the apex tracing unless exaggerated by slow heart rate or vagal stimulation.[9]

In summary, although the time of onset of the swift upstroke and the diastolic nadir of the left ventricular pressure pulse, as well as certain diastolic details, are accurately depicted in the apexcardiogram, the morphology of the tracings is extremely complex and as yet incompletely understood. Ballistic recoil of the heart, rotation, and manner of coupling with the chest wall, as well as technical factors in the method and equipment affect the curves that one obtains.

EQUIPMENT

In order to secure an informative apexcardiogram we assume that one will use a transducer-recorder system adequate for the purpose. Unfortunately, in much of the literature on the subject such an assumption is unwarranted.[10–12] The most common problem in instrumentation centers on the popular crystal transducers that have been widely used for the past 30 years.[20] In general, these have been used with amplifiers having inadequate characteristics for handling low-frequency signals from such a high-impedance source, resulting in a time constant too short for accurate recording of precordial movements. The principles of physics pertinent to this argument are beyond the scope of this chapter. However, a simple test of the time constant of one's apparatus can be provided by merely observing the effect on the oscilloscope of a sustained pressure on the funnel or tambour of the transducer. If, after a rapid rise of the signal on the oscilloscopic tracing, there is an immediate (0.3 sec or so) fall to the baseline despite continued pressure on the sensing head of the transducer, then obviously the apparatus is going to yield a systematic distortion of precordial movements. This distortion is equivalent to partial differentiation of the signal: a plateau will appear as an iceberg, and a shallow trough, as a deep crevasse. Temporal alterations of a subtle and misleading nature will also occur from the phase shifts that result from inadequacy of the system for recording the low-frequency vibrations constituting the energy of precordial movements.[21] Phase shifts are particularly treacherous as a source of erroneous conclusions from apexcardiography. A partially differentiated tracing taken with a transducer-recording system having too short a time constant will result in alterations in the apparent timing of significant peaks and troughs in the record. These alterations can lead to errors in attempts to relate these morphologic features of the curve to events displayed in a simultaneous phonocardiogram. For adequate recording of apex tracings, a time constant of approximately 3.0 sec is most satisfactory. An infinite time constant as might be obtained with a direct current apparatus is theoretically ideal but impractical, owing to wide swings in the baseline occasioned by respiratory movements. The expense of such equipment is another serious drawback. To keep distortion at 1 to 5 Hz (the range of most vibrations of precordial movement) within tolerable levels, the transducer-amplifier system should have a bandwidth down to at least 0.05 Hz. For years, attention has been drawn to problems of instrumentation.[1,8,10-12,21] The majority of publications on apexcardiography, however, continue to ignore the importance of instrumentation.

TECHNIQUE

Before taking an apexcardiogram, the physician should examine the patient to determine what pulsatile (and acoustic) phenomena are to be recorded. The most satisfactory arrangement is to have a knowledgeable physician placing the transducers in appropriate sites while a technician operates the recorder. The room should be sound-conditioned, and the patient relaxed on an examining table capable of various levels of elevation of the upper part of the body for maximal comfort. Combinations of tracings such as an apexcardiogram, phonocardiograms in two locations, a carotid pulse tracing, an echocardiogram, and an ECG provide maximal information. Temporal relationship and physiologic interpretations are made possible by this means; these interpretations would escape detection in an apex tracing made by itself or with merely an ECG for timing purposes (Fig. 1–2). The left ventricular apex tracing is best recorded with the patient in the left lateral decubitus at about 45 degrees. A wedge-shaped pillow, such as that used in radiographic positioning, is placed under the patient's back in order to ensure repro-

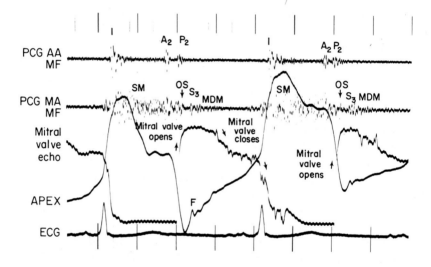

Fig. 1–2. A multichannel record of the interrelationships of the phonocardiogram, the apexcardiogram, and the echocardiogram of mitral valve movement. The patient has mitral stenosis and regurgitation resulting in systolic and middiastolic murmurs (SM and MDM). Phonocardiograms at the aortic and mitral areas (AA and MA) disclose the details of heart sounds. P_2 is widely transmitted. The opening snap (OS) occurs shortly before the early diastolic nadir of the apexcardiogram but precisely at the moment of full opening of the mitral valve as shown by echocardiogram. The third sound (S_3) is coincident with the exaggerated rapid-filling wave (F). The slow decline of the echo tracing in diastole is consistent with mitral stenosis. The middiastolic and the presystolic phases of the diastolic murmur occur while the valve is closing. (Time lines, 0.04 sec; time constant of the transducer-recorder system for the apexcardiogram, 11.0 sec; MF, medium frequency.)

ducibility of position and relaxation of the patient. The sensing head of
the transducer is held firmly over the point of maximal impulse, as
determined by palpation. The apparatus can be held by hand or by a
rubber strap. The exact site of maximal thrust can be located with some
practice and with the help of the oscilloscope. If the transducer is held
over a position away from the center of the maximal thrust, an inverted
or incomplete type of movement may be recorded, which will be misleading. Enlarged and hypertrophied hearts make contact with the inner
surface of the chest wall over a larger area and are thus easier to record.
Difficulty is encountered with obese or emphysematous patients. Probably about 15 percent of subjects encountered in clinical practice cannot
yield a satisfactory tracing.

Pulsations in other localities over the chest may be recorded in
similar manner. This method would apply to ectopic bulges resulting
from myocardial infarction, aneurysms of the aorta, right ventricular
hypertrophy, poststenotic dilatation of the pulmonary artery, or even
twitches of intercostal muscles due to pacemaker stimuli (Fig. 1–3).[22]

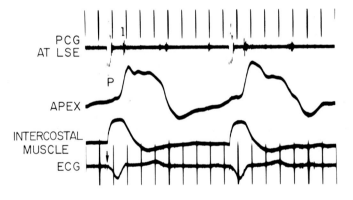

Fig. 1–3. A twitch of the intercostal muscles associated
with pacemaker stimulation of the chest wall. The phonocardiogram (PCG) records a pacemaker sound (P) which
is too early to be a first heart sound. Note that the pacemaker sound and the intercostal muscle twitch occur immediately with the pacemaker stimulus, whereas the apex
movement, which is coincident with the rise in left ventricular pressure, occurs 0.06 sec later because of the
electromechanical interval of heart muscle plus the conduction delay resulting from right ventricular stimulation
(LSE, left sternal edge; time lines, 0.1 sec). Arrow points
to the pacemaker artifact.

The position of the patient, just as during the physical examination, in general, can be altered to bring out the phenomenon under observation. Right ventricular thrusts are best appreciated to the left of the sternum in the third and fourth interspaces. Occasionally, in older individuals with chronic lung disease, the area just beneath the xiphoid may be the only site of palpable (and recordable) movement.

The transducer of the apexcardiogram senses the *relative* position of the diaphragm of the transducer with respect to its rim. Thus, ordinarily the rim of the sensing head of the transducer rests on ribs, and its diaphragm moves with soft tissues in the intercostal space. In this manner the apex transducer is capable of responding to the under-lying events producing soft-tissue movements.

Some situations exist in which the placement of the transducer on the chest wall by hand will not yield a useful tracing despite large obvious excursions of the chest wall. In severe tricuspid regurgitation, for in-stance, enormous alterations in right ventricular volume are reflected in large undulations of the whole chest wall. In this situation the rim and diaphragm of the transducer head ride up or down as a unit on the heaving chest wall, and there is no movement of the diaphragm of the sensor relative to the rim. Thus, little or nothing will be recorded by conventional technique. It is our practice under these circumstances to attach the transducer to a rod held firmly to a fixed point in space provided by a semicircular steel arch which goes across the chest and is screwed tightly at its base to a board on which the patient is lying. In most clinical situations, however, the hand-held apparatus is adequate and yields records which are satisfactory and, with practice, reproducible. In many clinical situations the diagnostic value of mechanocardiography can be enhanced by the production of physiologic alterations with isometric hand-grip exercise or pharmacologic interventions.[3]

UTILITY OF THE APEXCARDIOGRAM

Identification of Heart Sounds and Other Events of the Cardiac Cycle

In view of the close temporal relationship between the certain land-marks on the apex tracing and intracardiac events, the external record can be very useful in the identification of questionable heart sounds. The A wave of the apex tracing, for instance, is the palpable counterpart of the atrial, or fourth, heart sound (Fig. 1–4). These two phenomena,

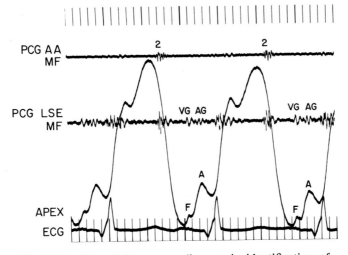

Fig. 1–4. Use of the apexcardiogram in identification of diastolic sounds. The ventricular gallop (VG) corresponds to the rapid-filling wave (F), whereas the atrial gallop (AG) is the audible expression of the low-frequency vibrations which constitute the A wave (A). The systolic movement is of the sustained variety in this 50-year-old man with severe left ventricular disease on a hypertensive and ischemic basis (AA, aortic area; MF, medium frequency; LSE, left sternal edge).

fourth heart sound and A wave of the apex trace, are of similar origin and are dependent on low-frequency vibrations resulting from distension of the ventricle following atrial systole.[23] Therefore, it is often helpful to have an apexcardiogram to sort out a complex of sounds in close proximity to the expected time of the first heart sound (S_1). The identity in timing of the systolic upstroke of the apex tracing and the left ventricular pressure curve makes it possible to dissect the preejection period (PEP) into its two major subdivisions—the electromechanical interval and the isovolumic contraction time (Fig. 1–5).[17,24] The possible advantages of measuring separately these fractions of the PEP in early systole are discussed in Chapter 6.

The first heart sound itself may, if accentuated, be indicated by a change in slope on the upstroke of the apex curve. This is best seen in mitral stenosis, in which a loud delayed mitral closure, coincident with the first heart sound, may be palpable and easily visible on the apex tracing (Fig. 1–6). The analogous event in the presence of left atrial

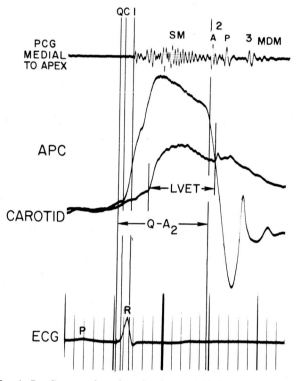

Fig. 1–5. Severe chronic mitral regurgitation in a patient
with a torn mitral leaflet resulting from trauma 8 years
prior to this test. The phonocardiogram shows a holosystolic murmur (SM) peaking in midsystole. S_2 is widely
split. A loud third sound (3) coincides with the peak of a
very large rapid-filling wave, and is followed by a brief
middiastolic murmur (MDM). The combination of apexcardiogram (APC), phonocardiogram (PCG), and indirect carotid tracing provides an opportunity to dissect out
the components of the preejection period into the electrical
mechanical interval (Q-C), the period from onset of ventricular pressure rise to first sound (C-1), and the period
from first sound to carotid upstroke. (See also Chapter 6.)

myxoma—the extrusion of the tumor into the atrium with ventricular
systole—leaves a deep notch on the systolic upstroke of the apexcardiogram, a useful clue in diagnosis of this rare, treatable condition (Fig.
1–7).[25] The midsystolic click and late systolic murmur syndrome, currently thought to represent late systolic mitral regurgitation, is often associated with a deep cleft in the apex tracing in midsystole at the time of the

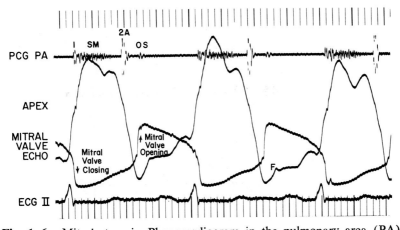

Fig. 1–6. Mitral stenosis. Phonocardiogram in the pulmonary area (PA) displays an opening snap (OS) 0.11 sec from A₂ (2A). The apexcardiogram shows a notch in the upstroke and change in slope at the time of S_1. The early diastolic trough has its nadir at approximately the time of the OS. The mitral valve echocardiogram reflects movements of the anterior leaflet. It demonstrates that the OS occurs at the precise moment of full opening of the valve. In diastole an abnormally slow closing movement of the valve is manifest by a sluggish downward slope. Full closure of the valve is achieved by ventricular systole and again the relationship of valve movement to S_1 and the notch on the apex is apparent. (From Fortuin NJ, Craige E: Echocardiographic studies of genesis of mitral diastolic murmurs. Br Heart J 35:75–81, 1973, with permission.)

click (Fig. 1–8).[26] This deformity in the apexcardiogram presumably occurs at the moment of eversion of the incompetent mitral valve leaflet. A prominent aortic closure sound (A₂) may be marked by a notch on the declining limb of the systolic excursion of the apex tracing. In early diastole, the nadir, or *o* point, occurs roughly at the time of mitral valve opening and so may be used to distinguish an opening snap from a broadly split second heart sound (S₂) or a prominent third heart sound (S₃). The S₃ occurs at the peak of the rapid-filling wave (F wave) of the apexcardiogram (Figs. 1–2, 1–4, 1–5, 1–9). The third heart sound has been attributed by Nixon to distension of the ventricle, with sudden tensing of the mitral cusps and chordae. Traction on these structures pulls the apex of the left ventricle inward and produces the rapid decline which follows and emphasizes the characteristic peaked appearance of the F wave in the apexcardiogram (Fig. 1–5).[27] If filling of the ventricle is impeded, as in severe mitral stenosis, the F wave will be diminished or absent and, of course, there will be no S₃ of left-sided origin.

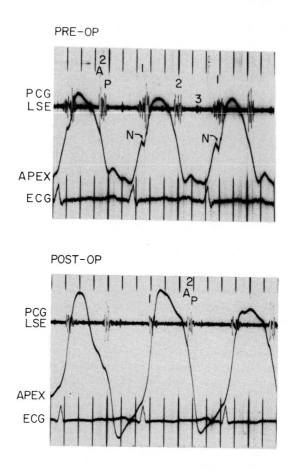

PRE-OP

POST-OP

Fig. 1–7. Left atrial myxoma. The preop (top) recording shows a prominent notch (N) deforming the upstroke of the apex tracing. A brief crescendo murmur precedes the loud delayed first sound (1). These palpable and auscultatory phenomena occur as the tumor is being extruded from ventricle to atrium. A third sound or "tumor plop" (3) is recorded in diastole. The postop record (bottom) shows a disappearance of the notch and abnormal sounds. (From Craige E, Algary WP: Left atrial myxoma, diagnosis with the help of the phonocardiogram and apexcardiogram. Arch Intern Med 129:470–474, 1972, with permission.)

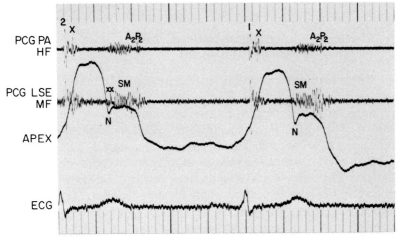

Fig. 1–8. Midsystolic click and late systolic murmur. There is an ejection sound (X) in the PCG taken in the pulmonary area. A midsystolic click (XX) initiates a late systolic murmur recorded at left sternal edge. The apex tracing shows an unusual notch (N) at the time of the midsystolic click and the remainder of the systolic portion of the apexcardiogram is low and deformed presumably due to alterations in ventricular dynamics resulting from regurgitation confined to the latter half of systole.

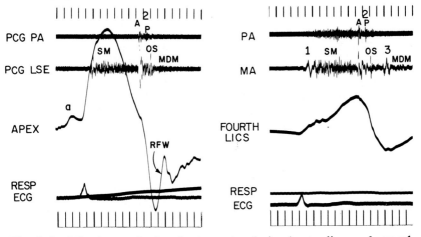

Fig. 1–9. Mitral regurgitation due to ruptured chordae tendineae of several months duration. *Left.* The systolic outward movement is hyperdynamic. In this patient the A-wave (a) is of normal dimensions and there is no atrial gallop. A very large rapid-filling wave (RFW) is noted. *Right.* Precordial movement at the fourth intercostal space (LICS) displays a gradual rise in systole to a peak at the time of S_2, reflecting expansion of the precordium due to a large V wave in the left atrium. Phonocardiographic findings include both an opening snap (OS) and a third sound (3), the latter being followed by a brief middiastolic murmur (MDM).

Physiologic Information Derived from Patterns of Systolic Movement

Three basic types of systolic curves are registered in the apexcardiogram: normal, hyperdynamic, and sustained.[16,28] Although the details of the morphology and height of these systolic excursions vary with the position of the patient and the type of equipment used, the following correlations have been found in the author's laboratory.*

The curves of *normal* subjects display an outward movement of modest amplitude in systole. The upstroke occurs during isovolumic contraction and reaches a peak at approximately the moment of onset of ejection, i.e., at the beginning of the carotid upstroke (Fig. 1–1).[30] A declining plateau is noted during systole, with a more rapid slope beginning just prior to A_2. A very steep decline is present during isovolumic relaxation, reaching a nadir at approximately the time of mitral valve opening. This is followed by a brisk rapid-filling wave of moderate proportions, then a slow-filling wave, and finally a small A wave following atrial systole,[19,31]

Hyperdynamic curves differ from normals in amplitude but not in basic morphology (Fig. 1–5). A much larger systolic rise provides a graphic counterpart to the hyperdynamic apical impulse which has long been known to be characteristic of conditions in which there is a large stroke volume such as mitral or aortic regurgitation.

Studies in the author's laboratory relating amplitude of excursion to ventricular volume measurements have demonstrated the close association between a hyperdynamic systolic tracing and a large stroke volume in valvular regurgitation.[32] These observations in man have been supported recently by the careful correlative studies in dogs of Willems et al.[15] An exaggerated rapid-filling wave in early diastole is an expected accompaniment of the hyperdynamic movement in systole.[27,31,32]

The *sustained* type of apex impulse is the third principal type encountered in clinical situations (Figs. 1–4, 1–10, 1–11). It is the graphic representation of a systolic "heave" or "thrust." The sustained type of apexcardiogram may display an exaggerated height in systole. A more important feature, however, is the plateau of horizontal or rising shape during systole. This type of movement may be found in aortic stenosis,

---

* Equipment consists of a Hellige pulse microphone transducer with an excellent frequency response in the low-frequency range (below 1 Hz).[29] The time constant should be 3 sec or more and is 11 sec for the transducer-recorder system currently in use in our laboratory. The transducer is combined with a Cambridge Multichannel Photographic Recorder for the illustrations in this chapter. Patients are studied in the left lateral decubitus.

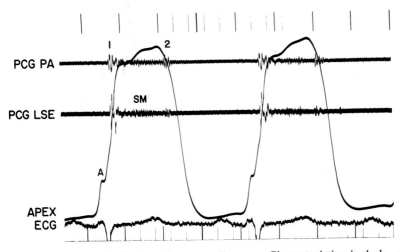

Fig. 1–10. A sustained type of apexcardiogram. Characteristics include a normal or exaggerated height and a horizontal or rising curve during systole. A prominent A wave (A) is a frequent accompaniment. In this case the A wave measures 20 percent of the total amplitude.

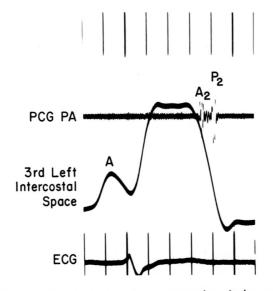

Fig. 1–11. Ventricular aneurysm appearing during convalescence from a large anterior myocardial infarction. The movement is in an unusual location medial to the apex. The bifid shape is typical though nonspecific. It consists of a huge A wave and a sustained bulge in systole over the site of the aneurysm.

systemic hypertension, or any condition characterized by hypertrophy of the left ventricle. In idiopathic hypertrophic subaortic stenosis (IHSS), or obstructive cardiomyopathy, a variant of this pattern is seen with a brisk initial upstroke followed by a larger sustained second hump during the remainder of systole.[33] In studies relating the various patterns of systolic pulsation to ventricular volume measurements, the sustained type of movement has also been found to be related to conditions of myocardial dysfunction and low ejection fraction, such as cardiomyopathy or late stages of valvular or coronary heart disease (Figs. 1–4, 1–10).[16] An explanation for this alteration in shape of the systolic outward movement in conditions characterized by poor myocardial function and low-ejection fraction is reported in the recent study of Hood and Rolett.[34] These investigators found that, in severe myocardial disease, the left ventricle did not maintain its elliptical shape but assumed a more spherical shape during systolic contraction. Since the "apex" transducer is not placed over the exact apex of the heart but rather nearer its equator, this modification in contraction pattern would be expressed in a domelike or *sustained* curve of outward movement in the apexcardiogram. A similar sustained curve in ectopic locations higher and more medial than the usual point of maximum impulse on the anterior chest wall is characteristic of ventricular aneurysm (Fig. 1–11). This type of tracing may be seen transiently during bouts of angina pectoris or in the early phases of an acute myocardial infarction, presumably owing to bulging of the anterior wall of the left ventricle. In all the situations characterized by a sustained movement in systole, a common accompaniment is an exaggerated A wave in presystole.

The A wave is due to displacement of the wall of the left ventricle in late diastole as a result of atrial systole. Exaggerated A waves of left-sided origin occur, as noted above, in a variety of conditions associated either with hypertrophied noncompliant ventricles (hypertension, idiopathic hypertrophic subaortic stenosis, aortic stenosis) or with the dilated malfunctioning ventricles of severe myocardial disease (coronary heart disease, cardiomyopathy, late stages of valvular heart disease). Among these apparently dissimilar groups of conditions the common denominator which appears to manifest itself in a large A wave (and accompanying atrial sound or gallop) is a rapid and disproportionate rise in pressure associated with the increase in ventricular filling occurring with atrial systole. Therefore, in order to produce a large A wave (or sound), the subject must have an atrium capable of adequate contraction and either a noncompliant or a distended ventricle.[23] An exaggerated A wave in the apex tracing provides a useful external clue to the presence of an increased peak A wave pressure in the left atrium.[35] An analogous explanation pertains to the genesis of right-sided A waves and atrial gallop sounds, and examples will be described below.

Unfortunately, the apexcardiogram can express itself, so to speak, in only a limited number of ways, as mentioned above. This limitation illustrates one of its shortcomings, i.e., the nonspecificity of its findings. Therefore, as mentioned in the introduction to this chapter, the diagnostic value of the apexcardiogram is enhanced when it is recorded in association with other graphic parameters, as we will illustrate below.

APEXCARDIOGRAPHY IN CLINICAL SITUATIONS

Coronary Artery Disease

Coronary artery disease exists in many individuals in a subclinical form. When complications result in clinically apparent disease, abnormal physical signs and their graphic counterparts may be discovered. During an attack of angina pectoris, for instance, there may be anterior bulging of the thoracic wall over an area of ischemia. This phenomenon and its almost invariable accompaniment, an atrial gallop, can be appreciated with a recording of pulsatile and audible events over the area where the bulge is palpated.[36,37] A similar type of curve is characteristic of ventricular aneurysm. Figure 1–11 illustrates a large, sustained systolic bulge over the site of an anterior left ventricular aneurysm. The bifid movement is the result of a very large A wave preceding the systolic expansion. This unusual physical finding overlying an area of characteristic QS waves in the precordial leads of the electrocardiogram led to appropriate investigations with confirmation of the diagnosis by angiography and successful surgical correction. The combined use of various noninvasive methods is illustrated in this case by the phonocardiogram (atrial gallop) and the measurement of systolic time intervals, which disclosed a greatly shortened left ventricular ejection time and lengthened preejection period, all of which confirmed the serious state of left ventricular dysfunction.

Studies by Benchimol and Dimond[36] and more recently by Voigt and Friesinger[38] have demonstrated the value of the large A wave (more than 15 percent of the total excursion of the apexcardiogram) as an indicator of elevated left ventricular end-diastolic pressure (LVEDP) in coronary heart disease. Exceptions have been noted in which a high LVEDP exists in the absence of large A waves, but the relationship is sufficiently reliable to be of clinical value.

Idiopathic Hypertrophic Subaortic Stenosis (Obstructive Cardiomyopathy)

The characteristic constellation of physical signs which now permit IHSS to be diagnosed at the bedside is well reflected in the apexcardiogram and associated graphic curves (Fig. 1–12). The carotid pulse exhibits a remarkably brisk upstroke and a subsequent dome-shaped curve during systole. The jugular venous pulse may show a large A wave indicative of altered right ventricular compliance. The phonocardiogram illustrates the ejection murmur simulating that of aortic stenosis but located maximally at the left sternal edge. The apex curve is a variant of the sustained type of impulse and displays a brisk initial rise during isovolumic contraction, followed by a longer convex upward bulge during the remainder of systole. Recently, studies of volume changes in the left ventricle by echocardiography have shown a remarkably rapid systolic ejection, as had been previously noted by cineangiographic methods.[39] Putting the information from all these graphic records together, one can obtain an accurate analysis of the anatomic diagnosis, as well as some of the details of the physiologic derangement.

Valvular Aortic Stenosis

Although the classical feature in palpation of the precordium in valvular aortic stenosis is the heaving or thrusting movement of the apical impulse, the graphic records obtained with apexcardiography are surprisingly varied.[40] The dome-shaped movement in systole or sustained type of impulse is most characteristic. In young subjects, however, a normal, or occasionally a hyperdynamic, impulse can be found. Attempts to discover physiologic variants of left ventricular outflow obstruction to account for these patterns in the apexcardiogram have not been successful. There is, however, in severe aortic stenosis an exaggerated A wave in presystole. This ancillary finding or its accompanying atrial sound has been found useful in predicting the height of the gradient across the aortic valve.[41] As with IHSS, the information from noninvasive techniques is best obtained from a battery of observations which can be obtained simultaneously in a cardiac graphics laboratory. These techniques should include the carotid pulse tracing, which in aortic stenosis is characterized by a slow upstroke in systole, with delayed peak and shudder (the graphic counterpart of a thrill) (Fig. 1–13). The prolonged left ventricular ejection time (LVET) is useful in predicting the severity of the stenosis. The phonocardiogram shows the characteristic murmur, and the second sound may demonstrate reversed splitting in severe cases. In congenital valvular aortic stenosis, an

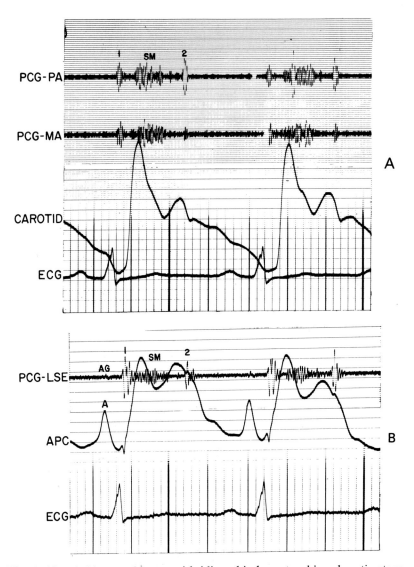

Fig. 1–12. A 20-year-old man with idiopathic hypertrophic subaortic stenosis. A. Carotid pulse tracing shows an abnormally fast upstroke and a second hump prior to the incisural notch. The murmur at pulmonic (PA) and mitral (MA) areas is midsystolic, ejection type. B. Phonocardiogram at left sternal edge (LSE) shows an atrial gallop (AG) and ejection systolic murmur (SM). The apexcardiogram (APC) includes a very large A wave (A) and a saddle-shaped systolic outward movement giving a triple-peaked effect which paralleled the palpable signs at the apex. Time lines equal 0.04 sec. (From Craige E: Gallop rhythm. Prog Cardiovasc Dis 10:251, 1967, with permission.)

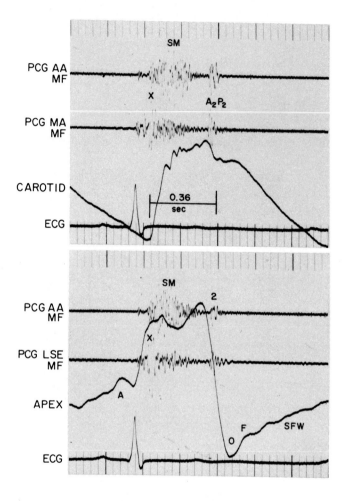

Fig. 1–13. A 15-year-old boy with severe congenital valvular aortic stenosis. A. The loud ejection systolic murmur (SM) is initiated by an ejection sound (X). The carotid tracing displays a delayed upstroke with a shudder. Ejection time is prolonged at 0.36 sec. B. The apexcardiogram is of the sustained variety in systole and is preceded by an A wave of only modest proportions, i.e., less than 15 percent of total amplitude of the apexcardiogram. Left-sided catheterization disclosed a peak gradient across the aortic valve of 125 mm Hg.

ejection sound is also noted. The apexcardiogram, as mentioned previously, may display a dome-shaped sustained movement in systole and, in severe cases, a large presystolic A wave.

Mitral Regurgitation

The apexcardiogram in mitral regurgitation (MR) reflects the increased left ventricular stroke volume. This is manifested by hyperdynamic movement in systole—normal in shape but exaggerated in amplitude.[32] In diastole, a large rapid-filling wave terminates in a sharp peak coincident with its acoustical counterpart, the third heart sound (Figs. 1–5, 1–9).[27,31]

In acute mitral regurgitation, as from trauma, infective endocarditis, or rupture of chordae tendineae or papillary muscle, quite a different constellation of findings is obtained with external graphic records (Fig. 1–14). The systolic movement may be similar—hyperdynamic in type —as in chronic mitral regurgitation (Fig. 1–5), and the rapid-filling wave may also be similar in both situations. The unusual features of acute mitral regurgitation are the large A wave in the apexcardiogram (and accompanying atrial sound) and the diamond-shaped silhouette of the systolic murmur (Fig. 1–14).[42] S_2 is usually broadly split with an accentuated P_2, the latter reflecting an elevation in pulmonary arterial pressure. In severe MR, whether acute or chronic, there may be a heaving movement of the whole precordium at the left sternal edge (Figs. 1–9, 1–14). This movement is wider in dimensions and later in its timing than the more discrete thrust of right ventricular hypertrophy.[28] The graphic record obtained from this type of movement in MR simulates very closely the exaggerated V wave in the pressure tracing from the left atrium, where figures of 50 to 60 mm Hg or higher may be recorded in late systole. This lifting movement of the whole precordium—both ribs and intercostal tissues—may be inadequately registered by means of the conventional hand-held apex transducer. A better tracing, reflecting more accurately the broad heaving movement, can be obtained with the transducer held to a rigid bar in space as was employed in the recording shown in Figures 1–9 and 1–14d.

Other noninvasive observations that permit a remarkably thorough appreciation of the disturbed hemodynamics of acute mitral regurgitation include the carotid pulse tracing, which demonstrates a short LVET, and the echocardiogram, which gives evidence of a very large stroke volume.[43]

Studies have shown midsystolic click syndrome with or without a late systolic murmur to be associated with late systolic mitral regurgita-

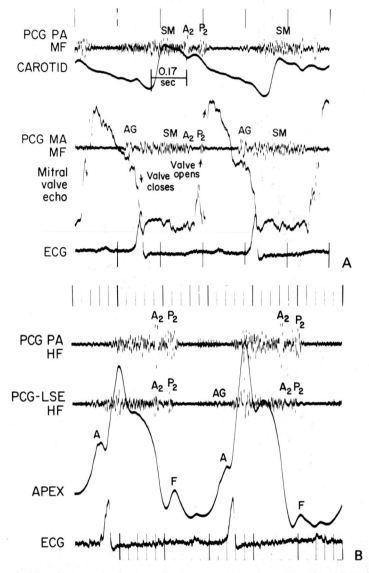

Fig. 1–14. Acute mitral regurgitation occurring in a 50-year-old woman with infective endocarditis. A. Carotid tracing with PCG in the pulmonary and mitral areas with a mitral valve echogram. There is a holosystolic murmur, widely split S_2 with accentuated and widely transmitted P_2, and an atrial gallop (AG). The ejection time is short at 0.17 sec. The echogram shows that the valve reopens only partially with atrial systole. B. Apex-cardiogram illustrates a hyperdynamic curve in systole preceded by a very large A wave (30 percent of the total amplitude of the apex tracing) and followed by an exaggerated rapid-filling wave (F). (AG, atrial gallop.) C. Jugular venous pulse (JVP) displays a dominant A wave (a) which,

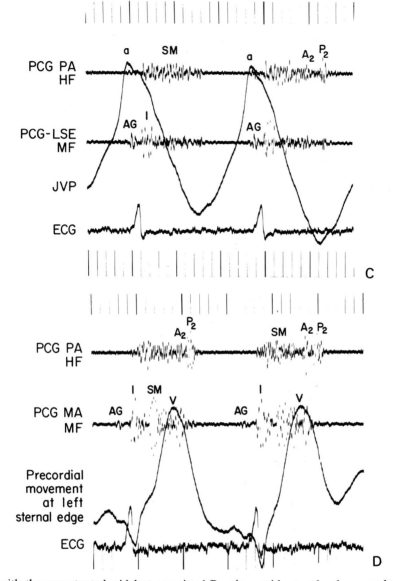

with the accentuated widely transmitted P_2, gives evidence of pulmonary hypertension. D. Precordial movement at left sternal edge. The expansile wave (V) in this location peaks late in systole coincident with the high-pressure V wave in the left atrium which in this patient reached 80 mm Hg. This movement of the precordium is a diffuse heave recorded by attaching the transducer to a fixed point in space (see text). It reflects the anterior displacement of the heart resulting from left atrial expansion and differs in morphology from a heave of right ventricular hypertrophy or the left ventricular apex curve in B.

tion.[44] An example of this is seen in **Figure 1–8**, in which a significant disturbance in ventricular physiology is suggested by the sudden alteration in the apical systolic pattern associated with the midsystolic click.[26] It is possible that this deformity represents late systolic decompression of the left ventricular chamber into the left atrium.

Mitral Stenosis

In mitral stenosis of mild-to-moderate severity, the left ventricular apexcardiogram may be of normal configuration and amplitude. The A wave is diminutive, as is the rapid-filling wave, since the stenotic valve impedes the movement of blood from atrium to ventricle. The *o* point is close in time to the opening of the mitral valve and may be used for timing purposes to distinguish the opening snap from a widely split second or third heart sound.[19] A more accurate reflection of the impaired motility of the valve as well as the temporal relationship between its opening and the snap is provided by the echocardiogram (Figs. 1–2, 1–6). When pulmonary hypertension complicates mitral stenosis, a heave of right ventricular hypertrophy (RVH) may be appreciated by palpation at the left sternal edge and may be recorded graphically with the transducer held over the point of maximal thrust, usually in the third or fourth left intercostal space at the edge of the sternum.

Aortic Regurgitation

Aortic regurgitation provides an unusual opportunity to study a wide spectrum of variations in stroke volume and filling pressure of the left ventricle and the reflection of these physiologic derangements on the apexcardiogram. In uncomplicated aortic regurgitation of moderate severity, the apex tracing may be of the hyperdynamic variety, as would be expected with the exaggerated stroke volume resulting from the aortic reflux.[16] With a more severe hemodynamic abnormality, as in chronic longstanding disease, the ventricle may dilate and its ejection fraction decline. Under these circumstances the morphology of the apex tracing may assume a sustained type of movement.[16] The elevated left ventricular end diastolic pressure, which is a characteristic feature of severe aortic regurgitation, is reflected in the apexcardiogram by an exaggerated A wave.[35,45] A large A wave, however, is not invariably present in severe aortic regurgitation. That is, there are occasional instances of high LVEDP without an increased A wave in the apexcardiogram. Recent studies by Fortuin and Craige using echocardiography to explain the genesis of the Austin Flint murmur in aortic regurgitation have demonstrated that, in very severe hemodynamic deterioration, the pressure in the left ventricle may rise so high in late diastole as to prevent the opening of the mitral valve with atrial systole. Since the valve does not open, no blood moves forward across the valve and, with no effective ventricular filling in this portion of the cardiac cycle, no A wave can occur.[3,46] The presence of a large A wave is also useful in differentiating an Austin Flint murmur from that of mitral stenosis, since if the valve is narrowed, there will be diminished flow into the ventricle with atrial systole, and no A wave will occur in the apex curve. Figure 1–15 illustrates the type of assessment that can be made using a carefully selected battery of noninvasive techniques in a patient with aortic regurgitation.

Right Ventricular Abnormalities

Normal right apexcardiogram. Normally in adults there is no perceptible movement of the chest wall over the right ventricle, and consequently no consistent movement can be recorded from the interspaces at the left sternal edge. In normal children, however, one can in most in-

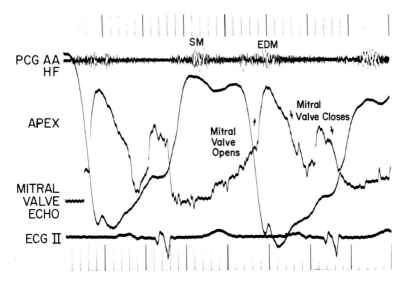

Fig. 1–15. Aortic regurgitation. Phonocardiogram in the aortic area (AA) illustrates the characteristic systolic ejection (SM) and early diastolic murmurs. The apexcardiogram and mitral valve echocardiogram demonstrate the interrelationship of the rapid-filling wave and the A wave of the apex to the two opening movements executed by the mitral valve in diastole. The closing movements of the valve are abnormally rapid due to the distension of the ventricle by the aortic reflux.

stances record a right apexcardiogram—a low outward thrust in early systole which is a miniature version of the systolic excursion customarily found at the left ventricular apex (Fig. 1–16).[10] This normal movement reaches its peak at the time of onset of ejection from the ventricle. There is a decline during systole as the right ventricle is losing volume and a rapid fall in early diastole to a nadir at the time of tricuspid opening. This is followed by a shallow rapid-filling wave, slow-filling wave, and low A wave as seen normally on the left.[10,47] That one is actually recording something different from merely a reduced version of the left apexcardiogram is suggested when a zone of inverted movement, i.e., a zone in which the familiar landmarks of the apex tracing are upside down, is recorded surrounding the optimal areas of the left apexcardiogram and separating it from the right-sided manifestations described above.

Right ventricular hypertrophy. Evidence of right ventricular hypertrophy can often be appreciated by palpation of a thrust or heave at the left sternal edge, usually in the third or fourth intercostal space. The patient should be studied in the supine position, and the exact site to be recorded should be determined by careful palpation. Occasionally in

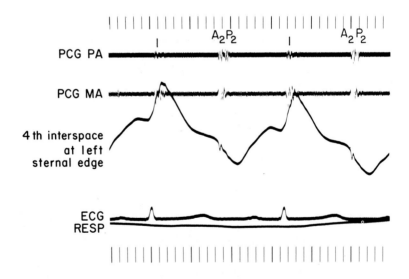

Fig. 1–16. Normal right ventricular movement in a child. The record is made at the left sternal edge in the fourth intercostal space with the transducer fixed to a hemispheric bar. The curve consists of a small A wave preceding a moderate outward movement in early systole. There is a notch at the time of A_2 and a trough coincident with tricuspid valve opening, followed by a filling wave in diastole.

emphysematous patients, the optimal site may be just beneath the xiphoid. At a slightly higher location (usually the second left intercostal space), a dilated pulmonary artery may occasionally be felt, as well as the shock of an exaggerated P_2. These phenomena can easily be recorded by the technique of apexcardiography and displayed along with other relevant graphic tracings.

Pulmonary hypertension. When severe pulmonary hypertension has been present sufficiently long to produce right ventricular hypertrophy, the right apexcardiogram demonstrates a sustained type of movement in systole.[47] This systolic thrust is usually preceded by a large A wave in presystole reflecting the altered compliance of the hypertrophied ventricle.[23] Not only the presence of pulmonary hypertension but also some estimate of its degree can be provided by a combination of pulsatile and phonocardiographic tracings (Fig. 1–17). The method of Burstin and Fishleder, using an externally obtained measure of right ventricular isovolumic relaxation time, makes it possible to obtain a rough approximation of right ventricular systolic pressure.[48] For this purpose the simultaneously obtained phonocardiogram is used to give the time of P_2, and the early diastolic trough of the right apexcardiogram gives the time of tricuspid opening. When pulmonary hypertension is severe, the duration of isovolumic relaxation is prolonged to 0.10 to 0.12 sec. In other cases, such as uncomplicated atrial septal defect, the time from P_2 to the trough that reflects tricuspid opening is negligible (0.02 to 0.03 sec), a figure associated with a low pressure in the lesser circulation. When complicating conditions such as tricuspid regurgitation are not present, this method may be quite useful in selecting patients whose disease is of such severity as to warrant further, invasive types of investigation.

Other manifestations of pulmonary hypertension may include forceful pulsations of the dilated pulmonary artery and increased force of P_2, which signs may be palpated and recorded at the upper left sternal edge. The arterial origin of the pulsatile tracing in this location can be determined by the delayed timing of its upstroke with reference to a simultaneously obtained electrocardiographic Q wave. This affords one of the rare opportunities to record externally the right ventricular ejection time. The heave of the right ventricle itself is perceived lower along the left sternal edge and follows the Q wave more closely, after a usual electromechanical interval of only 0.02 to 0.03 sec (Fig. 1–18).

Pulmonary stenosis. In children with valvular pulmonic stenosis, precordial movement over the right ventricle may provide a valuable ancillary method of estimating the severity of the obstruction. Where the

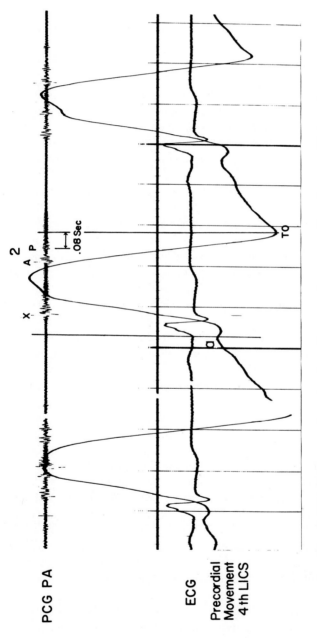

Fig. 1–17. Pulmonary hypertension of severe degree resulting from multiple pulmonary emboli. The phonocardiogram in the pulmonary area demonstrates an ejection sound, soft systolic murmur and widely split S_2. Precordial movement in the fourth left intercostal space (LICS) is a sustained heave of huge proportions. The duration of isovolumic relaxation measured from P_2 to tricuspid opening (TO) is prolonged at 0.08 sec, providing a rough measure of the degree of pulmonary arterial hypertension.[48]

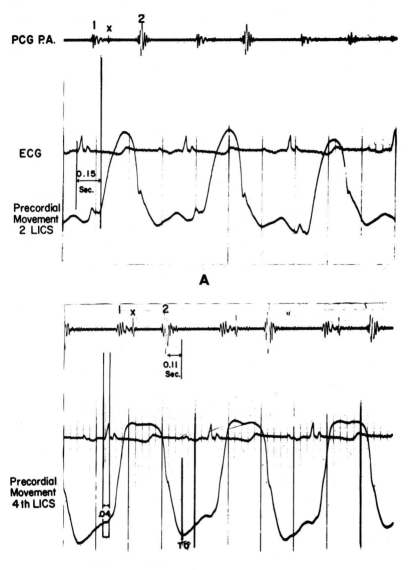

Fig. 1–18. Pulmonary hypertension, severe associated with a large atrial septal defect with right to left shunt. PCG displays a prominent ejection sound (X). Precordial movement at the left sternal edge is the result of pulmonary arterial expansion in the second left intercostal space (A) but reflects right ventricular systole in the fourth interspace (B). The morphology of the curves and the time of onset from Q reflects the differing origin of pulsations in the two localities. The prolongation of isovolumic relaxation time (P_2 to tricuspid opening) of 0.11 sec reflects the severity of the pulmonary hypertension.[48]

29

right ventricular systolic pressure exceeds approximately 60 mm Hg, one can usually record a convex or sustained systolic movement at the left sternal edge (Fig. 1–19).[49] Usually the systolic expansion is preceded by an A wave of increased size, reflecting the altered compliance of the hypertrophied ventricle. The accompanying phonocardiogram from the pulmonary area demonstrates a wide separation of A₂ and P₂. Measurement of the delay of P₂ provides probably the most sensitive noninvasive method of estimating the severity of the obstruction.[50]

Tetralogy of Fallot.   Although the degree of infundibular stenosis in this condition may be extreme, and right ventricular pressures equal to those in the left ventricle are to be expected, the precordial movement in cyanotic children with tetralogy of Fallot is extraordinarily quiet. There is usually a quick, very transitory thrust at the time of isovolumic contraction, followed by a plateau or even a concave movement in systole at the left sternal edge (Fig. 1–20). A second major vibration may be recorded at the time of the single second sound in the accompanying phonocardiogram. There is no atrial sound and no exaggeration of the

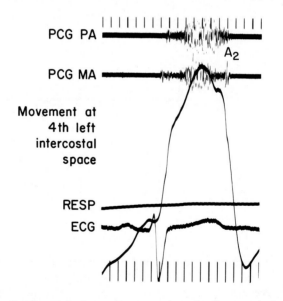

Fig. 1–19.   Valvular pulmonary stenosis. Severe obstruction in a child is reflected in the late peaking ejection murmur which runs into A₂. P₂ is not visible. Precordial movement is very abnormal and consists of a sustained outward thrust at the fourth left intercostal space, resulting from right ventricular hypertrophy.

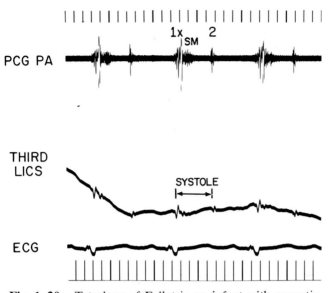

Fig. 1–20. Tetrology of Fallot in an infant with cyanotic congenital heart disease. The phonocardiogram illustrates an ejection sound (X), presumably aortic in origin. The systolic murmur is very brief as is characteristic in a severe disease. S_2 is single. Precordial movement over the right ventricle is minimal, and consists of brief shocks at the time of the heart sounds but no heave of right ventricular hypertrophy despite systemic pressures in that chamber.

A waves in the right apexcardiogram or the jugular venous pulse. These differences between the pulsatile records in cyanotic tetralogy of Fallot and pure valvular pulmonic stenosis probably result from the escape route afforded by the right-to-left shunt through the septal defect which may serve to decompress the right ventricle. In "pink tetralogy," in which the shunt is left to right, an altogether different picture is seen in graphic records. The right ventricular apexcardiogram is usually much increased in amplitude and sustained in its morphology. The accompanying phonocardiogram displays a widely separated S_2 with P_2 easily visible. In this situation one can estimate right ventricular systolic pressure roughly from the amount of separation of A_2 and P_2, and the pulmonary arterial pressure from the duration of isovolumic relaxation as described above in the section on pulmonary hypertension.[48]

Tricuspid regurgitation. Tricuspid regurgitation usually appears as a late manifestation of mitral stenosis when complicated by pulmonary hypertension, right ventricular hypertrophy, dilatation, and failure. In this situation there may be a significant heave at the left sternal edge. Graphic recordings are as described above under pulmonary hypertension. Tracings made over the jugular vein and liver will reflect characteristic systolic expansions.

In rare instances, however, as with trauma or infective endocarditis there may be isolated tricuspid regurgitation in the absence of pulmonary hypertension. Under these circumstances the right ventricular "heave" often reported on physical examination may be found, on graphic recordings, actually to be an expansion in early *diastole*.[28] In systole, the predominant movement at the left sternal edge in the presence of tricuspid regurgitation in the absence of pulmonary hypertension is an *inward* excursion. This movement reflects the loss of volume of the right ventricle and is practically a mirror image of the expansile tracings obtained over the great veins and liver (Fig. 1–21).

In constrictive pericarditis, a similar *inward* movement over the whole precordium may be appreciated by palpation and graphic records (Fig. 1–22). This movement is presumably due to widespread pleuro-

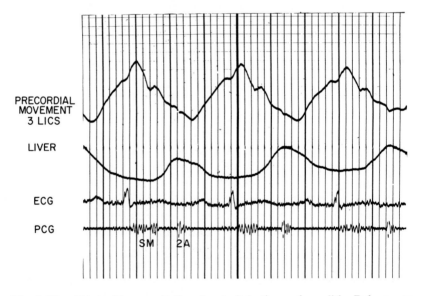

Fig. 1–21. Tricuspid regurgitation due to infective endocarditis. Pulmonary arterial pressure was normal. Massive regurgitation results in an inward movement during systole over the right ventricle, as it loses volume. A corresponding expansion of the liver and jugular venous pulse (not shown) is typical.

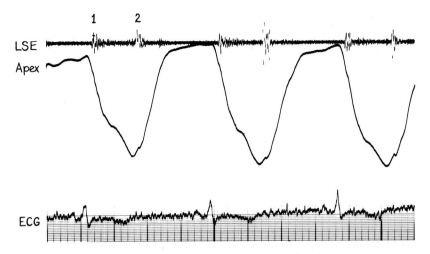

Fig. 1–22. Constrictive pericarditis. An inward movement over the precordium results from adhesive disease of precordial and pleural surfaces. The simultaneous phonocardiogram illustrates the usefulness of the heart sounds in avoiding confusion between systole and diastole in this situation in which the predominant "thrust" is diastolic.

pericardial adhesions. Palpation may be misleading, with inadvertent inversion of the phases of the cardiac cycle, unless one is careful to use the heart sounds or the carotid pulse as a temporal landmark.[28]

COMPARISON OF APEXCARDIOGRAPHY AND KINETOCARDIOGRAPHY

In Chapter 4 the technique of kinetocardiography (KCG) is described with illustrations of its usefulness in diagnosis. Since the KCG obviously is recording precordial impulses similar to those observed in apexcardiography (ACG), a few words may be in order to compare the two methods.

Kinetocardiography is recorded by means of a transducer attached to a fixed point in space. Thus it records "absolute" movement of the precordium in contrast to apexcardiography in which only the *relative* movement of the movable diaphragm of the transducer to the rim of the sensing head is registered.[51] In kinetocardiography the patient lies supine, and tracings are made from a series of fixed points at several intercostal spaces according to a prearranged protocol. In apexcardiography, the left ventricular impulse is usually recorded with the patient lying in the left lateral decubitus with the transducer applied to the point of maximum impulse as determined by palpation. Obviously, under these circumstances (patient on his left side) the impulse that is palpated and recorded will be exaggerated in amplitude as compared with standards obtained in the supine position. There is, however, ample precedent for feeling, hearing, and recording various physical findings in body positions known to "bring out," for example, a diastolic rumble, a gallop, or a spleen that is being looked for. Standards of normality are set up by experienced clinicians and recorders of precordial movement appropriate to the body position in which the patient is placed. Actually, none of the transducers in use for either KCG or ACG is ideal, for the "absolute" movement of the precordium is an elusive goal. The pressure of the transducer itself alters the vibrating characteristics of the chest wall on which it is pressed. Efforts to escape this distortion by means of electronic transducers that can be held just off the chest wall are satisfactory for appreciating systolic expansions but fail to provide faithful recordings of inward movements because of the interposition of loose fat over the chest wall.[52] Thus, events in diastole which mirror so accurately the morphology of the intraventricular pressure curve may be missed.[15] Of the several methods under consideration—ACG, KCG, and other techniques that do not touch the chest at all—only the ACG with the patient in the left lateral decubitus provides an adequate representation of diastolic events. With children or uncooperative patients who cannot remain quietly apneic for a short period, respiratory excursions may result in wide swings of the baseline when one is recording, as with KCG from a fixed point in space.

The most valuable information is derived from apexcardiography in the author's laboratory when the technique is used in conjunction with a battery of other graphic records, including echocardiography, as stressed earlier in this chapter. The most informative collection of graphic curves can be obtained by an experienced observer only after careful examination of the patient so that the appropriate choice of external recordings, frequencies, and positions can be selected for the particular diagnostic problem at hand. The same possibilities for combined recordings exist for kinetocardiography, and some published records of multichannel recordings are quite informative.[53] The majority of published KCG records, however, illustrate only the pulsatile chest wall movement in fixed prearranged locations without other simultaneous recordings. Such a record has the advantage that it can be made by a technician alone. This valuable method could be even more useful if combined with other graphic techniques. When any noninvasive technique—apexcardiography, systolic time intervals, echocardiography, or phonocardiography—is used as the *sole* method of external graphic recording, a whole host of exciting relationships may fail to come to one's attention.

SUMMARY

Apexcardiography has a useful role to play in the assessment of anatomic and physiologic abnormalities in heart disease. Its usefulness, long under a cloud because of the empirical nature of the method, is now being established, thanks to improved recording methods, including devices for quantitation, as well as more precise physiologic correlations in both man and experimental animals.

Apex tracings provide excellent temporal landmarks for the onset of the rise in left ventricular pressure and the early diastolic nadir in the intraventricular pressure pulse. Atypical sounds, third heart sounds, opening snaps, and pacemaker sounds can be identified in accompanying phonocardiograms with the help of the apexcardiogram. Apex tracings can be divided into three major types: normal, hyperdynamic, and sustained. The *normal* apex impulse is of relatively low height and tends to fall away in systole. It is accompanied by a small A wave in presystole and modest rapid-filling wave in early diastole. The *hyperdynamic* impulse is found in conditions characterized by a large stroke volume, such as mitral or aortic regurgitation. It is exaggerated in height but similar to the normal in morphology. The *sustained* record is marked by a domed or rising curve in systole, the graphic accompaniment of a heave or thrust. Such a movement is found in left ventricular hypertrophy or in the presence of a dilated ventricle with low-ejection fraction. Usually a large A wave precedes the systolic outward movement. The apex movement of idiopathic hypertrophic subaortic stenosis is a variant of the sustained type of tracing.

The technique of apexcardiography is quite versatile, more so than its name implies. The apparatus can be used to record movements of aneurysms, pulmonary arterial pulsations, thrusts or right ventricular hypertrophy, inward movements caused by tricuspid regurgitation or constrictive pericarditis, or even twitches of intercostal muscles stimulated inadvertently by pacemakers. The position of the patient and the location of the transducer can be varied at will by an experienced cardiologist in order to obtain the best tracing to illustrate the physical finding in question. The apparatus, however, must be appropriate for the purpose, and much instrumentation that is commercially available is not. The most informative records are those taken in conjunction with other external graphic methods. An apexcardiogram with only an electrocardiogram, for instance, is a feeble source of diagnostic data compared to a full panel of multichannel records especially selected for the problem at hand. A modern apexcardiogram then should be studied in the context of simultaneous phonocardiograms, cartoid pulse tracings, jugular venous tracings, and echocardiograms.

ACKNOWLEDGMENTS

The author is indebted to Dr. Nicholas J. Fortuin and Dr. David K. Millward for help with the figures illustrating the combined use of echocardiography and other graphic techniques and to Dr. Aubrey Leatham of St. George's Hospital London in whose laboratory the graphic records for Figures 1–1, 1–9, 1–16, 1–19, 1–20 were made. Invaluable technical assistance was provided by Mrs. Sally Moos.

REFERENCES

1. Kesteloot H, Willems J, Vollenhoven E van: On the physical principles and methodology of mechanocardiography. Acta Cardiol 24:147–160, 1969
2. Fishleder, BL: Exploracion cardiovascular y fonomecanocardiografia clinica. Prensa Med Mex: 1966, p 1
3. Fortuin NJ, Craige E: On the mechanism of the Austin Flint murmur. Circulation 45:558–570, 1970
4. Hope J: A Treatise on the Diseases of the Heart and Great Vessels. Philadelphia, Lea and Blanchard, 1842, p 427
5. Chauveau A, Marey EJ: Détermination graphique des rapports de la pulsation cardiaque avec les mouvements de l'oreillette et du ventricule, obtenue au moyen d'un appareil enregistreur. Gaz Med (Paris) 31:675–678, 1861
6. Potain C: Du rhythme cardiaque appelé bruit de galop. Bull Mem Soc Med Hôp (Paris) Ser 2, 12:137, 1875
7. Hartman H, Snellen HA: The apex cardiogram. Proc 3rd Eur Cong Cardiology (Rome, Pars Altera 2: (pt B) 711, 1960
8. Craige E: Clinical value of apex cardiography. Am J Cardiol 28:118–121, 1971
9. Willems JL, De Geest H, Kestleloot H: On the value of apex cardiography for timing intracardiac events. Am J Cardiol 28:59–66, 1971
10. Craige E, Schmidt RE: Precordial movements over the right ventricle in normal children. Circulation 32:232–240, 1965

11. Roberts, DV, Jones ES: A new system for recording the apex beat. Lancet. 1:1193, 1963

12. Mashimo K, Tanabe Y, Kinoshita S, Sakamoto S, Tsaushima N: An instrumental aspect of apexcardiography: Decay characteristic of transducers and its clinical implication. Jap Heart J 7:536–542, 1966

13. Deliyannis AA, Gillam PMS, Mounsey JPD, Steiner RE: The cardiac impulse and the motion of the heart. Br Heart J 26:396–411, 1964

14. Sutton GC, Craige E: Quantitation of precordial movement. 1. Normal subjects. Circulation 35:476–482, 1967

15. Willems JL, Kesteloot H, De Geest H: Influence of acute hemodynamic changes on the apex cardiogram in dogs. Am J Cardiol 29:504–513, 1972

16. Sutton GC, Prewitt TA, Craige E: Relationship between quantitated precordial movement and left ventricular function. Circulation 41:179–190, 1970

17. Bush CA, Lewis RP, Leighton RE, et al: Verification of systolic time intervals and true isovolumic contraction time from the apexcardiogram by micromanometer catheterization of the left ventricle and aorta (abstr). Circulation 41: (Suppl) 3:121, 1970

18. Hawthorne EW: Instantaneous dimensional changes of the left ventricle in dogs. Circ Res 9:110, 1961

19. Tavel ME, Campbell RW, Feigenbaum H, Steinmetz EF: The apexcardiogram and its relationship to hemodynamic events within the left heart. Br Heart J 27:829–839, 1965

20. Miller A, White PD: Crystal microphone for pulse wave recording. Am Heart J 21:504–510, 1941

21. Leech G: Measurement problems in external pulse recording. Annual Meeting of the Laenaec Society of the AHA. Anaheim, Calif. Nov. 10, 1971

22. Harris A: Pacemaker "heart sound". Br Heart J 29:608–615, 1967

23. Craige E: Gallop rhythm. Prog Cardiovasc Dis 10:246–261, 1967

24. Sutton R, Hood WP Jr, Craige E: Correlation of pre-ejection period with left ventricular ejection fraction (abstr). Clin Res 18:28, 1970

25. Craige E, Algary WP: Left atrial myxoma, diagnosis with the help of the phonocardiogram and apexcardiogram. Arch Intern Med 129:470–474, 1972

26. Lucardie SM, Durrer D: The late systolic murmur. Arch Kreislaufforsch 53: 174–192, 1967

27. Nixon PGF, Wooler GH: Phases of diastole in various syndromes of mitral valvular disease. Br Heart J 25:393–404, 1963

28. Mounsey JPD: Inspection and palpation of the cardiac impulse. Prog Cardiovasc Dis 10:187–206, 1967

29. Lohr HA, Vollenhoven E van, Rotterdam W van: Fundamentals in vibrocardiography. Precordial accelerography and acceleration ballistocardiography. Am Heart J 66:108–127, 1963

30. Rios JC, Massumi RA: Correlation between the apexcardiogram and left ventricular pressure. Am J Cardiol 15:647, 1965

31. Coulshed N, Epstein EJ: The apexcardiogram: Its normal features explained by those found in heart disease. Br Heart J 25:697–708, 1963

32. Sutton GC, Craige E, Grizzle JE: Quantitation of precordial movement: II. Mitral Regurgitation. Circulation 35:483–491, 1967

33. Benchimol A, Legler JF, Dimond EG: The carotid tracing and apexcardiogram

in subaortic stenosis and idiopathic myocardial hypertrophy. Am J Cardiol 11:427–435, 1963

34. Hood WP Jr, Rolett EL: Patterns of contraction in the human left ventricle (Abstr). Circulation 40: (suppl III) 109, 1969

35. Epstein EJ, Coulshed N, Brown AK, Doukas NG: "A" wave of apexcardiogram in aortic valve disease and cardiomyopathy. Br Heart J 30:591–605, 1968

36. Benchimol A, Dimond EG: The apexcardiogram in ischemic heart disease. Br Heart J 24:581–594, 1962

37. Eddleman EE Jr, Harrison TR: The kinetocardiogram in patients with ischemic heart disease. Prog Cardiovasc Dis 6:189–211, 1963

38. Voigt GC, Friesinger GC: The use of apexcardiography in the assessment of left ventricular diastolic pressure. Circulation 41:1015–1024, 1970

39. Fortuin NJ, Hood WP, Craige E: Evaluation of left ventricular function by echocardiography. Circulation 46:26–35, 1972

40. Tafur E, Cohen LS, Levine HD: The apex cardiogram in left ventricular outflow tract obstruction. Circulation 30:392–399, 1964

41. Goldblatt A, Aygen MM, Braunwald E: Hemodynamic-phonocardiographic correlations of the fourth heart sound in aortic stenosis. Circulation 26:92–98, 1962

42. Sutton GC, Craige E: Clinical signs of severe acute mitral regurgitation. Am J Cardiol 20:141–144, 1967

43. Fortuin NJ, Hood WP Jr, Sherman ME, Craige E: Determination of left ventricular volumes by ultrasound. Circulation 44:575–584, 1971

44. Barlow JB, Bosman CK: Aneurysmal protrusion of the posterior leaflet of the mitral valve. An auscultatory-electrocardiographic syndrome. Am Heart J 71:166–178, 1966

45. Parker E, Craige E, Hood WP Jr: The significance of the Austin Flint murmur and the a wave of the apexcardiogram in aortic regurgitation. Circulation 43:349–359, 1971

46. Dimatteo J, Lafont H, Hui Bon Hoa F, et al: La courbe mechanique ventriculaire dans l'insuffisance aortique. Arch Mal Coeur 60:1320–1333, 1967

47. Kesteloot H, Willems J: Relationship between the right apexcardiogram and the right ventricular dynamics. Acta Cardiol 22:64–89, 1967

48. Burstin L: Determination of pressure in the pulmonary artery by external graphic records. Br Heart J 29:396–404, 1967

49. Schmidt RE, Craige E: Precordial movements over the right ventricle in children with pulmonary stenosis. Circulation 32:241–250, 1965

50. Leatham A, Weitzman D: Auscultatory and phonocardiographic signs of pulmonary stenosis. Br Heart J 19:303, 1957

51. Bancroft WH, Eddleman EE Jr: Methods and physical characteristics of the kinetocardiographic and apexcardiographic systems for recording low-frequency precordial motion. Am Heart J 73:756–764, 1967

52. Valero A: Recording actual heart movements and arterial pulsations with a new electronic device. Am J Cardiol 19:224–230, 1967

53. Heikkilä J, Luomanmäki K, Pyörälä K: Serial observations on left ventricular dysfunction in acute myocardial infarction. II. Systolic time intervals in power failure. Circulation 44:343–354, 1971

N. Ty Smith

2

Ballistocardiography

"I am an old man and have known a great many troubles, but most of them never happened." (Samuel Langhorne Clemens, 1835–1910)

Ballistocardiography was born too soon. Born in an era of physiological and physical ignorance, it spent its childhood in obscurity. Yet because it was the only one of its kind, it was called upon at a young age to perform difficult tasks without proper preparation. Thus by the time it had reached maturity, its reputation was so tarnished that few physicians were willing to be seen with it; only an occasional research scientist would dare play with it, usually as a hobby.

The recent emphasis on noninvasive techniques in medicine has convinced many physicians to reconsider ballistocardiography as a possible method to fulfill the strict criteria imposed on these techniques. It is the purpose of this chapter to present enough background on the ballistocardiogram (Bcg) to put into perspective its present status and usefulness. This background includes history, development, theoretical considerations, laboratory and clinical investigations, and examples of established applications. Then I shall outline studies needed to improve

The author's studies outlined in this chapter were supported by Army Contract DA-49-193-MD-2135, Public Health Service Program Project GM-12527 and Computer Grant HE-07812, Grant FR 70 from the General Clinical Research Center Branch, Division of Research Facilities Resources, and NIH Research Career Development Award LK3-GM-31757. The literature search was completed July 1, 1971.

the understanding of the Bcg, as well as give practical suggestions for setting up a Bcg system in a physician's office.

Several excellent sources of information on the Bcg have accumulated. Scarborough undertook the publication of an extensive bibliography[1] providing more than 1500 references to papers, reports, monographs, reviews, and books, both domestic and foreign, which appeared during the period from 1877 to 1964. A Russian monograph by Baevskiy is now available in English.[2] The best of the recent reviews is in the French literature,[3] and is well worth the effort in translating. The outstanding single source in the field is the monograph by Starr and Noordergraaf,[4] the former the authority in the clinical area, the latter the authority in the theoretical area. Since the Bcg is so old, two research societies, American and European, are well established. The proceedings of ten of their meetings are available.[5-14] These provide most of the significant recent Bcg literature. Finally, a thesis by Verdouw provides valuable information.[15]

EARLY HISTORY

The Bcg is a record of the movements of the body caused by shifts in the center of mass of the blood and to a lesser extent of the heart. The first to notice these movements is lost in time. In 1786, Parry detected oscillations of the trunk synchronous with the heart beat.[16] The first recording was published in 1877 by Gordon.[17] The paper attracted some attention, for it was discussed by Trotter,[18] who suggested that the easiest approach to an understanding of the phenomenon would be through the study of the center of gravity (mass) of the body, an approach which was only verified 80 years later by Burger and Noordergraaf.[19-23] Gordon's paper was reviewed in 1880 by Landois,[24] who also made the first clinical observation. Patients with aortic insufficiency exhibit considerably greater ballistocardiographic amplitudes than do normal persons. After this brief period, interest subsided, and no mention of ballistocardiography can be found for 26 years.

The first physiologic application of the Bcg was attempted by Yandell Henderson, who had constructed an excellent Bcg in 1905.[25] Along with Douglas and Haldane,[26] in 1913 he hauled a much simpler and less reliable instrument to the top of Pike's Peak securing records on all personnel on the summit, in the valley, and at sea level. From these records they concluded that cardiac output was not altered by changes in altitude, a conclusion not supported by modern invasive or ballistocardiographic methods.[27] Three lessons can be learned from this early failure. (1) The desire for excessive simplification produced an inaccurate instrument. (2) The physiological knowledge of the time was not adequate to interpret the Bcg. (3) Far-reaching conclusions were drawn from uncertain methods.

Over the next 23 years, scattered attempts were made to investigate and to use the Bcg.[28-31] The most successful, significantly enough, was by the geophysicist, Angenheister,[30] who used his seismograph to secure surprisingly good Bcg's.

DEVELOPMENT

High-Frequency Ballistocardiography

Modern ballistocardiography began in 1936, when Isaac Starr became interested in the technique. In fact, it was Starr who gave us the name "ballistocardiography."* Starr, who was looking for a noninvasive method for determination of cardiac output, was stimulated by Henderson's reminiscenses on his experiences of 30 years before. He tried the same type of bed which Gordon, Landois, and Henderson had used—a very slowly swinging pendulum bed. As did the others, he recorded displacement of the bed. However, it soon became apparent that this instrument was not practical for clinical use. The respiratory amplitude was about 10 times greater than the cardiac amplitude. Asking a patient to hold his breath failed, because the pattern of breath holding was uncontrollable. Starr solved this problem by constructing a different type of bed. Instead of allowing it to swing freely like a pendulum, he opposed the motion of the bed with a stiff spring (Fig. 2–1). This changed the system from a simple pendulum to a giant strain gauge. Thus, although displacement was recorded, the system actually measured *force*. Since force equals mass times acceleration, acceleration was indirectly measured. As we shall see later, this has made it easy to compare Starr's early tracings with modern acceleration tracings.

Opposing the motion of the bed with a stiff spring changed the natural frequency† of the bed from a value less than the heart rate to

* Ballistocardiography: from the Greek *ballein*—to throw, hurl, or eject; *kardia*—heart; *graphein*—to write.

† Natural frequency can be understood best by a simple analogy. If one pushes a child on a swing gently on each descent, the swing will go back and forth easily at a certain frequency. One can *force* the swing so that it oscillates at a greater or lesser frequency for any given amplitude, but this requires considerably more energy, hence the term "natural" frequency for that frequency at which the least effort augments the excursion.

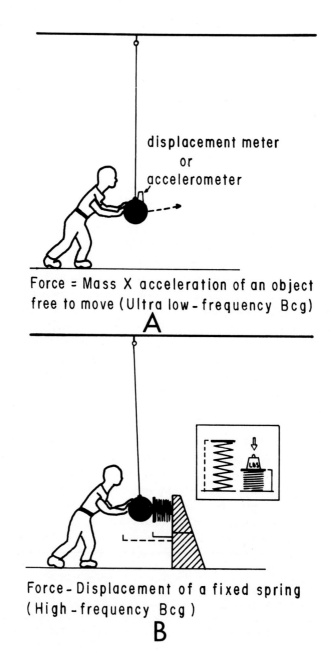

displacement meter
or
accelerometer

Force = Mass X acceleration of an object
free to move (Ultra low-frequency Bcg)

A

Force-Displacement of a fixed spring
(High-frequency Bcg)

B

one considerably greater, about 15 Hz. Thus began the era of *high-frequency* ballistocardiography, which lasted about 15 years. The contributions made by Starr, using this system, to cardiovascular physiology cannot be overestimated. However, although the bed proved convenient for clinical recordings on large numbers of patients, it did have three distinct disadvantages which Starr realized but decided to tolerate. First, the natural frequency was taken from outside the range of interest of the Bcg and placed into this range. This resulted in distortion of the waveform.*

Another disadvantage of Starr's system was the necessity for strong coupling, or attachment, of the subject to the heavy bed. Since very strong coupling was usually not used, further distortion occurred. High natural frequency and loose coupling resulted in late systolic and diastolic after-vibrations which Hamilton and Dow[32] incorrectly attributed to standing waves in the blood vessels. This coupling requirement retarded the progress of ballistocardiography for another reason; experimentation in dogs was virtually impossible. One can couple the skin of a dog to a bed, but not the skin of a dog to the dog. His skin is too loose.

The third major disadvantage of the high-frequency bed resulted from the strong coupling of this heavy instrument to ground, or the

---

* This distortion is analogous to that occurring in a stereo set. If by misfortune the speakers have a broad band natural-frequency peak in the range of, for example, 1,000–1,100 Hz, the speakers will sound too loudly each time an instrument plays a note in that range. What sounds unpleasant to the ears can also look unpleasant to the eyes.

Fig. 2–1. Diagrams of Starr's conversion of his system from ULF to HF which also illustrate the principles behind the two systems. In both A and B, the man represents the blood which, by moving, exerts a force on the body-bed system—the ball. The movement of the bed can be determined in one of several derivatives, in A, it is displacement or acceleration. B. The man pushes the ball against a strong spring, which in turn is compressed a short distance. Calibration is accomplished by turning the spring upright and adding weights until the spring is compressed the same distance. The system acts essentially like a giant strain gauge, or force gauge. Force and acceleration are easily convertible. Hence, the main difference between the two systems is the distortion seen with the HF system. (From Starr I, Noordergraaf A: A comparison between ultralow-frequency ballistocardiograms and those secured by an improved high-frequency technique, with studies to explain remaining differences, Am Heart J 64:79–100, 1962, with permission.)

building. This meant that someone walking down the hall, a truck passing outside, or any other inevitable building vibrations would clutter and interfere with the tracing.

Starr appreciated these problems, but decided to continue to work with the high-frequency system because of its clinical usefulness. Nickerson also understood the problems and realized that a very low-frequency bed was desirable. However, he too had to compromise, and with Curtis[33] he constructed a low-frequency bed, with a natural frequency of about 1.0 to 1.5 Hz. To circumvent respiratory artefacts, appropriate damping was necessary.

Direct-Body Ballistocardiography

Nickerson's bed was too complicated for clinical application, and very few physicians had the tenacity to use his or Starr's system. The breakthrough for the clinician was the development of the direct-body, or shinbar, method by Dock in 1949.[34, 35] In this technique, body movements were recorded with a velocity transducer placed across the shins of the patient. The method was so simple that the Bcg was finally available to every physician. The blessing, however, was mixed, and the temporary boon eventually proved to be disastrous for ballistocardiography. The direct-body method had one important difference from all of the previous methods; it recorded the displacement of the body moving across a *fixed* surface. This meant that the properties of the body tissues seriously warped the tracings, and since these properties vary from patient to patient, neither this effect nor the coupling between body and bed could be predicted precisely. The recording was therefore subject to distortion, and large and inconstant errors; it could not be calibrated, so that amplitude had little meaning, and judgment had to be based on contour alone; and it probably recorded only gross abnormalities, with many false-positives. But it was inexpensive and seemed simple, and everyone tried it. Its apparent simplicity was its downfall. Many of those using this method did not recognize the need for care and the strict attention to details and recording technique necessary to attain reliable and reproducible records even under the best of circumstances. Furthermore, there emerged a confusing diversity of hybrid types of direct-body instruments which produced such a perplexing variety of records as to make comparison of results difficult or impossible. Finally, many reports of inferior quality were published, reports based on scientifically unsound studies from which extravagant claims and sweeping generalizations were made.

The Decline

During the mid and late 1950s the great enthusiasm for ballisto-cardiography which the direct-body device had generated turned into disenchantment. This attitude developed particularly among cardiovas-cular investigators who were not using the Bcg. Other factors besides the inconsistencies of the direct-body device were responsible for this attitude. For example, the Bcg was a premature innovation, and many physicians expected more from this method than it could provide. They became impatient with what they considered to be the relatively slow progress in defining the clinical value of the method. The few available investigators were becoming preoccupied with the invasive methods which were just beginning to appear. The ostensibly greater accuracy of these new methods was alluring. Assistance from bioengineers was not available either to help discriminate the good from the bad and the simple from the complex or to construct reliable ballistocardiographic systems. The wrong physiological variables were compared with the Bcg, since the true significance of the Bcg was not understood. Finally, and ironically, many investigators observed that the Bcg's of a substan-tial number of apparently normal persons in the middle and older age groups were "abnormal." Hasty conclusions were made that any method that yielded so many false-positives could not be clinically useful.

The Modern Era

Unnoticed during this adverse reaction, the turning point in ballisto-cardiography was occurring: the entrance of physicists and engineers into the field. Four groups simultaneously and independently decided that the Bcg needed a new foundation.[31-42] More importantly, they were able to outline a precise procedure for this revision. The fundamental tenets were (1) The bed supporting the subject must be extremely light. Heavy beds create serious distortions. (2) The coupling of subject to bed should be as tight as feasible. Requirements 1 and 2 combined suggest that, ideally, subject and bed should float in space as a unit. (3) Coupling of bed to ground should be minimal. (4) The natural frequency of the system should be as low as possible, preferably less than 0.3 Hz. One of the benefits of this very low frequency, that is, ultralow frequency (ULF), is that it helps to realize requirement num-ber 3. (5) Acceleration of the bed, rather than velocity or displacement, is the measurement of choice. These ostensibly simple objectives proved difficult to achieve, but the vast improvement in ballistocardiography has rendered the effort more than worthwhile.

SYSTEMS AND EQUIPMENT

Standardization

Thus far I have emphasized the disadvantages of ballistocardiography's prematurity. There has been, however, one distinct advantage. The initial period of difficulty has been traversed, and physicians, physicists, and engineers have had time to help develop an excellent set of standards, which are not only rigid but also practical for the practicing physician. Some of the former deficiencies of the Bcg, as with most other clinical tests, were related to the lack of adequate quality control. Each laboratory had its own unique instrumentation, testifying to the rugged individualism which seemed to be the hallmark of those engaged in the field.

Recently, however, ballistocardiography has been well disciplined with respect to nomenclature, conventions, and terminology. The first committee on standardization (1953) laid the essential groundwork for later development.[43,44] This committee labeled axes in three orthogonal and three rotational directions, established signs, labeled wave forms in the recordings, defined terms, and specified calibration techniques and publication formats. It also discussed the measurement of displacement, velocity, and acceleration, and the relationships between these quantities (see below). In 1956, a second committee[45,46] provided a comprehensive extension, comparing various Bcg systems, as well as defining principles of vibration theory, electric filtering, integration, and differentiation. Also, recommendations were made concerning the desirable characteristics of the various types of Bcg suspension systems. Initially, American investigators seldom felt it necessary to take any actions on these recommendations aside from acknowledging their existence. The European Society of Ballistocardiographic Research followed suit and published its own set of standards in 1961.[47] In all important respects, its recommendations were identical with those published by the American Committee, thus providing a certain degree of uniformity. Despite the usefulness of the standards, the individual investigator remained free to adopt or to ignore the proposals as he wished.

Enough research was conducted between 1956 and 1969 to require a further extension of the earlier recommendations. It was also apparent that more stringent physical specifications for current and future Bcg's were necessary. Frankly, however, the main impetus to change was commercial. Manufacturers of newly designed Bcg's wished to make sure that their new instruments would meet at least minimal official specifications. Accordingly, a joint committee of the American and European societies published still another extension of Bcg specifications.[48] This report dealt only with the most generally accepted type of Bcg, the ULF suspension type. The original drafts of the reports gave detailed specifications for three classes of Bcg's: clinical, clinical research, and laboratory research, in order of increasing stringency. However, this convenient arrangement was abandoned because it was felt that the standards should be kept high for all types of Bcg's. Specifications were given for body position, bed weight and stiffness, frequency bandpass, signal-to-noise ratio of the recording, chart speed, transducer location, quantities to be recorded, body restraints, calibration procedures, and the provisions for use of other physiologic transducers. The intent of the committees was to provide minimum specifications that would ensure good results from any group entering the field. In fact, all investigators who follow the composite recommendations of the committees should be able to record similar Bcg's from the same subject. The Bcg is like a fingerprint: it is precisely reproducible in any given person, but each person's is distinctly different. All of the specifications mentioned in the rest of the chapter are taken from these committee reports.

Natural Frequency System

One of the major goals in the design of any system is to achieve as low a natural frequency as possible, 0.3 Hz or less. Anything in that range is called ultralow frequency (ULF). The only disadvantages to ULF systems are their relative complexity and the interference of respiratory movements with displacement and velocity recordings. If the natural frequency is much higher, however, distortion results. The greater accuracy of the ULF system and its elimination of many of the old objections to the Bcg exceed any disadvantages and have assured its predominance. Therefore, much of the remaining chapter will center on the ULF system. The exceptions are the early observations, which come from systems other than ULF.

Equipment

A complete Bcg system consists of a bed on which the subject lies in the supine position; a means of suspending the bed and of achieving a very low frequency, a means of isolating the bed from the environment, a transducer for measuring the movements of the bed, electronic amplifiers, filters, differentiators and integrators, and a recorder. With the highly developed electronic equipment of today, the only potential problems for the physician are the bed and the transducer.

Beds. One of the nonnegotiable requirements placed on the Bcg is that the mass of the bed should be extremely low. The lightest patient should weigh at least 10 times more than the bed. Several materials have been used to make beds light. These include balsa plywood, aluminum honeycomb, and aluminum tubing and canvas.

The Starr high-frequency (HF) bed weighs 24 kg; with accessories the weight is 36 kg. The system has been refined to a considerable degree.[49] Most of the improvements involve means of coupling the subject more tightly to the heavy bed, occasionally to the point of discomfort. This of course belies the very rationale for noninvasive testing, and for this reason the HF bed will never be ideal. The new Starr table has one outstanding advantage; it can be tilted up to 60°. This can be useful for orthopneic patients.

The simplest of the ULF beds, and the one which we use frequently, is the pendulum bed (Fig. 2–2). Canvas or dacron sail cloth is stretched over a very light aluminum frame. The frame is suspended from the ceiling by four or eight braided, thin airplane cables. Adjustable turnbuckles are used to level the bed. The total weight is 4.5 lbs, light enough for a large dog. A practical disadvantage of this bed is that the wires must be at least 3 meters long to achieve the required natural frequency of 0.3 Hz or less. Unfortunately, since the natural frequency of a pendulum is inversely proportional to the square root of the length, to halve the natural frequency it is necessary to quadruple the length of the wires. Although suspending the wires at a more acute angle can decrease the necessary height of the ceiling, many laboratories or offices do not have ceilings and areas large enough for this bed. To make a bed for a lower ceiling, Rappaport[49] and Starr[48] devised systems very much like the one used by Henderson 70 years ago. The bed is displaced laterally by two pins (Fig. 2–3). When these pins are in place, the point of support of the suspension on this same side is not directly over the end of the pin, but over a point 1.5 cm from this base. This is analogous to offsetting the hinges on a door so that it swings to a preferred position. The natural frequency is dependent on the offset. The bed is somewhat tricky to use, and with its additional contact points, is more sensitive to building vibrations.[51]

Talbot devised an interesting bed which, although not clinically useful, deserves mention because it approached the most nearly ideal ULF system then attainable.[52] A light wooden platform was floated on a 188-kg pool of mercury. Building vibrations were poorly transmitted.

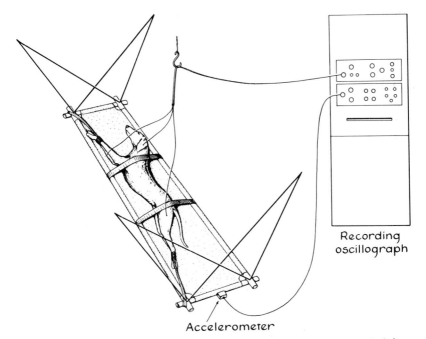

Recording
oscillograph

Accelerometer

Fig. 2–2. A simple ULF bed. An aluminum-canvas bed is suspended from eight long cables attached to the ceiling (see text). Notice that major electrical cables are brought to the bed from above in order to minimize damping of the bed. The suspending wires are arranged so that head-foot motion only is allowed. The hip and shoulder straps are used in both dogs and man to increase coupling between subject and bed. The straps must be placed so that they do not interfere with the subject's ventilation. The paw straps are not used in awake dogs (length of wire suspension, 3 cm; length of Bcg, 180 cm; width, 50 cm).

The bed was aperiodic, that is, it had a natural frequency of zero. This meant that there was no restoring force and the slightest touch could send the bed skittering against the side of the pool. Soft springs can take care of this difficulty; however, under such circumstances the natural frequency of the bed is no longer zero.

One of the many benefits of the space program was the development of the air bearing for guidance systems. This was soon transferred to ballistocardiography as a possible means of solving many of its problems, particularly those of suspension. Using the air bearing, the bed literally floats on a thin film of air. Nyboer and Sharp[53] were the first to exhibit a working model of an air-supported ballistic system. Martin[54] assembled a sophisticated bed floating on a single large

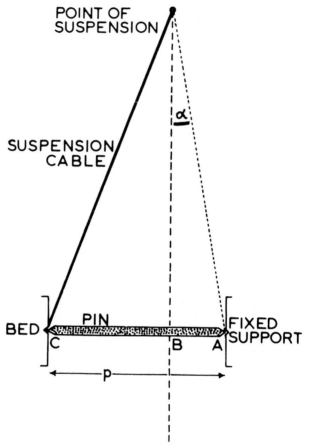

Fig. 2–3. Diagram to show the lateral displacement of a ULF bed (see text). To conserve space, the vertical dimension has been reduced in respect to the horizontal (AB, 1.5 cm; angle α, 0.5 deg). (From Starr I, Noordergraaf A: A comparison between ultralow-frequency ballistocardiograms and those secured by an improved high-frequency technique, with studies to explain remaining differences, Am Heart J 64:79–100, 1962, with permission.)

bearing. Its main problems were its expense and the difficulty of leveling the bed on a single bearing. Cunningham[55,56] has developed a system in which the bed floats on three air bearings, thus making leveling easier. Figures 2–4 and 2–5 show the basic design of such a bed. An aluminum honeycomb frame, weighing 3 kg is supported by three small air bearings. The air bearings can be seen in Figure 2–4, which

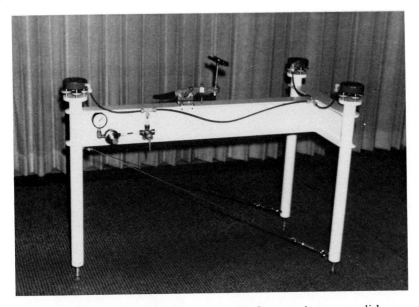

Fig. 2–4. The heavy supporting frame. All three steel concave disks can be seen with their air supplies. The lever arrangement in the center is for clamping the bed.

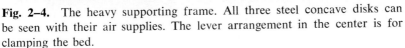

shows the supporting structure. The disk itself is slightly concave, with the center about 0.004 in. below the edge. It is essentially a segment of a sphere with a 36-ft radius. Thus, it is analogous to a pendulum with 36-ft wires. The natural frequency is accordingly about 0.14 Hz. Figure 2–5 shows the entire assembly. Some of the advantages of the system include a light yet stiff frame, good coupling of subject to bed, portability, relatively small size, ease of operation, and the ability to record the Bcg in more than one direction. Building vibrations are still noticeable, although the system is superior to most in this respect. Cunningham is grappling with this problem by designing a bed which floats on air in three dimensions.[57] This assures virtually complete isolation from ground.

A group of Scottish bioengineers[58] has suspended a plywood bed over two rails, using six pressure-fed orifice-controlled air bearings. The bearings and rails are arranged to constrain motion to the head-foot direction.

Harrison and Talbot[59] have designed an air-bearing bed which is now commercially available,* although it could be built by anyone with a good workshop and considerable patience. The bed is made of

* Royal Medical Corporation, 110 Wynn Drive, Huntsville, Alabama.

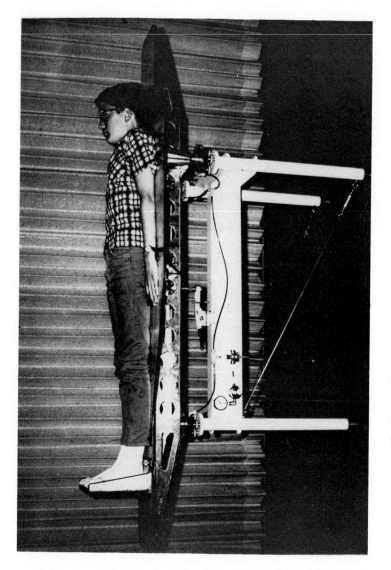

Fig. 2–5. The entire assembly of the Cunningham system.

aluminum and styrofoam and floats on one large air bearing, which is positioned under the entire bed. Air flow comes from a special silenced "reverse" industrial vacuum cleaner. The advantages of the bed are its portability and relatively low cost if made in a workshop. In addition, it can be used with an x-ray table, thus permitting simultaneous Bcg recording and cardiac catheterization.*

A disadvantage of most air-bearing beds is that the patient-contact surface is often too smooth, with resulting poor subject-bed coupling and distortion. The solution can be lateral clamps, an extremely light-weight bed, or a rougher surface.[60]

Three interesting beds are currently under investigation and may help simplify matters for the physician. The servo-counterforce bed of Nyboer uses an opposing force to nullify the Bcg forces acting on the bed and to keep the bed in one position.[61,62] Although the bed is aperiodic, it has many of the properties of an HF instrument. Tolles[63] designed a bed which rests on several springs. Although complex in design, it is easy to operate, inexpensive, and portable. A German ULF model uses four leaf springs to support the bed from underneath.[64,65] All of these beds need further independent evaluation.

Transducers. Although a multitude of transducers have been devised for Bcg's, some of them quite ingenious, I shall confine myself to describing two types: the linear variable differential transformer (LVDT), or bar magnet-coil transducer, and the accelerometer. The LVDT is simply a transformer with a moving core. The soft iron core is usually attached to the Bcg bed, and the coil is fixed in relation to ground. As the core moves back and forth through the coil, a signal proportional to the displacement of the bed is generated when the core is unmagnetized. Velocity is measured when the core is magnetized.

Some of the physicists who defined the requirements for the ideal Bcg in the early 1950s also recommended that acceleration be measured. Until recently, however, satisfactory accelerometers have not been available commercially. We have used an inexpensive variable capacitance accelerometer designed by Dr. Walter L. Gamble. Again the space program has aided ballistocardiographic technology by developing light-weight, sensitive, yet rugged accelerometers. A detailed description of the theory and construction of the accelerometers available at the time has been given in a previous publication,[66] and will not be repeated

---

* We solved this problem with our pendulum bed simply by inflating an air mattress between the x-ray table and the Bcg bed during catheterization and deflating it for recordings.

here. In brief, an accelerometer is constructed on Newton's second law: force equals mass times acceleration. Theoretically, attaching a mass to any force gauge (strain gauge) converts the gauge to an accelerometer. However, the old bonded strain gauges were much too stiff, and it was not until Statham invented the unbonded strain gauge that an acceptable accelerometer became possible. Since then, many accelerometers have become commercially available, but few are suitable for the Bcg. The specifications for a Bcg accelerometer are simple, but not easy to meet. The instrument must be small,* rugged, durable, and yet have a high sensitivity for the very low magnitudes recorded. It must have uni-directional sensitivity; it must be insensitive to temperature changes; it must have a flat-frequency response from direct current to 0.2 Hz up to 100 Hz; it must be easy to use, reliable, and reasonably priced. The best combination of these properties, particularly lightness, rug-gedness, sensitivity, and more than adequate frequency response, can be found in accelerometers based on the piezoresistive principle.† A piezoelectric crystal produces a current when distorted; a piezoresistive (semiconductor) crystal changes its resistance when distorted. This is the principle behind many implantable and catheter-tip pressure trans-ducers.

Differentiators and integrators. As described later, valuable infor-mation can be obtained from the Bcg by simultaneously recording several tracings, or derivatives: displacement, velocity, acceleration, and jerk, which is the first time derivative of acceleration. It is possible to record each of these derivatives with a different transducer, but it is easier and less expensive to record directly any one and obtain the others by processes called *differentiation* and *integration*. Differentiation measures the slope of a curve; integration, the area under a curve. To derive acceleration from displacement requires differentiating circuits; to obtain displacement from acceleration requires integrating circuits. Each method has its own advantages and disadvantages. Differentiation accentuates HF noise, whereas integration reduces it. On the other hand, differentiation attenuates LF noise, such as that arising from respiration, whereas integration accentuates it. The author prefers to measure ac-

---

* The mass should probably be less than 100 gm, especially if three or more are to be used: the mass of the accelerometer must be added to the mass of the bed.

† In addition to the variable capacitance accelerometer, we use piezoresistive accelerometers manufactured by Endevco Co. These accelerometers were selected after a long search.

celeration, and if desired integrate to obtain velocity and displacement and differentiate to obtain jerk.

Filters. Considerable unwanted noise can be attenuated with filters. A set of filters should pass frequencies between 0.3 Hz and 50 Hz. Often such filters are available on modern recorders. If not, they can be purchased or easily assembled using a few resistors, capacitors, and two potentiometers. If 50- or 60-Hz noise is a problem, a notch filter, one which almost selectively eliminates the unwanted frequency, can be constructed.

THE BALLISTOCARDIOGRAPHIC WAVEFORM

Ballistocardiographic derivatives. The contemporary cardiovascular physiologist measures as many variables as he can, hoping for a complete description of the cardiovascular system. The Bcg has the advantage of being able to measure at least four variables simultaneously. With proper analysis many more can be extracted. The four variables include the motion derivatives: displacement, velocity, acceleration, and jerk, each with a totally different pattern. The first three are the most commonly used and are shown in Figure 2–6. The relation between displacement, velocity, and acceleration can best be understood by the analogy first proposed by Starr.[67,68] Each automobile has two motion indicators—a displacement meter (odometer) and a velocity meter (speedometer). A third, an acceleration meter (accelerometer) could be added. Which meter is most useful depends on the information one wishes to obtain. Measurement of distance between towns is simple. Estimation of gas consumption is not so simple. For the latter, the odometer provides the most information, but it is also useful to know the velocity over that distance. If a record is kept of the acceleration, an even more precise answer can be obtained; the greater the accumulated accelerations and decelerations, the greater the gas consumption. The odometer of a car, the displacement Bcg, and stroke volume are all analogous; that is, they measure similar functions. The speedometer, the velocity Bcg, and aortic flow measured by a flow meter are similarly analogous. Finally, the acceleration meter, the acceleration force Bcg, and the acceleration of aortic blood flow are all analogous. Stroke volume gives some information about the circulation as a whole, but by itself is not very useful in evaluating myocardial function. Systolic acceleration tells much about the heart but

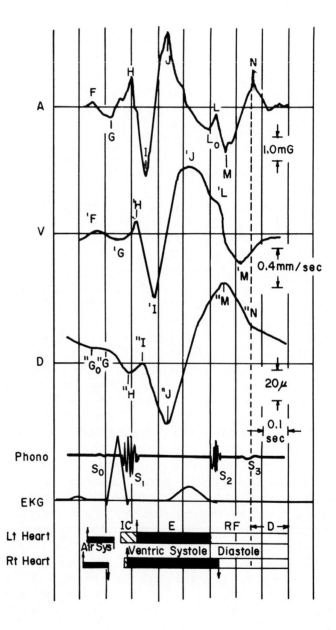

little about the peripheral circulation. The automobile-heart analogy can be carried one step further. If a minor problem arises with the engine, the first sign is a decrease of the car's ability to accelerate properly after stopping or its ability to climb a hill, rather than its ability to cover the customary distance or achieve a maximum velocity. The same is true of the heart; the first function to decline is often its ability to accelerate blood into the aorta.[69–72] In addition, acceleration is relatively insensitive to preload or afterload.[70,73,74] Thus, acceleration is one of the most useful variables with which to evaluate myocardial performance. Estimating myocardial oxygen consumption is analogous to estimating gas consumption; one should measure cardiac output, peak and mean flow velocity, and acceleration. All of these are reflected in the different ballistocardiographic derivatives.

There are other advantages to acceleration besides its ability to evaluate myocardial performance: (1) Acceleration needs no reference to ground. Displacement and velocity must be measured relative to some point, and that point must be isolated from ground as carefully as the Bcg bed itself. (2) Respiration does not affect acceleration nearly so much as it does velocity and displacement. Thus breath holding is not necessary. (3) Recording acceleration and then integrating produces much quieter records than recording displacement and differentiating twice. (4) Acceleration apparently has little relation to body mass. As discussed later, the magnitude of body acceleration for mice, men, and whales is surprisingly close.

Some ballistocardiographers have computed *jerk*, the first derivative of acceleration.[75,76] With this derivative, body mass is a somewhat less important consideration. Jerk is more sensitive to changes in myo-

---

Fig. 2–6. Ballistocardiogram. Examples of normal ULF acceleration (A), velocity (V), and displacement (D). An ECG, phonocardiogram, and the events of the cardiac cycle are given for reference (1.0 mG = 1/1,000 the acceleration of gravity). Do not be discouraged by all of the waves and labels. For most purposes, the most important waves are H, I, and J. Wave L (acceleration) is equivalent to the K wave of the HF system. This wave is usually not nearly so prominent in ULF recordings and was probably artifact in the former. (From Scarborough WR, Folk EF, Smith PM, et al: The nature and records from ultralow-frequency ballistocardiographic systems and their relation to circulatory events, Am J Cardiol 2:613–641, 1958, with permission.)

cardial function than any other variable yet measured. But thus far it cannot be recommended for the clinician or for most researchers. The record is very noisy and sensitive to building vibrations. Therefore measurements of amplitudes can be variable. In one study performed by an outstanding group of engineers,[77] technical difficulties precluded measurement of jerk in three out of seven catheterized subjects. This is rather discouraging for most of us. Talbot et al[76] measured the slope of acceleration manually and thus eliminated most of the artefacts caused by random noise. This is not, however, an easy method for studying a large number of patients. Jerk may prove useful in detecting the onset of ejection. In the acceleration Bcg, the onset often coincides with a slur or notch, which would become a peak on differentiation.

Origin of the Bcg

Until recently there has been much controversy concerning the origin of the Bcg. In discussing the origin of individual waves, one must remember that a number of events act simultaneously throughout the cardiac cycle, and that a wave tip merely means that the sum of several events is maximal or minimal. Therefore a tip or inflexion of the record cannot, in general, be attributed to a single physiologic event, although one event may be the major contributor. This is in contrast to the ECG.

Since acceleration is the most useful motion derivative, to simplify the discussion of the generation of the Bcg, only the acceleration Bcg will be considered. The most important factor is the acceleration of blood from the left ventricle. Movement of blood in the pulmonary circulation plays a lesser role, partly because of relatively low acceleration, partly because the pulmonary arteries are short and partly because of symmetrical flow distribution after branching. Acceleration of blood in the veins contributes little because it is very low and much of it takes place in opposite directions. Other factors that contribute in a minor fashion are motion of the heart, movement of blood into the heart in diastole, stroke volume, pulse wave delay, and the state of the vessels with regard to radius, resistance, and rigidity.

The Bcg waves can be divided in general into three groups: preejection (FGH), ejection (IJK), and diastolic (LMN). The preejection waves are thought to be caused either by venous return to the heart, plus atrial filling,[78] or by atrial contraction.[79] That the latter mechanism is the dominant one is suggested by two pieces of information. First, West and Corbascio[79] demonstrated a prominent GH wave during pure atrial contraction, as recorded by pressure and strain-gauge measurements along with a P wave, and absent QRS complex. Second, the GH wave is often absent during atrial fibrillation. Left ventricular ejection begins about 10 msec after the H wave.[73] The I wave corresponds to rapid acceleration of blood in the ascending aorta, around the aortic arch, and into the carotid arteries (body moves footward),[15,80] a very important fact. Indeed, the tip of the I wave coincides with maximal acceleration of blood in the aortic root.[81,82] The J wave represents acceleration of blood in the descending and abdominal aorta, and iliac and femoral arteries, plus initial deceleration of blood in the ascending aorta (body moves headward). The KL waves reflect the deceleration and cessation of flow and closing of the aortic valve. The MN waves correspond to blood flow in peripheral arteries as well as to ventricular relaxation and initial passive ventricular filling. Thus, the late systolic and the diastolic waves are more diagnostic of peripheral vascular disease, but this phenomenon is more prominent in displacement Bcg's than in acceleration. For example, a marked change in the displacement Bcg is produced by flexing the knees, whereas velocity and acceleration tracings are much less conspicuously affected.[31,83] These observations had been predicted in advance by a computer model.[84]

Ballistocardiographic Criteria of Normality

To be able to interpret and analyze the Bcg, one must have standards of "normality." Many have been published, but unfortunately most were set up when Bcg techniques were below current quality. Comparison between sets of results is handicapped also by differences in apparatus and technique, in the age and sex of the populations, and in the physiologic conditions under which the records were taken— body position, phase of respiration, state of fasting, or recent activity.

Age is an important variable affecting the normal Bcg. The ballistocardiographic amplitudes decline with age, as do many other physiologic functions.[85,86] Standards for different age groups have been published,[87-89] the best coming from Moss.[88] Rigid standards can only be attained retrospectively, however. Over the age of 40, the number of abnormal tracings in apparently normal people increases. When no previous standards are available, it can be difficult to determine which patients on the borderline are normal and which are abnormal. Smith[89] suggests that a 3-year followup may be necessary to determine which subjects are normal and which have developed overt coronary artery disease. Even more than 3 years may be required.

In addition to age, several other factors can influence the Bcg.

Two of the most important of these are body position and respiration. Body position would be expected to influence the Bcg, since it affects the circulation in general.[59,70,90] Several systems have been constructed for recording the Bcg in the sitting[70,91,92] or quasi-standing position.[93,94] Only one of these, a sitting bed, uses the ultralow-frequency principle.[59] Changing position from lying to standing could serve as a stress test. Indeed, Starr and Rawson[94] noted that a patient may have a borderline Bcg in the supine position but a definitely abnormal one when standing up. One advantage claimed for sitting or standing Bcg's is that they permit the study of cardiac performance with a bodily orientation more closely resembling that during daily activities. Coupling of subject to instrument is obviously better in the sitting position. On the other hand, head–foot skeletal coupling (hip and knee joints) may be better with the legs extended. Two earlier problems with Bcg's obtained in the sitting position include the greater disturbance by building vibrations and the more prominent muscle tremor, with the latter especially noticeable in elderly or seriously ill patients. The former has been eliminated by the bed of Harrison and Talbot,[59] but the latter will probably always remain.

The influence of respiration is a more serious matter. It was this problem that turned Starr to the HF system and kept him there for many years despite its disadvantages. The ULF system may be the most nearly perfect system theoretically, but respiratory wander in the displacement and velocity ULF Bcg is so great as to make acceptable recordings almost impossible to obtain during breathing. This is no problem with the acceleration Bcg. Several methods have been used to try to eliminate respiratory interference, each with only moderate success. These techniques include computer-constructed filtering[95-97] and signal averaging.[98] In one unique attempt, Josenhans used a compensating mass which was actuated by a Collins respirometer to slide back and forth on the bed.[99] Winter et al[100] used an analog computer to eliminate some of the respiratory signal. A cancellation signal was derived from a displacement signal obtained from the abdominal wall. Holding the breath might be a solution, but many patients cannot do it properly and reproducibly. The influence of different breath-holding patterns is considerable.[101] This author would ask a patient to watch an oscilloscope screen and superimpose two lines, one a fixed volume line, the other the patient's volume. The glottis must be kept open so that pressure is not a factor.

One can only speculate on the cause of the respiratory variation in amplitude and form. Some of it may be caused by a change in cardiac position,[102] but this is a minor factor in the longitudinal Bcg.[103]

Most of the variation probably stems from the same factors that create respiratory variation with any cardiovascular measurement: changes in venous return, chamber filling, heart rate, and autonomic influences on the myocardium. We have devised analog computer programs for the calculation of the preejection period, isometric time-tension index, and $\dfrac{dP/dt}{KP}$ and extrapolated V_{max}. All of these variables show noticeable respiratory variation during intermittent positive pressure ventilation in the dog. Since ballistocardiographic respiratory variation is significantly greater in patients with heart disease (see later section), it would be interesting to determine if this phenomenon occurs with some of the invasive variables, such as left ventricular dP/dt max. Also, a respiratory fluctuation in myocardial synergy might be expected in these patients.

The respiratory variation can be used to advantage. This is the basis of Starr's qualitative method of analysis, which has been used with considerable success to detect latent coronary artery disease and to predict life expectancy.

ANALYSIS OF THE Bcg

The complexity of the ballistocardiographic tracings and the availability of so many different modes of recording have discouraged many physicians. However, analysis is possible and relatively simple. The following sections describe some basic approaches to extracting information from the Bcg. The type of analysis the physician uses will depend on his time, patience, and facilities. Three major types are available: qualitative, manual quantitative, and computer quantitative. Unfortunately, the greater the sophistication of a method, the less has been the validation of the usefulness of that method.

Qualitative Analysis

The first step in any analysis is to record a simultaneous ECG to help identify the proper waves. Once they have identified the waves, many ballistocardiographers, especially those using the direct-body Bcg, have simply examined the waveform. Certain conditions, such as idiopathic hypertrophic subaortic stenosis[104-107] and abdominal aortic aneurysms[108] produce virtually pathognomonic patterns. Another form of qualitative, or semiquantitative, analysis has been in use for 30 years, and has proved its usefulness in the field of prognosis. Brown et al[109] described a simple system for analysis, subsequently improved by Starr.[110] This

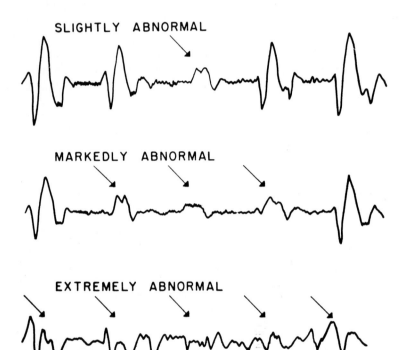

Fig. 2–7. Ballistocardiogram. Examples of the four groups in the Starr qualitative classification, chiefly based on the proportion of normal to abnormal complexes. The tracings correspond, from top to bottom, to Groups I to IV. Actual ULF acceleration records were traced and adjusted to permit vertical alignment of the respiratory cycles. Arrows point to complexes abnormal in form. (From Starr I: Proc First Congress Ballistocardiography and Cardiovascular Dynamics, Amsterdam, Karger; New York, 1966, pp 7–20, with permission.)

system is based on the variation in ballistocardiographic form and amplitude seen during a respiratory cycle. In the Brown system, high-frequency force or ULF acceleration records* are divided into five classes or groups; in the Starr system they are divided into four groups. In the Starr classification (Fig. 2–7) records normal in form during the entire respiratory cycle are placed into group I. Group II includes those records in which a minority of complexes during the respiratory cycle are abnormal. In group III, the majority of complexes are abnormal. In group IV, complexes may be so disorganized that the position of systole cannot be identified with certainty from the Bcg alone. Starr[110] has given rules for classifying these abnormalities.

Some will object that Starr's classification contains an element of subjectivity. To evaluate the importance of this objection, three investigators independently classified HF force (Starr) and ULF acceleration Bcg's obtained from patients with known coronary artery disease.[111] The three examiners interpreted and applied the Starr criteria with considerable uniformity to records from both types of systems. Repeated classifications of the same record by the same reader at widely separated intervals were also highly consistent.

Simple Manual Quantitative Analysis

It is beyond the scope of this chapter to describe in detail all of the quantitative methods proposed. The simplest methods involve the measurement of wave amplitudes and slopes, or time intervals between the ECG and Bcg wave tips and between Bcg wave tips (Fig. 2–8). Since the acceleration I wave amplitude reflects peak aortic flow acceleration most closely in theory[80] and since the IJ amplitude does in practice,[81] it would seem wise to concentrate on these measurements. The H wave has too much preejection information to be useful. The I and IJ amplitudes are useful for detecting subclinical and early abnormalities in large populations, in testing the effects of drugs and other therapy, in evaluating certain diseases, such as aortic valvular disease, in detecting the presence of coronary artery disease, and in predicting life expectancy. Of all the systems of measurement that of Moss[88] is drawn from the largest group of subjects, and is recommended reading.

---

* Except for the distortion in the HF force records, the two are fairly similar. This follows from the relation force equals mass times acceleration, with mass essentially a constant (see Fig. 2–1).

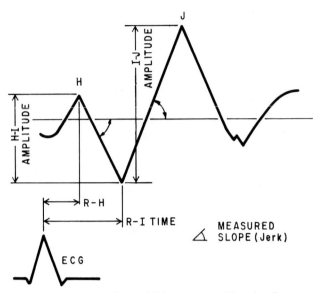

Fig. 2–8. Some of the variables measured for simple quantitative analysis. Schematic drawing of the major systolic complex, consisting of the H, I, and J waves. Notice that with a Bcg normal in form, measurement of amplitudes and time intervals is easy, and measurement of slopes is not too difficult. (Adapted from Harrison WK, Talbot SA: Discrimination of the quantitative ultralow-frequency ballistocardiogram in coronary heart disease, Am Heart J 74: 80–87, 1967, with permission.)

Computer Analysis

In clinical work, the ballistocardiographic morphology may be so grossly distorted that simple quantitative analysis is prohibitively difficult. In extremely abnormal records, confusion reigns; the absence or distortion of individual waves and the alteration in their relative magnitude and duration may make it difficult or impossible to identify either the waves themselves or the position of systole. In such cases, if quantitative analysis is desired, a digital computer must be used. The computer approach to Bcg analysis should be imaginative; the computer should not only be used to do more rapidly what a human can already do but also to do what no person could possibly do. An excellent example of the latter is the electrocardiographic analysis developed by von der Groeben.[112]

One of the most commonly used techniques to bring order out of apparent chaos is signal averaging. If a repetitive signal occurs among

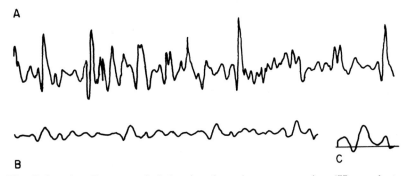

Fig. 2-9. A. Bcg recorded 1 min after vigorous exercise (Harvard step test, 3 min at 20 steps/min). Paper speed was 50 mm/sec. Note wide variation and bizarre configuration of some complexes. B. Control Bcg from same patient as in A. C. Control Bcg from same patient as in A and B, but after averaging 13 complexes with a computer of average transients. (From Jackson DH, Molina E: The postexercise ballistocardiogram. A study method utilizing average transient computing, Bibl Cardiol 20:35–38, 1968, with permission.)

random noise, and several cycles are superimposed beat after beat, the repetitive signal will emerge, and the noise will be cancelled out. The result is a clean, easily read Bcg. Laverman[113] has used this technique with the ULF Bcg when building vibrations, muscle tremors, rapid breathing, or inability to breath hold renders accurate recording otherwise impossible. Signal averaging can also extract the acceleration Bcg from the chaotic tracings obtained in congestive heart failure[114] and after exercise,[115] when muscle tremor and panting are particularly annoying (Figs. 2–9 and 2–10). Finally, transient averaging has been used to resolve the displacement ULF Bcg into cardiac and respiratory components.[98]

Transient averaging suffers from some disadvantages. Since the time interval of the Bcg after the Q wave varies during respiration, loss of detail and decrease in amplitude are inevitable in the averaged signal. The effect of respiration on the Bcg also disappears, and along with it any chance for the Starr qualitative analysis. The final result is a complex which does not really exist.

By using communications theory and constructing autocorrelograms (transient averaging and autocorrelograms are both used in electroencephalographic analysis) subtle Bcg changes, undetectable, or at least unquantifiable, by standard techniques can be evaluated.[116–120]

Other computer techniques* have been used to automate simple

* Reitan JA: unpublished data.

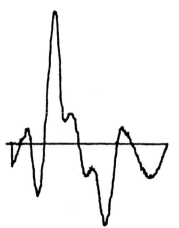

Fig. 2–10. X-Y plotter reproduction from 13 complexes. Recording was made from the same patient as in Figure 2–9A, 1 min after exercise during respiration. (From Jackson DH, Molina E: The postexercise ballistocardiogram. A study method utilizing average transient computing, Bibl Cardiol 20:35–38, 1968, with permission.)

manual analysis by identifying and measuring waveforms.[121,122] Harrison et al[122] have made a significant advance by automating the processing of the Bcg and carotid pulse. A small digital computer implements measurement of intervals and amplitudes by detecting local maxima and minima of cycles which are first smoothed and leveled. Correlation of wave forms of subdivisions of the cardiac cycle are made by comparing with an ideal Bcg. At the moment, the printout is in a complex form which would have meaning primarily to those familiar with ballistocardiography. However, Harrison* has suggested a format for a Bcg cardiac function report, which is in understandable terms and is excellent for patient evaluation (Table 2–1). This evaluation would permit a useful assessment of the physiologic status of the patient regardless of the anatomical lesion.

Additional computer uses have been proposed for statistical or "number crunching" purposes. Proper[123] has used computer techniques to sort out correlations among disease, age, and 400 variables (990 correlation coefficients). Freiman and Steinberg[124] evaluated the separate discriminatory power of four measurements, with the conclusion that in distinguishing aortic insufficiency from other conditions, the Bcg was the most useful, followed by the ECG, arterial pulse, and phonocardiogram. Talbot et al[125,126] used manual quantitative, rather than

* Harrison WK: personal communication.

Table 2–1
Bcg Cardiac Function Report

PATIENT: JOHN D. SMITH
NUMBER: 130529

                          DATE OF TEST: 25 December 1971
                          TIME OF TEST: 1030

CONDITION: Resting, regular clinic visit

AGE: 50 years   BLOOD PRESSURE: 165/90 mm HG
HEIGHT: 170 cm   WEIGHT: 72 kg

HEARTBEAT SAMPLE: 10 beats, eupnea
HEARTRATE: 75 BPM, regular

1.0   Cardiac strength
    1.1   Initial blood acceleration is below normal for age 50 years
    1.2   Blood acceleration as a whole is below normal
    1.3   Wave timing is retarded
2.0   Cardiac coordination and filling
    2.1   Record pattern is abnormal during ejection
                           abnormal during filling
    2.2   Record pattern is highly variable
    2.3   Cardiac filling acceleration is below normal

---

qualitative analysis, to separate patients with known coronary artery disease from normal subjects. With the aid of automatic data processing methods, 75 percent of the entire group was classified correctly.

VECTORBALLISTOCARDIOGRAPHY

One of the factors impeding the progress of ballistocardiography has been the difficulty of investigating the vector Bcg. The heart operates electrically in three dimensions. It should come as no surprise that the circulation should also operate three dimensionally. Until the vector Bcg is fully analyzed, the final decision on the Bcg cannot be made; it is no more rational to judge the Bcg on the basis of one dimension alone than it would be to judge the usefulness of the ECG on the basis of a single lead.

Four difficulties have slowed the development of the vector Bcg: (1) constructing proper beds, (2) obtaining proper recordings, (3) analyzing the signal, and (4) performing proper animal experiments.[127–130]

The most progress has been made in the area of constructing beds. Two-dimensional beds are becoming more common. The original Nickerson LF bed was two dimensional. Baan and Noordergraaf[131] have arranged the suspending wires of a ULF pendulum bed in such a way that it allows two-dimensional recordings. Most air-bearing beds[54,56,59] can record in two dimensions (three modes).

Several three-dimensional beds have been constructed, but with one exception they are of the Starr[132] or the shin-bar type.[133-177] The exception is a differential pendulum, a formidably complex instrument built by Talbot[138] purely as a research tool and a standard reference. Cunningham[57] has laid the plans for an ingenious three-dimensional air-bearing bed. When completed, the bed will constitute a significant advance in ballistocardiography. Not only will it allow a definitive evaluation of the vector Bcg, but also it will virtually complete the isolation of the Bcg from the ground.

With two-dimensional beds, lateral recordings can be difficult. The lateral frequency response of the body is not as good as the longitudinal.[56] Furthermore, body roll, when the bed is not free to roll, theoretically could overshadow the lateral Bcg.[138] By clamping the shoulders and hips firmly, body roll is prevented, and the resultant lateral recordings are excellent.[139] These recorded curves agreed with simultaneously but independently published theoretical curves.[140] With a three-dimensional bed, body roll is no longer a problem, and severe clamping is not necessary.

The position of the heart and the geometry of the ascending and descending aorta influence the lateral Bcg much more than they do the longitudinal Bcg. This can be a disadvantage, since it means that the lateral Bcg is more sensitive to the degree of inspiration, intrapleural pressure, and exact orientation of the heart. However, it is of diagnostic importance, and in cases of increased load, such as hypertension or aortic stenosis, the lateral Bcg increases moderately, coinciding with the more lateral ejection of blood.[141] These findings again were predicted with a computer model.[140]

Since asymmetric lateral displacement of blood is quite small compared to head-foot movement, cardiac motion plays a more important role in the origin of the lateral Bcg.[140] Furthermore, the amplitude of the lateral displacement Bcg is very sensitive to the degree of eccentricity in the position of the heart.

One of the complicating factors in vector ballistocardiography is that the measurement of six "leads" or degrees-of-freedom is required. If one records in three dimensions, he must record in three orthogonal directions and three rotational directions (Fig. 2–11). That there *is*

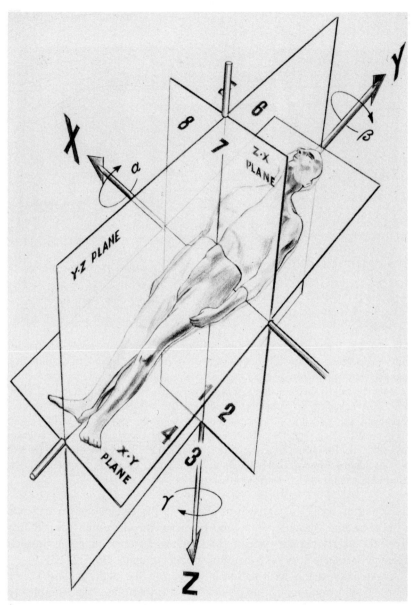

Fig. 2–11. The six "leads," or degrees of freedom, in which a 3-D Bcg can be recorded (*Y*, head-foot; *X*, lateral; *Z*, anteroposterior). In addition, three rotational directions can be recorded. For the sailors among the readers: α, pitch; β, roll; and γ, yaw. These can be measured from special accelerometers. (From Scarborough WR, Talbot SA: Proposals for ballistocardiographic nomenclature and conventions: revised and extended report of Committee on Ballistocardiographic Terminology, Circulation 14:433–450, 1956, with permission.)

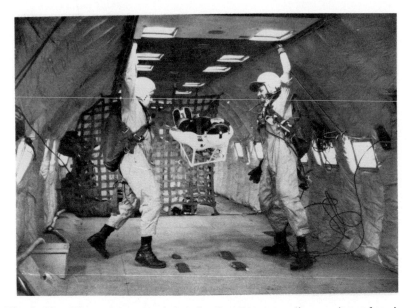

Fig. 2–12. View of an actual free-floating Bcg recording session taken in-side an airplane during a brief period of 0-gravity. Triaxial ECG and Bcg signals were telemetered to an on-board receiving station. This system rep-resents the nearly perfect Bcg system—aperiodic, with no coupling to ground and firm coupling of subject to bed because of the custom-molded bed. However, the bed and accelerometers did have a mass of 23.5 lb. (From Hixson WC, Beischer DE: Biotelemetry of the triaxial ballistocardiogram and electrocardiogram in a weightless environment, in: Monograph 10. US Naval School of Aviation Medicine, Pensacola, Fla. US Naval Aviation Medicine Center, 1964, with permission.)

information in all six degrees was shown by the fascinating experiments of Hixson and Beischer,[142,143] who recorded the three-dimensional Bcg from the nearly perfect system: the inside of an airplane going through a Keplerian trajectory and therefore at zero gravity (Fig. 2–12).*

Analysis of this information is staggering. To plot standard vector loops would require 15 combinations. Furthermore, the complexity of each loop is overwhelming (Fig. 2–13 and 2–14). A possible ap-proach is to use the orthogonal electrocardiographic analysis of von der

---

* A rather imaginative engineering friend, not content with somebody else's evidence that a rotational Bcg existed, decided to try for himself. He anesthetized a mouse with chloroform and suspended it by its tail. Sure enough, the mouse rotated slightly with each heart beat.

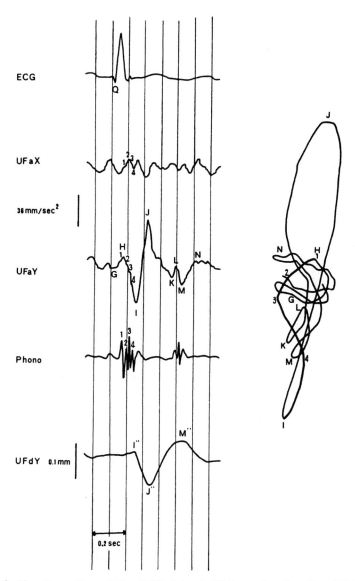

Fig. 2–13. Recording of the ECG, lateral ULF acceleration Bcg (UFaX), head-foot ULF-acceleration Bcg (UFaY), phonocardiogram, and head-foot displacement Bcg (UFdY). The tracings are said to be normal, although UFaX appears low in amplitude. The complexity of the vector plot (UFaX versus UFaY) is sobering. (From van der Linde J, Knoop AA: Proc 1st World Congr Ballistocardiography, Karger, Basel, 1966, pp 78–84, with permission.)

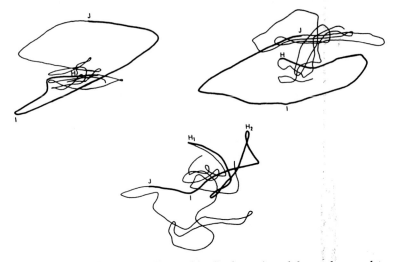

Fig. 2–14. Vectorballistocardiographic displays plotted from abnormal tracings. These certainly do look different from the display in Figure 2–13, but the difference is difficult to describe in quantitative terms. (From van der Linde J, Knoop AA: Significance of the frontal vector ultralow-frequency acceleration ballistocardiogram of man, Proc 1st World Congr Ballistocardiography, Karger, Basel, 1966, pp 78–84, with permission.)

Groeben,[112] who retains time as a variable and plots it against magnitude and two angles (alpha and tilt, or "latitude and longitude").

The difficulties of vectorballistocardiography are compounded in the dog because of the easily changed and unpredictable heart orientation.[127–130] These are the only conclusions possible from the few animal experiments which have been performed.

MATHEMATICAL AND ELECTRICAL MODELS

A considerable body of knowledge on the Bcg has developed through the construction of mathematical and electrical models of the circulation. One series of models originally designed by Noordergraaf and his group to examine the Bcg, has made a major contribution to cardiovascular physiology. The early models[144,145] suffered from a lack of proper knowledge of physiology. The first major model was the one proposed by Noordergraaf's group. It began as a mathematical model and was extended to an analog computer model because of its complexity. They approached the problem with the assumption that the Bcg reflected a shift in the center of mass of the body, caused by shifts of blood in the opposite direction.[146–149] Figure 2–15 demonstrates this

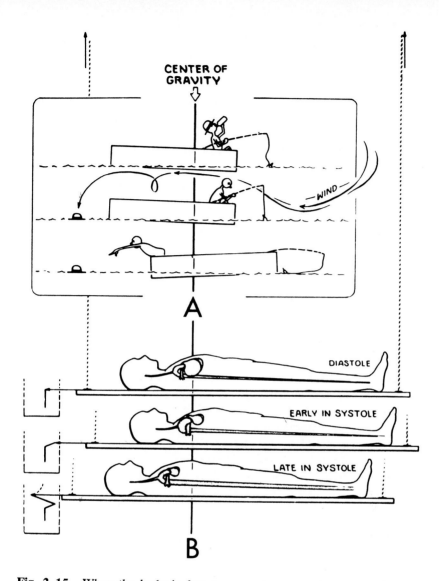

Fig. 2–15. When the body is free to move in space, the center of mass (gravity) will remain constant. This is the basic principle behind ULF ballistocardiography. A. In the top 3 pictures, the fisherman has difficulty in recovering his hat because of this principle: the common center of mass of boat and fisherman keeps a constant position with respect to the bottom of the lake. B. In the bottom pictures, again the common center of mass of blood and body remains constant when the distribution of blood changes. Thus, with the ULF Bcg, the subject's body moves in the opposite direction to the blood, i.e., initially footward, then headward. (From Noordergraaf A: Further studies on a theory of the ballistocardiogram, Circulation 23:413–425, 1961, with permission.)

principle so important to ballistocardiography. The Bcg, then, is a special kind of whole-body plethysmograph. The redistribution of blood brought about by the pumping action of the heart results in periodic changes in volume, and in mass content of many parts of the body such as the heart, the thoracic and abdominal blood vessels, and the extremities.

For the mathematical model they therefore divided 31 arteries, with an internal radius of more than 0.11 cm, into 115 small segments. The mass of blood in excess of the end-diastolic value was calculated in each successive segment as a function of time with intervals of 20 msec. This was done by accepting an average for arterial distensibility, a normal aortic pressure, and a normal pressure contour. These excess masses were then multiplied by the distance from the heart. They also calculated the contributions of the filling of the heart, contractions of the atria, movements of the heart itself, and the effects of soft-tissue motion. Algebraic summation of these calculations gave an estimate of the displacement of the center of mass. The final result represented the change in the center of mass of *blood* throughout the cardiac cycle; the change in center of mass in the *body* was set to be equal in magnitude but opposite in direction. The predicted displacement Bcg thus calculated showed a close resemblance in form and amplitude to the records obtained experimentally. We must emphasize that Noordergraaf performed his calculations before ULF tracings were available, thus eliminating an important source of bias.

Over a period of 15 years, the analog model has been expanded and improved so that it is now of great size, complexity, and sophistication.[150-153] In fact, for years it stood by itself as the best model of the circulation. The model now includes adjustable peripheral resistances, plus the viscoelasticity, stiffness, radius, and wall thickness of each segment, viscous properties of the blood, tapering in radius and elasticity, and frictional losses. The simulated arterial tree gives an accurate representation of reality when tested by pulse wave velocity and input impedance. Recently, the pulmonary circulation has been added.[154,155] The model also has a "heart," which can pump blood at any volume, velocity, and acceleration, in any waveform. Pressure and flow can be "measured" in any of the arterial segments. Abnormalities such as aortic stenosis,[156] aortic insufficiency,[156] idiopathic hypertrophic subaortic stenosis,[157] and atrial septal defect[158] have been simulated, and the resulting Bcg's evaluated.

Several important conclusions have been drawn from studies on these models. Most of the ULF Bcg can be accounted for by the redistribution of blood in the systemic arterial circulation. The relative contributions to the systolic Bcg of the pulmonary circulation,[80] venous circulation,[159] movement of blood into the heart,[147] and movement of the heart itself[147] are considerably less. The flow pattern of blood in the aorta and major arteries is the prime determinant of the early systolic Bcg. Specifically, the greater the peak aortic flow acceleration, the greater is the amplitude of the I wave. This is a constant, close and linear relation.[80] Later waves, particularly KL and MN, reflect the state of the peripheral circulation. No FGH complex is present in the Bcg's calculated from ejection phenomena only. The amplitude of the I wave is virtually insensitive to changes in peripheral resistance, radius of the arteries, and distensibility of the arteries, provided ejection flow remains the same.[80] Of these factors, arterial wall distensibility has the greatest influence on the Bcg. Thus, conditions such as arteriosclerosis and hypertension have less influence on the early systolic Bcg than was formerly believed. As one progresses in time to the LMN waves, the influence of peripheral resistance and arterial wall stiffness increases. Not only can an excellent Bcg be derived from an input of an aortic flow curve but also the opposite is true: given a Bcg, a good aortic flow curve can be constructed. The implications for deriving important information from this noninvasive technique are exciting.

It is clear that theoretically, at least, many of the old objections to the Bcg have been removed by studies on these models. Also, the Bcg emerges as a powerful physiologic tool. The confirmation of these findings by investigations in other areas will be discussed later.

Several other models have appeared recently.[160–162] Baan's model[161] uses a continuum approach, in which the mass increase of blood in the vessels is a continual, rather than an incremental, function of time. Two models were evaluated, pressure and flow. The flow model was felt to be superior. The models predicted a linear relation between aortic flow acceleration and the HI jerk (slope) and between jerk and the aortic pressure derivative. A model by Harrison[162] uses instantaneous flow patterns in eight areas: left ventricular outflow tract to the proximal aortic arch, distal arch, descending thoracic aorta, abdominal aorta and iliac arteries, pulmonary artery, superior vena cava, inferior vena cava, and intracardiac tract.[162] The theory allows predictions of the effects on cardiovascular force of alterations in peak flows, accelerations, velocity profiles, pulse wave velocity, blood viscosity, and wall friction. The Bcg derived from typical flow patterns strongly resembles a normal Bcg in most respects, except amplitude (Fig. 2–16). The uniqueness of this model is that testing and validation in man are at least possible, although still difficult.

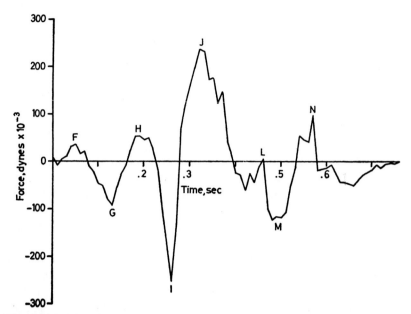

Fig. 2–16. Cardiovascular force calculated from the combined flows and mass motion outlined in the text. Remembering that this is a straight line approximation, one can see a strong resemblance in form to the ULF Bcg of a young normal subject in Figure 2–6. (From Harrison WK: Calculation of cardiovascular force from phasic regional blood flow, Bibl Cardiol 26: 262–268, 1970, with permission.)

STUDIES ON CADAVERS

The same conclusions drawn from the mathematical models have been drawn from experiments of a totally different nature. Beginning in 1950, Isaac Starr performed a series of ingenious experiments probably unique in medicine.[163–172] In these meticulously designed experiments he attempted to substitute his arm for the heart by using large syringes to inject blood into the aorta or pulmonary artery, or both, of fresh cadavers. Well-controlled protocols were used. Only one item, such as arterial pressure or stroke volume, was changed in any given injection. The results of these experiments led eventually to a new viewpoint from which to judge the performance of the heart.

Starr made some very revealing observations in these studies:

1. The influence of the pulmonary circulation on the Bcg was relatively small.[163]

2. With a standard systole, effects of differences in arterial pressure were small but noticeable when water was used; as arterial pressure increased, the ballistocardiographic amplitude decreased slightly. Only when diastolic pressure was twice normal did its effects on the Bcg become significant. When blood was used, the effects of arterial pressure were negligible.

3. The size of the subject made considerably less difference than had been predicted. With larger subjects, the Bcg did become slightly smaller.

4. Blood flow in the veins exerted little influence on the force Bcg.

5. Excellent correlations were found between the force Bcg amplitude and the maximum velocity of ejected blood,[165] as well as between the initial force and the HI slope.[172] The excellence of these correlations is particularly impressive when one realizes that stroke volume ranged from 19 to 83 ml, arterial pressure from 42/29 to 282/139 torr, left ventricular stroke work from 13 to 109 (10^5 ergs), the cross section of the aorta from 2.5 to 10.8 cm^2, pulse wave velocity from 3.1 to 13 m/sec, and body mass from 47 to 63 kg.

6. The presence of arteriosclerosis made little difference in amplitudes.

7. The most significant finding was that the force of Starr's arm could not imitate the heart. Even when a normal stroke volume was injected at a normal mean velocity, the Bcg was not normal in amplitude or form. He solved this problem by using a 30-lb mallet, swung from a fixed jack to strike the barrel of the syringe.[158,164] Now he could calculate the energy imparted to the blood. When the energy delivered by the mallet was altered, the IJ amplitude changed correspondingly. More importantly, when total energy was kept constant, but *initial* energy, and thus force or acceleration, of blood, was modified by changing the amount of padding on the mallet, the IJ amplitude closely reflected the magnitude and direction of this change. Thus originated the concept of ventricular impulse.

SELECTED ANIMAL STUDIES

As stated above, animal studies were virtually impossible with the HF system because of the difficulty in coupling the animal to the bed. With the ULF system, this problem was solved, provided the bed was extremely light and the animal was tightly strapped to the bed. Other problems soon appeared, however. Only rarely would a conscious animal lie quietly on its side while strapped to the bed. Respiratory interference in an excited animal, especially a dog, was frustrating. The only alternative seemed to be to anesthetize the animal. This did immobilize him and provide quiet respiration, but it caused still other problems. With morphine-barbiturate anesthesia, for example, the Bcg was acceptable initially but deteriorated with time.[173] Thiopental[174] or pentobarbital[175,176] proved to be no better. These observations are fundamentally important. This was the first time it had been pointed out that anesthetized animals, in general, are not satisfactory for physiologic or pharmacologic studies. This conclusion was made possible by the marked sensitivity of the Bcg to changes in cardiac function. To solve the problem we drew on a background of decades of practice in patients and devised a satisfactory method for anesthetizing animals and maintaining a normal Bcg for an indefinite period.[174] Just as important as the anesthetic agents in this technique is the provision or ventilation adequate to maintain a normal arterial blood pH and P_{CO_2}. This is a difficult lesson for some physiologists to learn.

The range of animals studied with the Bcg is incredible, from chicken embryos to whales. This represents a body mass ratio of 1/6,000,000. The animals include chicken embryos, mice, frogs, guinea pigs, rabbits, cattle, sheep, goats, baboons,* a young California gray whale, and, of course, dogs. Some studies will be described in the appropriate sections. Several miscellaneous studies deserve mention here.

In the rabbit,[190] digitalis increased IJ amplitude. Doses of digitalis, small enough to affect only the acceleration Bcg, and not arterial pressure, could be administered. Elzinga and Knoop[193] found an increase in the HI and IJ segments of the ULF acceleration record after administration of ouabain in the dog, but the displacement record showed no consistent changes. Left ventricular and aortic pressures increased rapidly. Thus the Bcg was able to demonstrate with one noninvasive technique what otherwise required extensive invasive measurements: digitalis increases the contractility of the normal heart, but cardiac output is not predictably affected.

Rademeyer[188] investigated the effect of age on the Bcg in rats, whose life span is 700 days. Older animals showed decided effects of cardiovascular aging, such as decreased HI and IJ amplitudes and slopes, as well as increased Q-H and Q-J time intervals. Unfortunately, sequential measurements were not taken. In this type of model, an easy, nontraumatic technique such as the Bcg would be ideal for a large number of serial measurements over a long period of time, using each animal as his own control.

Juznic[181] investigated five species, mice, rats, guinea pigs, rabbits, and man, and found an interesting relation between body weight and "total cardiac force," measured either as the product of the internal surface area of the left ventricle and mean arterial pressure or as the mean amplitude of the three systolic Bcg waves multiplied by the heart rate. Plots on a double log scale produced straight lines, the Bcg force curve parallel to and slightly below the invasively calculated line.

* Chicken embryos, Ref. 177; mice, Refs. 178–182; frogs, Refs. 178, 182, 184, 185; guinea pigs, Refs. 179–182, 186; rats, Refs. 179–182, 187–189; rabbits, Refs. 179–182, 190; cattle and sheep, Ref. 175; goats, Ref. 176; baboons, Refs. 81, 182, 191, 192.

More interestingly, maximum body acceleration, as measured by the Bcg, and aortic flow acceleration, as estimated by the Bcg, were very similar in mouse and man.[183]

During the preparation of this manuscript, we recorded the ULF Bcg on a young, California gray whale. The ballistocardiographic amplitudes in this 5-ton animal were in the same range as a normal man or a mouse. The comparison between the acceleration values in these extreme species shows an interesting similarity in the design of the cardiovascular system in mammals (Fig. 2-17). Not only do they have a similar aortic pressure[194] but also a similar peak aortic flow acceleration. Thus myocardial wall tension and force of ejection vary linearly with body mass.

To test some theories of the origin of the Bcg, West and Corbascio devised a new technique which was subsequently widely adopted by other cardiovascular physiologists—selective intracoronary artery administration of drugs. Small amounts of drugs were injected by catheter into the right coronary, circumflex, or the anterior descending branch of the left coronary artery. Stimulating or depressant drugs, such as isoproterenol, epinephrine, or acetylcholine, produced selective stimulation or depression of the Bcg without changing arterial or right atrial pressures.

THE Bcg FOR INVESTIGATIONS IN NORMAL HUMAN SUBJECTS

A just criticism leveled against the Bcg-cardiac output method and the simple IJ amplitude analysis has been that they are inapplicable in some critically ill patients. Yet these methods are unequivocally useful for studies in normal volunteer subjects, where noninvasive techniques are particularly desirable. The stimulus being investigated may actually be so subtle that any disturbing factor induced by the measurement could invalidate the experiment. During one such study, the Bcg was able to distinguish among a subject's cardiovascular responses to different colored lights.[197]

More hazardous experiments such as those concerning blood volume, inspired oxygen tension, or digitalis have been conducted. No changes in the Bcg were seen in normal subjects[198] on withdrawal of 500 ml of blood. After withdrawal of 1000 ml, the force Bcg decreased, while arterial pressure and heart rate showed variable changes. The changes were immediately reversed on reinfusion of blood. Hypoxia under most conditions causes an increase in the Bcg amplitude,[199–202]

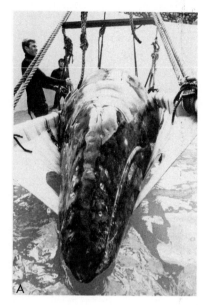
A

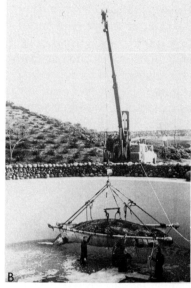
B

MOUSE

An.17.25; R.19h, 27.04g; 16.8.68

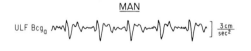

$I \dfrac{2\,cm}{sec^2}$

$I\,0.1\,mV$

0.2 sec

MAN

ULF Bcg$_a$

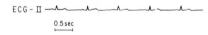

$]\dfrac{3\,cm}{sec^2}$

ECG - II

0.5 sec

WHALE

ECG - II

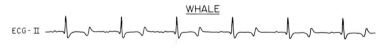

ULF Bcg$_a$

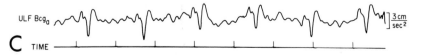

$]\dfrac{3\,cm}{sec^2}$

C TIME

80

whereas hyperoxia produces a small but definite decrease.* These consistent results can be contrasted with Henderson's early studies in which a much more crude Bcg system was used.

Zöllner et al in normal subjects noted an increase in the Bcg IJ amplitude and a decrease in the "preejection" period (Q-H interval) with Lanatoside C, a decrease in IJ and an increase in the preejection "PEP" with propranolol, and no influence by propranolol on the digitalis effect.[206]

The Bcg as a pharmacologic technique. The author has conducted many investigations in normal human subjects using the Bcg as a pharmacologic technique. It is in this area that the Bcg has one of its simplest and most valid applications. Being able to use the Bcg for noninvasive evaluation of cardiovascular function has been of inestimable value. We have used two forms of analysis, measurement of amplitudes and calculation of stroke volume by an analog computer.[207,208] The latter method was developed in 1964 for the noninvasive beat-to-beat calculation of stroke volume, cardiac output, left ventricular work, and systemic vascular resistance. Although the Bcg-cardiac output method may be of doubtful value in sick patients, it is very reliable in normal subjects given drugs. We have performed 7 series on 55 subjects, for a total of 1200 dye-dilution cardiac outputs for validation,[209,210] and

* Refs. 200, 203, 205.

Fig. 2–17. A. Gigi the whale in her bed. She is being prepared for her ULF Bcg by members of the staff of Sea World, Inc., San Diego. She ultimately resigned herself to the situation. The bed, although weighing 500 lb, was small by Gigi's standards; her weight was 9,950 lb. (Photo courtesy of Sea World, Inc., San Diego, Calif., with permission.) B. Gigi and her custom-made Bcg system. The reasonable leveling of the bed can be attributed to the ingenuity of the staff in arranging Gigi on the bed. The truck was rather small for the task, but the tires and hydraulic lift mechanism supplied a nearly ideal isolation from the ground. The accelerometer is being attached to the bed. C. ULF Bcg tracings from a mouse, a man, and a whale. These tracings were recorded in animals of different masses (ratio of about 160,000:1), body configurations, and fat distribution. The Bcg systems were of different designs and, in the case of the whale and mouse, were situated over 7,000 miles apart. In spite of this, the records are remarkable for their similarities, being more similar than a normal and abnormal human Bcg. (Mouse Bcg is from Juznic G: The ultralow-frequency ballistocardiogram of the mouse, Bibl Cardiol 26:280–291, 1970, with permission.)

we have found correlation coefficients between the Bcg and dye-dilution methods of 0.85 to 0.94.* These results compare favorably to those obtained when the dye-dilution and direct Fick techniques are correlated.[211,212] The method has been particularly useful for detecting rapid changes in cardiac output, changes which would have been missed by the dye-dilution method. Some of the observations which we have made in these studies are described in the succeeding paragraphs.

We have studied the effects of halothane anesthesia on the diving reflex in man.[213,214] The diving reflex, initiated in diving animals by immersion and apnea, consists of intense bradycardia, markedly decreased cardiac output, and profound vasoconstriction with selective perfusion of the brain and heart. The bradycardic response is present in man, although considerably attenuated.[214-218] We were able to show that a vasoconstrictor response is also induced in man[212] (Fig. 2–18). The reflex was altered by light halothane anesthesia, so that increased cardiac output and heart rate occurred (Fig. 2-19); it was abolished by deep anesthesia[214] (Fig. 2-20).

Isorhythmic dissociation is a form of AV dissociation in which the ventricles and atria beat at the same rate from independent pacemakers. It is fairly common during anesthesia, although rare in conscious patients. In halothane-anesthetized subjects, stroke volume and cardiac output decrease after conversion to isorhythmic dissociation and increase on reconversion to normal sinus rhythm.[220] More interesting are the changes observed during conversion. As the P wave slowly marches into or out of the QRS complex, stroke volume decreases to an even lower level, the minimum occurring when about half of the P wave is visible on the QRS. Analogous observations have been made in patients by Winer with his direct-body apparatus.[221]

Two pressor agents were compared in man: methoxamine, an agent with a "pure" vasoconstrictor effect, and mephentermine, with a mixture of cardiac and peripheral effects. The changes induced by methoxamine were much more rapid in onset and far more profound[209,222] (Fig. 2-21). Systemic vascular resistance increased while heart rate, stroke volume, and cardiac output decreased. Atropine, 1 to 2 mg intravenously, abolished the chronotropic effects, without affecting the negative inotropic effects of methoxamine. After mephentermine, the changes were more gradual and less drastic[210,222] (Fig. 2–22). Heart rate and cardiac output did decrease slightly at first, but rose after several minutes. Atropine administered 1–1.5 hr after initial injection of mephentermine restored the pressor effects of mephentermine, and increased

* Smith NT: unpublished data.

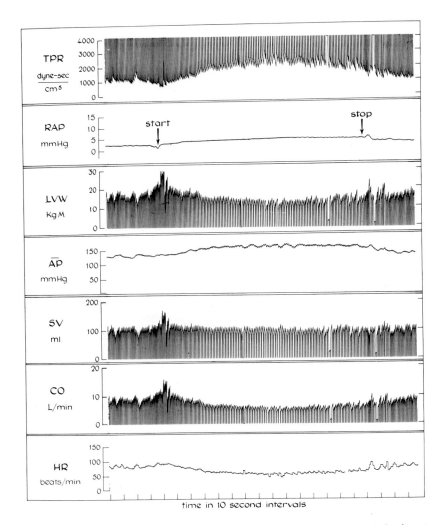

Fig. 2–18. Recording from a study on a 21-year-old man. Part of the input (Channels 2, 4, and 7) and output (Channels 1, 3, 5, and 6) of the analog computer (TPR, total peripheral resistance; RAP, right atrial pressure; LVW, left ventricular minute work; AP, mean arterial pressure; SV, stroke volume; CO, cardiac output; and HR, heart rate). This demonstrates in a conscious subject the diving reflex, initiated by apnea and placement of a cold, wet towel over the face ("start"). "Stop" indicates the resumption of ventilation and removal of the towel. The sharp peaks are caused by movement of the bed during placement and removal of the towel. Note the increase in resistance and decrease in cardiac output and heart rate, typical of the diving reflex. (From Smith NT, Eger EI II, Kadis LB: Progress in Anaesthesiology, Amsterdam, Excerpta Medica, 1968, pp 597–605, with permission.)

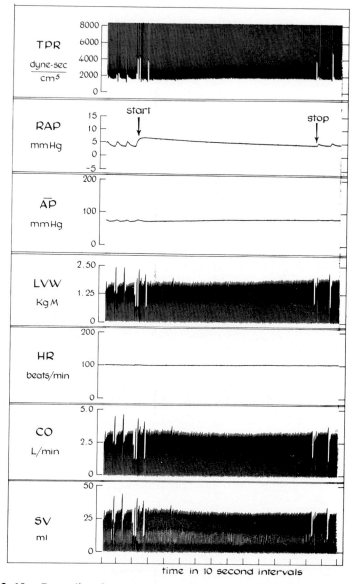

time in 10 second intervals

Fig. 2–19. Recording from the same subject as in Fig. 2–18. The diving reflex has been qualitatively altered by light, halothane anesthesia. Note change in gain early in recording (SV, CO, LVW). (From Smith NT, Eger EI, Kadis LB: Analogue computers in the study of anaesthetic and ancillary agents. In, Boulton TR, Bryce-Smith R, Sykes MK, Gillett GB, Reoell (Eds): Proc Fourth World Congr Anaesthesiologists. Amsterdam, Excerpta Medica, 1968, pp 597–605 with permission.)

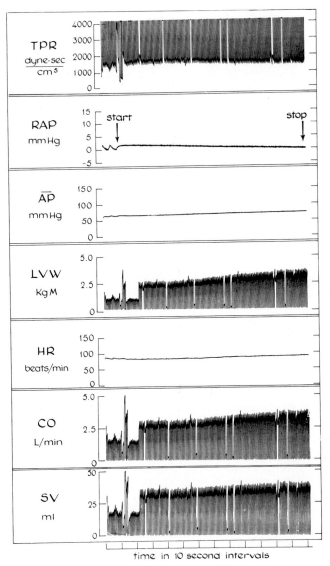

time in 10 second intervals

Fig. 2–20. Recording from the same subject as in Figures 2–18 and 2–20. The diving reflex was abolished by deep anesthesia with 1.6% halothane. (From Smith NT, Eger EI, Kadis LB: Analogue computers in the study of anaesthetic and ancillary agents. In, Boulton TR, Bryce-Smith R, Sykes MK, Gillett GB, Reoell (Eds): Proc Fourth World Congr Anaesthesiologists. Amsterdam, Excerpta Medica, 1968, pp 597–605 with permission.)

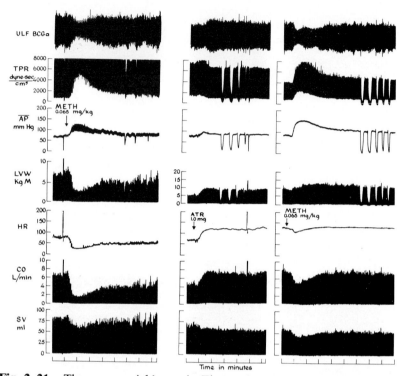

Fig. 2–21. The same variables as in Figures 2–18 to 2–20 except that an additional part of the input is shown (ULF BCG$_a$, ultralow-frequency acceleration ballistocardiogram) and part of the input has been omitted (right atrial pressure). The occasional sharp depressions in blood pressure and the corresponding changes in total peripheral resistance and left ventricular work are caused by inflation of a blood pressure cuff proximal to the arterial cannula. A. Methoxamine 0.065 mg/kg was injected intravenously. B. Atropine 1.0 mg was injected intravenously 90 min after injection given in A. C. The same injection of methoxamine was repeated 7 min after injection given in B. (From Smith NT, Whitcher CE: Monitoring of hemodynamic parameters by BCG in conscious man, Bibl Cardiol 19:36–42, 1967, with permission.)

heart rate and cardiac output strikingly. Further administration of mephentermine produced minor additional changes, suggesting that atropine had brought out the peak effects of mephentermine, 1.5 hr after administration.

The cardiovascular effects of two anesthetic agents have been compared in normal subjects. Although all inhalation anesthetic agents depress contractility in isolated hearts, not all depress the circulation

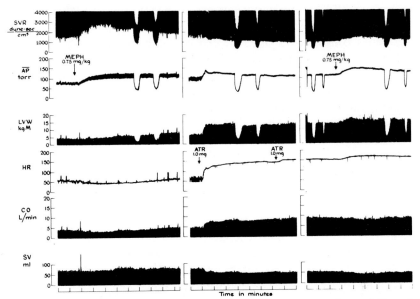

Fig. 2–22. A study on a 23-year-old man. The same protocol was followed as in Figure 2–21, except mephentermine 0.75 mg/kg was used instead of methoxamine. (From Smith NT, Br J Anaesth 44:452–459, 1972, with permission.)

in man. Fluroxene induces sympathetic stimulation, which compensates for the depression, so that no decrease in IJ amplitude is seen, whereas arterial pressure and cardiac output actually increase at higher concentrations.[223] With halothane, considerably less sympathoadrenal discharge occurs, hence there are profound decreases in stroke volume, cardiac output, mean arterial pressure, and IJ amplitude.

For decades, nitrous oxide has been considered to be merely a pleasant diluent in anesthetic mixtures, one without effect on the circulation or respiration. In dogs, Eisele[224] noted a sharp drop in stroke volume and maximum aortic flow acceleration after inhalation of a few breaths of nitrous oxide. This observation was confirmed in man with the Bcg.[225] An interesting side light of these studies was the usefulness of the Bcg in evaluating the validity of the protocol. The definitive study included arterial and right atrial catheterization. Before performing this study, we administered nitrous oxide on several separate days to accustom the subjects to the gas, the mask, and the strange surroundings. We dropped several subjects from the study because inhalation of nitrous oxide was an unpleasant experience for them. We retained only those in whom it was well tolerated. It could be argued that in addition to their psychologic responses, the two groups also differed in their circulatory responses to nitrous oxide and that the last series constituted a different experiment because of the catheterizations. However, we measured the Bcg and heart rate in all studies and could demonstrate that the two groups were similar. In addition, in the last experiment, when the selected group had recovered from the catheterizations, they were the same subjects as they were on other occasions, with identical ballistocardiographic reactions to nitrous oxide.

Nitrous oxide, when added to a more potent agent, such as halothane, fluroxene, or ether, may actually produce cardiovascular stimulation. In combination with halothane or ether, it behaves as an alpha-stimulating agent; that is, it increases arterial pressure, systemic vascular resistance, forearm vascular resistance, and decreases forearm venous compliance, without changing IJ amplitudes, ejection time, or heart rate.[226,227] With fluroxene, addition of nitrous oxide produces a mixture of alpha and beta effects.[228] If ganglionic blockade is produced by hexamethonium, the N_2O-induced alpha effect seen with halothane is converted to a beta effect—decreased systemic vascular resistance and increased heart rate, cardiac output, stroke volume, and IJ amplitude.[226]

RELATION OF THE Bcg TO
OTHER CARDIOVASCULAR MEASUREMENTS

In the next section I shall describe the relation between Bcg wave forms and some cardiovascular measurements obtained by invasive methods. The most important of these measurements for our purposes are cardiac output, aortic flow, and peak aortic flow acceleration. These are the variables which contribute more than any other to the systolic components of the respective motion derivatives of the Bcg.

Cardiac Output

The relation between cardiac output and the Bcg is of historical interest. The initial attempts to examine this relation had a considerable impact on the development of cardiovascular physiology. Starr first became interested in the Bcg because he wanted to develop a noninvasive technique for the measurement of cardiac output;[229] Cournand first became interested in cardiac catheterization to use the direct Fick method to validate Starr's Bcg formula.[229] He soon was immersed in the fascinating potential of this invasive technique.

The first series of formulas for computing cardiac output from the Bcg, all developed by Starr, were partly empirically and partly theoretically derived.[167,215] Since he was recording the force Bcg, he used integration and square root extraction to convert to a quasi-displacement function. These formulas have received extensive evaluation[209,210,231] by dye dilution,* direct Fick,[231-233] and even by exactly known stroke volumes.[167] As long as the Bcg record was normal, all formulas agreed to within 10 to 25 percent with the reference values. Stroke volume values obtained from grossly abnormal Bcg's, such as those from patients in shock or congestive heart failure, deviated greatly, and interest in this technique as a clinical method declined. However, the formulas remain valuable for pharmacologic studies in normal subjects and patients as discussed later. Thirty years after Starr's original publication, Burkhart[234] published a reasonable theoretical verification of Starr's formulas.

In spite of the strongly empirical and statistical characteristics of Starr's work and the disappointing results obtained from abnormal tracings, numerous formulas were developed subsequently. It seemed to many to be logical to use the displacement Bcg, since this derivative most directly reflects stroke volume. The simple formulas of Klensch and his students[235,250] have received the most extensive use and evaluation. One of the major disadvantages of these methods has been the need for breath holding during recording. The manner of breath holding influences stroke volume variably enough to render difficult comparison with "referee" values obtained during spontaneous respiration. Burger and van Brummelen[251] pointed out that to estimate accurately stroke volume from the displacement Bcg, four different characteristic times should be taken into account: ejection time, transmission time, which is related to pulse wave velocity, run-off time of the arterial tree, and the R-R interval. By incorporating two of these times, transmission and run-off, into an hydraulic model, van Brummelen[252] significantly improved the estimation of stroke volume. Later, van Brummelen and Josenhans[253] used the other two, ejection time and R-R interval, with equally good results. Rödenbeck[254] and Nickerson[28,255-258] also worked extensively with formulas for calculating stroke volume from the Bcg. Nickerson used the LF Bcg, which was ultimately overshadowed by the ULF system. However, he did develop a complex formula which was satisfactorily accurate.[258]

Several factors make it difficult to establish from the literature the validity and usefulness of most of these formulas. First, formulas were obtained using Bcg's with different physical properties. Second, the

* Smith NT: unpublished data.

determination of cardiac output by either the dye-dilution or direct Fick method is fraught with pitfalls which only recently have become apparent. Presently a 5 to 10 percent accuracy is the best to be expected with these methods under optimal conditions. Third, duplicate determinations were rarely performed in these studies. Finally and most serious, in very few circumstances were Bcg and reference cardiac output studies done simultaneously. The artificially high output to be expected during invasive catheterization would certainly account for much of any systematic discrepancy. In addition, the phase of respiration influences stroke volume considerably.

Despite all these difficulties, the lure of an accurate noninvasive method for cardiac output determination lingers. Two new approaches to stroke volume estimation from the Bcg have appeared recently.[259,260] Harrison in his derivation concluded that absolute values for stroke volume cannot be determined from the displacement ULF Bcg alone.[260] If measurement of changes only is desired, the technique is potentially useful, provided the changes do not result in a significant redistribution of blood.

Aortic Flow

There are two possible ways to compare the Bcg and aortic flow: either by measuring peak flows and Bcg amplitudes or by comparing the entire curves. The former task is simple, being analogous to the comparison with stroke volume, where only one value per beat is used. Smith et al have shown a good correlation between the ULF Bcg and peak ascending aortic flow in baboons.[191] Comparing phasic flow and the Bcg is considerably more difficult, since an infinite number of values are possible. Hence, only one group has attempted to correlate the early systolic Bcg with instantaneous aortic flow. You will recall that Noordergraaf in his model of the circulatory system used an aortic flow to generate a Bcg. On the computer, at least, the reverse is possible; a Bcg can be used to generate a typical flow curve.[80,261] It would be very useful to be able to synthesize an aortic flow curve from a patient's Bcg.

Aortic Acceleration

The most important and potentially useful relation is that between the acceleration Bcg and ascending aortic flow acceleration. Ascending aortic acceleration is probably one of the most valuable indicators of myocardial function available today, certainly among the beat-to-beat variables.[262] Rushmer[69] proposed the initial ventricular impulse (IVI) as a potential indicator of myocardial function in 1964. He originally intended to use the ascending slope of aortic root pressure as the IVI, but peak aortic acceleration is probably superior. Noble, Guz, Winter, and other workers have done considerable work on peak aortic acceleration, observing that this variable is more sensitive to changes in myocardial performance than other variables derived from flow measurements, and that it seems to be relatively insensitive to preload or afterload.[70,73] The latter fact implies that peak aortic acceleration measures true myocardial function, rather than any changes which might be induced by extraneous factors such as venous return or mean aortic pressure. Other studies* have confirmed this relative insensitivity to preload and afterload.[74]

That a close relation exists between the early systolic acceleration Bcg and peak aortic acceleration is undeniable. Studies in animals confirm those performed with analog computer models and in cadavers. Honig and Tenney[263] in early animal experiments measured aortic blood flow and estimated peak acceleration, finding a good relation between acceleration and the I and J Bcg amplitudes. Winter et al[71,72] studied dogs with electromagnetic flow probes implanted around the ascending aorta and catheters implanted in a coronary artery. Quantities of calcium or pentobarbital too small to affect stroke volume, peak aortic flow, or peripheral resistance altered both the Bcg and peak aortic acceleration. When the left anterior descending coronary artery was ligated, peak aortic acceleration and the Bcg dropped sharply, while stroke volume and peak aortic flow remained unaffected. Smith et al have found an excellent correlation between the acceleration HI or IJ amplitudes and peak aortic acceleration in baboons[81] and in dogs.† The correlation coefficients range from 0.79 to 0.90.

Direct confirmation of this relation in humans has not yet been established. Deuchar[264] derived instantaneous aortic flow acceleration by the pressure-gradient method in a small number of patients with aortic stenosis. He was able to find good correlations between Bcg amplitudes and peak acceleration. The only other relevant investigation was reported at a Bcg meeting[265] and mentioned in another publication.[266] It was said that there was an excellent relation between aortic acceleration as measured by the Fry differential pressure method and the acceleration HI amplitude.

* Reitan JA, Smith NT: unpublished data.
† Smith NT: unpublished data.

Other Variables

It is not surprising that the acceleration Bcg also correlates well with other invasive measurements than aortic acceleration. There are many ways to estimate myocardial performance, particularly when drugs are given. Although they measure different facets and are influenced differently by external factors, such as preload or afterload, they usually change in the same direction with a given stimulus. In dogs, Darby[267] found a reasonable correlation between the acceleration ULF Bcg and myocardial contractile force. In a more recent study, during simultaneous left heart catheterization and ballistocardiography in man, Harrison[77] noted a good correlation over a twofold range between left ventricular dP/dt and the Bcg IJ wave, although as might be expected, the correlation was not as good as that between IJ amplitude and ascending aortic acceleration.[81]*

Most studies correlating the Bcg and other noninvasive techniques have been limited to using the Bcg to estimate the time intervals of the cardiac cycle. Because of the many events contributing to a given portion of the Bcg, the technique is probably not reliable for this purpose. It must be admitted, however, that there is an inverse relation between the Q-H interval ("preejection period") and the peak velocity ULF Bcg.[206,268]

One interesting relation deserves mention, that between the systolic complexes of the force or acceleration Bcg and the first derivative of an aortic,[171,264,269] carotid,[270] or brachial pulse.[271-273] Similar abnormalities of form are often seen in the force Bcg and in the derivatives of the pulses.[270-274] Juznic[275] suggested that it would be logical to record simultaneously a headward and footward pulse. Cunningham[276] in a significant study, recorded the acceleration ULF Bcg, plus carotid and radial pulse derivatives in normal subjects and a few patients. Except on rare occasions, the important parts of the Bcg could be synthesized from the two pulses in normal subjects. In only 50 percent of patients with valvular disease did the synthesis succeed. This suggests that the three measurements could be used for mass screening, selecting for further study those patients in whom synthesis of the Bcg is not possible. We must remember that the first derivative of an externally recorded carotid pulse suffers from the same theoretical objection as that of an internally measured pressure—the pressure wave is very sensitive to vascular stiffness.[279] In addition, external carotid pulses in

---

* Smith NT: unpublished data.

particular can be very difficult to record, so that absolute amplitudes and slopes are not reliable. Winer[277,278] has used the second derivative of the direct-body Bcg and of the carotid pulse. The two resemble each other closely. This correlation has enabled more accurate notation of the Bcg segments and has enabled sharper delineation of the three phases of systole: isovolumic, early ejection, and "dominant" ejection.

SOME CONCEPTS DEVELOPED DURING
THE EVOLUTION OF THE Bcg

Because ballistocardiography is so old, there has been considerable time to speculate on the generation of normal and abnormal waveforms. As a result of the experimentation induced by this speculation, some important physiologic concepts have been advanced. These advances were initially unnoticed by those unacquainted with ballistocardiography and subsequently accepted without an awareness of their background. The three most important concepts brought to the attention of physicians are ventricular impulse, myocardial asynergy, and noninvasive evaluation.

The importance of the ventricular impulse was first realized by Starr as a result of his cadaver experiments.* After observing that he had to strike the injecting syringe sharply with a heavy mallet in order to simulate a normal Bcg, and that the Bcg became abnormal if the mallet was excessively padded, he began to concentrate on the meaning of this phenomenon. His observations were later confirmed by computer model and animal experiments relating IJ amplitude to peak ascending aortic acceleration, or ventricular impulse.

An important consequence of these observations was Starr's emphasis on the physiologic status of the heart, as opposed to its *anatomic* status. He has cautioned that the Bcg may provide few hints concerning the etiology of the abnormal waveforms.[282] For example, increased systolic amplitudes can be found during excitement[283] and in most patients with hyperthyroidism, aortic insufficiency, patent ductus arteriosis, or large peripheral AV shunts.[284] Probably because of the relative difficulties inherent in its concepts and measurements, cardiology has consistently lagged behind pulmonary medicine in its attention to physiologic diagnosis. Pulmonary medicine has already undergone

* Refs. 163–165, 172, 280, 281.

its period of skepticism about the value of some functional laboratory tests which were difficult to perform and even more difficult to interpret. Currently, however, instead of emphasizing "chronic bronchitis" or "silicosis," diagnoses coming from *routine* noninvasive pulmonary function studies include chronic obstructive disease, restrictive disease, or ventilation/perfusion abnormalities—functional rather than anatomic characterizations.

The concept of myocardial asynergy, or as he describes it, incoordination of myocardial contraction, was first advanced by Starr[230] in 1930. In dogs, destruction by cautery of part of the ventricular wall so that it bulged with each systole, changed the form of the Bcg. Since that time, Starr has tried to relate certain abnormal ballistocardiographic patterns to this incoordination. In 1958, he was able to reproduce these waveforms in cadavers by jerky, discontinuous "contraction" of the ventricles, as simulated with the syringe.[285,286] Later, using the Bcg combined with the brachial or carotid pulse, he suggested that in those patients in whom similar notching and slurring were detectable on both records, left ventricular incoordination was probably responsible.[270,286] These waveforms were also quite similar to those produced by incoordinate injection in cadavers. Recently, Noordergraaf's model[287,287a] has been used to demonstrate that incoordinate ejection could reproduce Bcg's typical of myocardial asynergy. Asynergy of contraction has received much attention lately.[288–291]

Perhaps one of the most important concepts arising from the Bcg is that of noninvasive evaluation of cardiac function. Starr turned to the Bcg in 1936 in his search for a noninvasive method for determining cardiac output. Thus Starr's work preceded by some 30 years the recent popular emphasis on noninvasive evaluation. It was the hope for noninvasive information that kept the interests of ballistocardiographers alive during the long period of skeptic latency.

Although ballistocardiography cannot assume credit for the concept and development of bioengineering, there is a connection between the two. One of the men responsible for the development of the ULF concept, Talbot, was chairman of the first Division of Biophysics and Bioengineering, which was founded at Johns Hopkins Hospital in the late 1940s. This was probably the first mention of the term bioengineering. The work in the late 1940s and early 1950s performed on the Bcg by Talbot's and other groups was certainly one of the first applications of true bioengineering: "a science [using] engineering concepts and methods in the study of living things," and in practical applications a science concerned with "the design and construction of instruments for biological research [and] in the practice of medicine."[292]

SOME CONCEPTIONS AND MISCONCEPTIONS
ABOUT BALLISTOCARDIOGRAPHY

As stated earlier, one of the prime handicaps of the Bcg's pre-maturity was that physicians expected more from the Bcg than it was designed to perform, and thus its reputation suffered. In this section I shall discuss some of the prevalent conceptions about the Bcg, many of which have justifiably caused physicians to hesitate to use the technique. Although in other sections we have discussed the resolution of some of these problems, it would seem advisable to group them into one section, so that the reader can gain a full appreciation for the many misguided criticisms and misconceptions which still plague bal-listocardiography.

The Bcg is excessively influenced by body mass. This is far less true than is generally believed. Body mass and total ejection force plot in a straight line, so that the difference in blood and body acceleration between mice, men, and whales is very small.[183,*] This constancy is analogous to arterial pressure, which is similar in most mammals, whereas ventricular wall tension varies enormously according to animal size. If one computes the derivative of acceleration, jerk, body mass is even less important as a consideration.[162]

The Bcg is influenced by loosely coupled masses such as the liver and other abdominal contents. Some distortion occurs because such masses resonate at a different frequency from that of the bulk of the body. However, the distortion produced by this effect is small,[36,49] and would be important only when subtle differences in waveform are being taken under consideration. Cunningham[37] states that *if* the transducer measures the true motion of the "dynamic" center of gravity of the body, it does not matter whether the body moves as a rigid unit. If the support is light enough and its restoring forces small enough, the true motion of the "dynamic" center of gravity is the true Bcg for all the coupled masses, the body acting as a mechanical filter damping out the major portion of the distortion. Recent unpublished evidence indi-cates that a head-foot accelerometer strapped between the shins pro-duces a better frequency response than one attached to the bed.†
Steps have been taken to eliminate even this small influence of loosely coupled body masses. Analysis has shown that a single loosely

---

* Smith NT: unpublished data.
† Cunningham DM: personal communication.

coupled abdominal mass is the most important component.[293] Franke and Braunstein[294] have therefore slightly modified Noordergraaf's model by using two body masses instead of one. They recently reported that by using their two-mass model, they could partially make the small corrections necessary in obese people, so that inexplicably abnormal Bcg's with peculiar notches were rendered more nearly normal.[295] The method seems deceptively simple: once the transfer function of the body is known, a recorded Bcg can be reduced to a pattern which would be produced by a rigid, that is, single-mass body.

The influence of the characteristics of body tissue such as fat and muscle is considerable. This is true for the direct-body Bcg except under optimal circumstances. However, the ULF bed, because of its light weight and strong coupling between subject and bed, has eliminated most of this inaccuracy. Furthermore, the fundamental natural frequency of the body ("bowl-of-jelly" phenomenon alluded to by some in reference to the Bcg) does not depend on body mass, amount of fat, or age.* Some of the higher mode frequencies may depend on the amount and distribution of body fat.

The coupling of the heart and blood vessels to the body frame is so loose and variable that much of the information is lost or distorted. Not satisfied with theoretic considerations, Nickerson[300-302] has attacked this problem from an engineering approach. He bolted the spinal column of dogs to a movable table, after implanting a radiopaque marker on the heart at the apex or base. Thus he could produce movements of the heart by moving the body. By shaking the table, he could calculate the distortion from the transmission between heart and body. In the first study,[300] he concluded that the amplitude distortion is minimal except at externally impressed frequencies close to the natural frequency of the Bcg suspension system, and therefore that distortion of this type will be minimal in a ULF system. The distortion which does occur lies in the range 0.2 to 0.3 Hz and can be filtered, since it is not important information. In the second study,[301] he concluded that the acceleration mode was the best for eliminating any distortion caused by coupling. Using the equations which had been validated by the shaking experiments, he computed the motion of the ballistic bed produced by the heart. He concluded that the ULF low-mass Bcg minimizes transmission distortion from heart to Bcg bed.[302]

Other investigators have suggested that even if coupling between

* Refs. 31, 32, 296–299.

the heart and body were perfect, the contribution of heart motion to the Bcg would be minor[147] except perhaps with massive cardiac hypertrophy. Little significant cardiac movement occurs during the very early part of ejection when acceleration is at its maximum, and only 5 percent of the stroke volume has been ejected. Movement of blood in the vessels, particularly the arteries, makes the preponderant contribution to the systolic Bcg. The arteries of the extremities and the aorta where it is adjacent to the spinal column, are relatively immobile.[303] For example, the longitudinal movement of the femoral arteries is of the order of micra. Such tight coupling should produce an extremely small amount of distortion in the Bcg. Only the proximal aorta has not been investigated. However, if Nickerson's studies on the importance of coupling apply equally well to this segment, as they probably do, the degree of tethering should not substantially affect ballistocardiographic amplitude or morphology.

In addition to myocardial performance, vascular tone influences the Bcg. Vascular tone influences the acceleration Bcg only to the degree that it influences peak aortic acceleration, on which the Bcg depends. On Noordergraaf's computer model, if aortic acceleration remains constant, peripheral resistance does not affect the Bcg and aortic compliance must change to physiologic extremes before an effect on the Bcg is noticeable.[80] In a study using cadavers, in only one subject with very severe atherosclerosis was the Bcg significantly different when a standard total energy and initial energy of injection were imparted to the blood.

The "normal" Bcg changes with age.[88,305-308] So does "normal" arterial pressure. However, ballistocardiographic amplitude declines while arterial pressure increases. The effect of age on the displacement ULF Bcg is more striking than that on the acceleration Bcg,* but the effect on the latter cannot be ignored. The reduction of the acceleration Bcg with increasing age cannot be attributed to arteriosclerosis, since the effect, if any, is a slight increase in amplitude.[313]

The variation with age can be used to advantage, provided normal values are established for each age group. One of the unique contributions of the Bcg to cardiovascular physiology has been the concept of the *physiologic age* of the heart. With the aid of regression equations, Starr[314,315] was able to determine that the hearts of certain persons are older physiologically than chronologically. In one longitudinal study,

---

* Refs. 123, 304, 305, 309, 312.

the Bcg actually provided more information reflecting physiologic age than all the other variables recorded—400 items in all.[123]

The contribution of venous flow to the Bcg is unknown. This is not true for acceleration recordings. It is known that venous flow contributes a very small amount, since it has a relatively low acceleration. Furthermore, much of the flow is in opposite directions.

The Bcg is too sensitive to preload and afterload. It is too sensitive to the same extent that maximum aortic acceleration is—minimally under physiologic conditions. Noble et al[70,73] and Sutherland et al[74] have presented evidence that maximum aortic acceleration is relatively insensitive to preload and afterload. In addition, Harrison et al[77] could demonstrate in man no correlation between the acceleration Bcg and minimum, end-diastolic, or maximum left ventricular pressure.

The Bcg is less reliable at faster heart rates.[316] This is true, particularly for displacement and velocity recordings. With acceleration recordings, however, the heart rate must be above 90 beats/min before the influence of a previous beat becomes noticeable.[317]

The influence of the right and left ventricles is inseparable in the Bcg waveform. They are in fact separable, but even if they were not, the contribution of the left ventricle to the Bcg dominates that of the right.[318]

The Bcg may be too sensitive an indicator of myocardial function. The Bcg declines so rapidly with the onset of poor myocardial function, that the margin may be slight between severely and catastrophically depressed function. This is still speculation and is of concern mainly with beat-to-beat monitoring. However, it should be considered seriously with any sensitive indicator of myocardial performance.

The Bcg does not correlate with anything yet measured. This was often true until recently, usually because the wrong variable, such as blood pressure or the electrocardiogram, was chosen for comparison. As our insight into the Bcg increases, the Bcg is beginning to demonstrate its usefulness in reflecting the more important cardiovascular variables, for example, peak aortic acceleration and maximum left ventricular dP/dt.

A major error has been the attempt by some to use the Bcg alone to arrive at an anatomical diagnosis such as aortic stenosis or anterior myocardial infarction. As with any other mechanical technique, only rarely can this be accomplished. Many have felt disillusioned that the Bcg does not correlate perfectly with the extent of coronary artery disease. It is becoming increasingly clear that the degree of coronary artery obstruction does not correlate well with myocardial damage, and that there can be "infarction without obstruction and obstruction without infarction."[319,320]

The Bcg does not measure cardiac output. This is a corollary of the preceding item that the Bcg does not correlate with anything yet measured. The Bcg can measure cardiac output as long as the systolic complex is nearly normal in form.

The Bcg is impossible, or at best difficult, to calibrate. This was certainly true of the direct-body Bcg. However, the HF force or the displacement ULF Bcg systems are extremely easy to calibrate. Accelerometers may be calibrated in two ways. Provided the amplifier is direct-current coupled, tipping the accelerometer a known angle from the horizontal axis provides satisfactory calibration. For example, tipping 90°, or to the vertical axis, will cause a-l-g deflection in the pen, since g represents the acceleration of gravity. As an alternative, one may use a mass moving at a known acceleration. A motor whirling an eccentrically placed weight can be assembled. A typical "shaker" would rotate a mass of about 150 gm and at a frequency of about 3 Hz and an amplitude of about 25 mm.[321] Such a combination of mass, amplitude, and frequency permits simultaneous dynamic calibration of acceleration, velocity, and displacement.

The ballistocardiogram is difficult and laborious to record. Our Cunningham air-bearing bed requires 15 to 45 min for initial set-up. However, if the bed remains permanently positioned, it takes only 1 min to prepare for each patient. After several weeks or months some readjustment may be needed. Modern circuits and oscillographic recorders have solved most other technical difficulties that plagued earlier systems. Actually, operating the bed is so simple that any physician can record a Bcg on himself.

The Bcg is such a sensitive instrument that it is almost impossible to obtain a record without artifacts, such as building vibrations. This still does present a problem, although some of the commercial beds, such as that built by Royal Medical Corporation, provide excellent isolation. It is advisable to select a quiet room, far from traffic, and as low in the building as possible—the basement is ideal.

The Bcg is not reproducible from patient to patient and in the same patient. The latter is true only for the older systems, especially the direct-body Bcg. Starr, by paying close attention to critical details, could reproduce a patient's record very well. Anyone today with currently available equipment can do likewise with far less effort. It is true that each person's Bcg is different. But many important measurements, such as IJ amplitude, fall within a relatively narrow range.

The Bcg is intolerant of poor technique. Yes it is. It does require care and attention to details.

The waveform is too complex to be of any use. We have already outlined two simple techniques of analysis (Starr's qualitative analysis and measurement of IJ amplitudes) which can provide considerable information. As soon as an appropriate technique of computer analysis is developed, a blackbox giving at minimum a simplified analysis and ultimately a differential diagnosis will be available.

The Bcg is too expensive. Our original ULF pendular system cost $350, including accelerometer, but not including labor or an already available recorder. A more realistic figure, including a recorder and amplifier suitable for additional noninvasive techniques such as the phonocardiogram or carotid pulse, is about $2000 to $2500, excluding labor. The commercial bed manufactured by Royal Medical Corporation costs $5800. This price includes accelerometer, amplifiers, filter network, and a built-in mechanical calibration system.

CLINICAL STUDIES WITH THE Bcg

Prognosis

Many people over 40 with no other evidence of cardiac disease have an abnormal Bcg. Formerly considered a drawback of the Bcg, it is now obvious that it is a distinct advantage. The phenomenon has been used to detect subclinical coronary artery disease and to predict the risk of acute coronary occlusion. In fact, the most impressive application of the Bcg in the clinical area has been that of prognosis, both short term and long term. All of the studies on prognosis have used semiqualitative analytic methods. That such singular successes have been gained with these ostensibly crude methods is remarkable. The new computer techniques should improve these results significantly.

Several reports on short-term prognostic studies have appeared. Recently Fischer[322] outlined the results of a study using the Bcg to predict the course of patients undergoing all types of surgery. In this large study, 1468 patients were grouped by the Starr Bcg classification and by electrocardiographic diagnosis. In none of the 608 patients in the normal or slightly abnormal ballistocardiographic groups (I or II) were there any incidents of major cardiovascular complications or deaths. In patients with group III abnormalities, the incidence was 12 percent, in group IV, it was 28 percent. A separation between no complications and minor cardiovascular complications was possible in the normal and slightly abnormal groups—2.6 percent versus 20 percent. The standard 12-lead ECG with visual interpretation proved worthless in this study. These results suggest that the Bcg could be used to screen presurgical patients in order to detect those who might need invasive monitoring during surgery. Talakov[323] studied 71 patients undergoing surgery for mitral stenosis. All six patients with very abnormal Bcg's ("inverted 3") died postoperatively. Seven out of 21 (33 percent of patients) in Brown's class 4 died; 3 of 23 (13 percent) patients in class 3 died; and 0 of 23 in class 0, 1, or 2 died. In the immediate survivor group, 43 percent of patients in class 3 or 4 survived 6 years, whereas 89 percent of those in class 0, 1, or 2 survived. In another series of patients with mitral stenosis, mitral insufficiency, or both, the Bcg was also able to predict the outcome of surgery.[324] None of the 37 patients in Brown's class 0, 1, or 2 died. All three patients in class 3 died. Kliorina[325] studied 60 patients with acute myocardial infarction. In the postinfarction period, seven showed ballistocardiographic changes of Brown's third or fourth degree. Only two of these patients were able to return to light work.

The results in the long-term prognostic studies are equally impressive. The requirements for such a study are very exacting, and difficult to follow. (1) The investigator, to collect his groups of normal and abnormal subjects, must be able to convince a large number of friends, relatives, and patients that they should have frequent Bcg's. (2) No matter what the study, Bcg or otherwise, the technique must be several years in advance of anything possible. This particularly includes statistical planning. When the results are published 5, 10, and 20 years later, the question will inevitably arise why a certain measurement or analysis was not performed. By definition, a long-term study will be out of date by the time it is published. (3) Finally, the investigator must plan to outlive all of his subjects in order to make the final analysis.

Starr used the qualitative analysis described on p. 62 for all of his studies. He began his long-term studies in 1937 with a series of ostensibly healthy subjects. He concluded, after 17- to 23-year followup periods, that those with an IJ amplitude of less than 275×10^3 were very much more likely to develop and die of cardiovascular disease.[326] The amplitude separation between those who developed and those who remained free of cardiovascular disease was very sharp. This was true even when Bcg amplitudes were adjusted for age and sex.

In the next series, he reported a 5-year followup on 221 hospital patients. When compared with insurance actuarial tables, the life expectancy of patients in the normal and slightly abnormal groups (I and II) was the same as predicted; that of groups III and IV was strikingly less.[327] Pooling data from healthy and hospital groups yielded even more striking results. Taking the age factor into account, Starr plotted the years of survival against the Bcg grade. In groups I and II there was a scatter of life expectancy from 0 to 25 years, with a some-what greater number of people dying from cardiovascular disease than from other causes. In class 3, only 2 of 31 lived longer than 17 years, but again a significant number died of noncardiovascular causes. In group IV, however, only 1 of 24 survived more than 4 years and 13 died within 1 year.[327] To diminish bias, Starr tried to pair his patients by age, sex, race, diagnosis, and duration of disease; only the Bcg was different. Since few perfect pairs were available, Starr formed some pairs in which the bias was slightly against him; for example, the abnormal Bcg belonged to the younger member of the pair. In the 18 pairs thus obtained, the mean duration of life in the patient with a normal Bcg exceeded that with an extremely abnormal Bcg (group IV) by 6.8 years. With the eight perfect pairs, the difference in life duration was 7.9 years. When group II and group III were compared, the dif-ference was 4.5 years. Many of the patients in the normal groups had not died at the time of publication; most of those in the abnormal groups had. Thus the differences in survival times can only grow.

Starr has been criticized in these studies because he did not have available the powerful statistical tools now in use. Baker did, however, and the long-term study conducted by him and his colleagues at Johns Hopkins has confirmed and expanded Starr's conclusions. Baker et al[328–330] were able to follow for 9 years 262 of 265 initially normal subjects and 259 of 309 patients with known ischemic heart disease.* Again, a qualitative evaluation of the Bcg was used. To eliminate the influence of age, multivariate logistic function analysis was used. The basic measurement of the study was an *event*. An event was defined as either a myocardial infarct, the onset of angina pectoris, or sudden death attributable to coronary artery obstruction.

The results were the most dramatic in the group classified normal by history, ECG, arterial pressure, and chest radiograph. Subjects whose Bcg's were abnormal at the onset developed an event six times more frequently than those with normal Bcg's. In the "young" group (third to fifth decade) the incidence of events in those with abnormal Bcg's was an astonishing 12 times that in the normal Bcg group. In older subjects the difference was 3.1.† The Bcg was a consistently better predictor than age. The risk that a 40-year-old male control would suffer an event attributable to coronary artery disease in the next year was 0.0046 if the Bcg was normal (Framingham risk 0.01), but 0.023 if it was abnormal. Put another way, a 40-year-old male control with an abnormal Bcg faces approximately the same risk as a 70-year old man with a normal Bcg. The results in patients with diagnosed coronary artery disease were not so consistent; the frequency of a recurrent event was only twice as great in patients with abnormal Bcg's as those with normal Bcg's. However, age disappeared as a predictor in this group. Using multiple regression analysis they evaluated a third group of control subjects with a minor abnormality in arterial pressure, heart size, or ECG. Compared to any combination of the other variables, the Bcg was a superior predictor of events. This was true even though hypertension is accompanied by slightly greater Bcg wave amplitudes, while decreasing life expectancy.[313]

What does all this mean to the physician? It would seem that the Bcg should be added to the list of predictive factors such as arterial pressure, serum cholesterol or lipids, blood sugar or uric acid, smoking, and body weight. Excess risks of 2- to 12-fold are impressive. What does one tell the individual patient? Statistics are considerably more useful for the group than for the individual. What would you do if

---

* An intensive followup was made on a random sample of the 50 patients lost from the second group. Contact was made with the entire sample, and extrapolation from their results did not alter the substance of the overall results.

† Another similar shorter term study[331] also suggested that the Bcg was a better predictor of the onset of manifest coronary artery disease between the ages of 30 and 50 years, rather than over 50 years.

tomorrow you were given not only a simple way to determine V_{max}*
but also the normal values and ranges? Would you alter the life pattern
of a patient with a low V_{max}? I would suggest that a patient with a
Starr grade III or IV Bcg be given the same advice concerning diet,
smoking, drugs, and stress as any other patient with an increased risk
of coronary occlusion.

Monitoring

Although the Bcg is sensitive to changes in myocardial function,
it is not appropriate for beat-to-beat monitoring in the operating room,
intensive care unit, or coronary care unit. In the operating room the
reason is clear; the Bcg is measured in millig's, whereas our surgical
colleagues work in megag's. However, by obtaining intermittent tracings,
the Bcg can be used for hour-to-hour or day-to-day monitoring. For
example, one could follow individually the course of digitalization and
select a dose of digitalis which produces satisfactory myocardial function, yet is less than the standard digitalizing dose.

Screening

The Bcg should be used for mass screening of patients, with an
abnormal record indicating a more extensive workup. This has not yet
occurred. Perhaps physicians would be willing to use the Bcg for screening purposes if convenient beds were made available. Standing[93,94] or
sitting[59,91,92] beds may meet such a need.

Physical Conditioning

The high predictive value in events connected with coronary artery
disease makes one ask about the effects of physical training on the Bcg.
The acceleration Bcg of athletes is indeed greater than that of sedentary
persons.[332-336] More meaningful are the ballistocardiographic changes
induced by training. The amplitude of the displacement Bcg can almost
double after 3 weeks training, while heart rate decreases from 78 to
55 beats/min.[318] This increase in amplitude is not surprising, since
the displacement Bcg amplitude approximately reflects stroke volume.
It is now well established that after vigorous physical training, the
acceleration Bcg can undergo a remarkable improvement (Figs. 2–23 &

*V_{max} is the maximum velocity of a muscle fiber or contractile element.

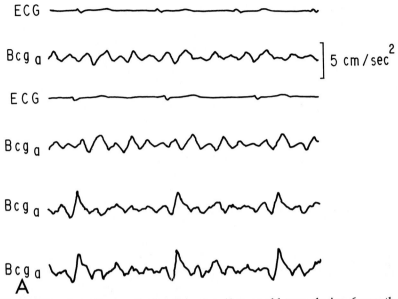

Fig. 2–23. A. Changes in the Bcg of a 43-year-old man during 6 months of training. He had a history and electrocardiographic evidence of an old myocardial infarction. Record 1 (top record) was taken at the beginning of the period and is grossly abnormal. The simultaneously recorded ECG is almost necessary to help identify the proper complexes. Records 2, 3, and 4 were taken after 2, 4, and 6 months of training, respectively, and show a progressive increase in force and normalization of waveform. Record 4 falls within the normal range. (From Holloszy et al: Effect of physical conditioning on cardiovascular function, Am J Cardiol 14:761–770, 1964, with permission.)

2–24).[337,338] This change is particularly marked if the Bcg was abnormal at the beginning of the training period. Not only are amplitudes increased but also wave forms are improved (Figs. 2–23 & 2–24). There is also a strong correlation between the maximum oxygen uptake, which is a generally accepted index of cardiovascular and respiratory fitness, and improvement in the Bcg.[337] In the careful, but small, study of Holloszy et al,[338] 5 of 15 subjects evidenced an abnormal Bcg at the beginning of training; four of five of these reverted to normal by the end of the 6-month period. In the sedentary control group, Bcg amplitudes actually decreased and two of the normal subjects developed abnormal Bcg's.[338] Elsbach et al suggest that if the preconditioning Bcg shows only slight abnormalities, conditioning should be just strenuous enough to abolish the abnormality.[337] If severe preconditioning

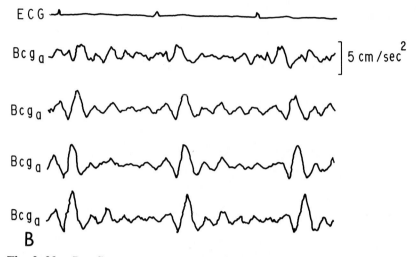

Fig. 2–23. **B.** Same sequence as in Figure 2–23A, in a 55-year-old man, who had no other evidence of cardiovascular disease. In this patient, the improvement in form is more spectacular than the increase in amplitude. One can see evidence of myocardial asynergy in Record 1. (From Holloszy et al: Effect of physical conditioning on cardiovascular function, Am J Cardiol 14:761–770, 1964, with permission.)

anomalies are found, conditioning must proceed cautiously and the Bcg must be checked frequently. One of the interesting features of these studies is that they give the same information as invasive studies,[339,340] or perhaps even more. For example, the Bcg predicts that physical training improves synergy of cardiac contraction in some patients.

Stress Tests

To try to extract even more information from the Bcg, several investigators have used stress tests. Many of these tests, such as exercise, anoxia, food, and smoking, are discussed extensively by Starr.[341–342] Exercise is not an ideal test for the Bcg. It is impossible to record the Bcg during vigorous exercise. Therefore the patient must climb onto the Bcg as quickly as possible after exercise. This maneuver is performed easily and quickly with a standing Bcg. Muscle tremor and panting distort the Bcg, requiring signal averaging for analysis.[329] Abnormalities are often brought out by exercise, but in some patients the Bcg actually improves, presumably as a result of release of catecholamines.

The smoking test has long been used by ballistocardiographers since the observation in 1951 in Dock's laboratory that smoking induced

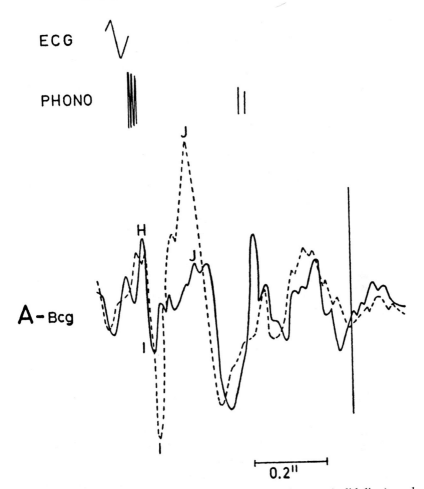

Fig. 2–24. Drawing of superimposed ULF Bcg's before (solid line) and after (dashed line) conditioning. The solid vertical line corresponds to an acceleration of 4.2 cm/sec². The difference between the two Bcg's in amplitude and coordination, or synergy, is striking. (From Elsbach H et al: The ballistocardiogram in selection for and assessment of physical conditioning in patients with ischemic heart disease, Bibl Cardiol 26:49–51, 1970, with permission.)

Bcg abnormalities, especially in patients with overt cardiac disease.[343] This has been confirmed countless times, the incidence of abnormalities in diagnosed coronary artery disease ranging from 50 to 90 percent. In young healthy subjects, abnormalities occur extremely rarely. Nitroglycerine prevents the Bcg abnormality of smoking. This, together with the observations that anginal pain occasionally accompanies the smoking test and that the Bcg wave form resembles that of patients undergoing a spontaneous anginal attack, suggests that the smoking is causing coronary artery insufficiency.[344] Indeed, it has recently been hypothesized that smoking may induce coronary insufficiency through two mechanisms: increased myocardial oxygen requirements from nicotine and decreased myocardial oxygen availability from carbon monoxide.[345,346]

Buchanan has performed the smoking test in control subjects and in patients with coronary artery disease, diabetes, thyrotoxicosis, and myxedema. No patient in the last three groups had a diagnosis of coronary artery disease. The test was positive in 16 of 19 patients less than 40 years of age and affected with coronary artery disease, and in 21 of 26 with thyrotoxicosis.[347] This suggested that the coronary circulatory reserve may be borderline in thyrotoxicosis. Nine patients euthyroid after therapy and 27 normal subjects showed no abnormalities with smoking. Only 1 of 18 patients with myxedema manifested a positive test.[348] In diabetic patients, 9 of 25 developed abnormalities during smoking, suggesting latent coronary artery disease.[349]

Evaluation of Therapy

As described above, the Bcg is useful for evaluating drugs in normal subjects. One might also suspect that it would be useful in evaluating therapy in patients. Again, this area is well covered by Starr,[350] and several articles are available from a recent symposium.[13] Only a few important examples will be discussed here.

In general, digitalis improves the Bcg in both normal and diseased hearts,[109,351-358] but the latter are frequently not completely restored to normal. Occasionally, digitalis produces a deterioration in function.[269] More importantly, one can demonstrate with the Bcg that subdigitalizing doses often produce optimal improvement. In contrast, in 11 extremely elderly women,[74-95] Starr and Luchi were unable to demonstrate with blind techniques any effect of digitalis on the heart.[359] Yet the hearts of the majority of these subjects were stimulated by mild exercise. This established clearly that the failure to observe digitalis action could not be attributed to incapacity of elderly hearts to respond to stimulation and that the techniques used were fully capable of demonstrating cardiac stimulation when it did occur.

Warembourg showed that although amyl nitrite increased Bcg amplitude in normal subjects, it usually decreased or did not change the amplitude in patients with angina pectoris.[360] Nitroglycerine, on the other hand, improves the Bcg in more than half of patients with documented angina pectoris (Fig. 2–25).[361,362] The improvement lasts

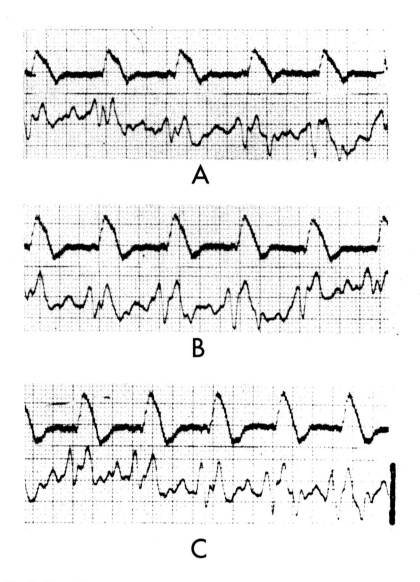

A

B

C

Fig. 2–25. Effect of nitroglycerine on a man aged 52 with occasional attacks of chest pain. The first derivative of an externally recorded brachial pulse is above the ULF acceleration Bcg. A. Before administration of nitroglycerine. B. Two minutes after 0.6 mg nitroglycerine had been placed under the tongue. C. Eight minutes after administration. (From Starr I, Noordergraaf A: Ballistocardiography in Cardiovascular Research, Philadelphia, Lippincott, 1967, p 325, with permission.)

only about 15 min. If the patient has a spontaneous or smoking-induced attack while lying on the Bcg, nitrites effect a marked improvement in the Bcg.[361,363,364] Klensch[235] and Juznic[365] concluded that the improvement in cardiac function which follows nitroglycerine is caused by a sharp decrease in left ventricular work, rather than by coronary dilation. Nitroglycerine worsens the Bcg in some patients with coronary artery disease.[361] One should probably approach vasodilator therapy with caution in these patients, since they may have extremely narrow, fixed coronary arteries.

In most patients with severe hyperlipemia and evidence of coronary artery disease, an improvement in the Bcg occurs after a prolonged low-fat diet.[366,369] In one patient the improvement was short lived. Within six months the Bcg deteriorated, and the patient soon died following a myocardial infarction.

Cardiovascular Surgery

The Bcg would also seem to be a useful technique for evaluating the efficacy of various cardiovascular surgical procedures. Immediately after surgery, a temporary but considerable deterioration in function is seen, both in aortic stenosis and aortic insufficiency.* If cardiac surgery for mitral stenosis is established to be successful by independent means, the Bcg soon shows a striking improvement over preoperative tracings[352,373,376] (Fig. 2–26). Unsuccessful surgery is also reflected in the Bcg (Fig. 2–26).[373] The lack of success may be due not to surgical techniques but to irreversible myocardial or systemic damage.[377]

Results after surgery for coronary artery disease are not as clear cut. After internal mammary artery ligation, two observers reported no ballistocardiographic improvement.[378,379] Unfortunately, one of the studies was misinterpreted by the authors as showing improvement,[378] and the other was never published,[379] unfortunately because the operation later proved to be worthless. Results have been mixed with the Harken,[369] Beck I,[380] and Vineberg[381,382] operations. After the Vineberg operation, 7 of 16 patients showed improvement in the Bcg, and three patients deteriorated.[381,382] Many patients with improved symptoms did not show Bcg improvements. No patient with a nearly normal preoperative Bcg died immediately after surgery, but the two patients with extremely abnormal Bcg's died. A disturbing finding in this series was the considerable variability in successive recordings in a given patient. Occasionally, the Bcg changed drastically during a recording.

---

* Aortic stenosis, Refs. 264, 370–372; aortic insufficiency, Refs. 264, 372.

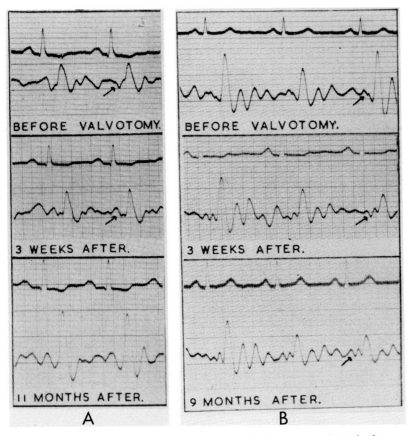

Fig. 2–26.   A.   An HF (force) Bcg before and after successful valvulotomy for mitral stenosis. Before surgery mean pulmonary arterial pressure was 40 torr; 11 months after, it was 18 torr. The improvement in the Bcg is obvious. (From Henderson CB: The ballistocardiogram in congenital heart disease, Am J Cardiol 3:799–810, 1959, with permission.)   B.   An HF (force) Bcg before and after an unsuccessful valvulotomy for mitral stenosis. Mean pulmonary arterial pressure was 26 torr before surgery, but rose to 43 torr 9 months after surgery. The Bcg has deteriorated somewhat. (From Henderson CB: Am J Cardiol 3:799–810, 1959, with permission.)

This variability is encountered so frequently in patients with severe coronary artery disease that it suggests that any invasive test infrequently performed might not give the complete picture.

The Bcg has also been used to evaluate patients after cardiac transplantation. One of the major problems in transplantation of any organ has been the planning of suitable immunosuppressive therapy. Therapy which protects the graft against rejection may allow infection in the patient. The physician walks a tight rope between too much and too little therapy. In dogs after cardiac transplantation, the cause of death was usually neither infection nor massive rejection, but rather progressive disability from multiple minor rejection crises. The goal therefore is to detect the onset of rejection before it produces irreversible damage, yet to avoid premature therapy. The need for a simple, daily measurement of cardiac function is obvious.[383,384] The relatively normal appearance of Bcg's after cardiac autotransplantation in dogs[385] suggested that the Bcg could be used to monitor the progress of animals after allotransplantation. In 16 dogs the Bcg was very effective in detecting the onset of early rejection, in assessing the efficacy of therapy, and in predicting life expectancy (Fig. 2–27).[386] In 11 patients studied subsequently, the success was not so striking, although the Bcg was useful in several areas.[387,388] It could detect when additional therapy was *not* indicated. For example, one patient showed clinical signs of rejection plus superimposed infection, although the Bcg was steadily improving. The patient nevertheless received additional immunosuppressive therapy and within 1 month died from pulmonary aspergillosis. During a similar episode in another patient, therapy was withheld on the basis of the Bcg, and a satisfactory recovery from that episode followed. Three patients died during the study; in all three, autopsy confirmed the Bcg diagnosis of rejection versus no rejection. The clinical diagnosis of rejection was often uncertain, and when it contradicted the Bcg diagnosis, a dilemma arose. One patient was treated twice during the study for "rejection" episodes, which consisted of weight gain and "logginess." Immunosuppressive drugs, diet, and fluid restriction improved the patient. Thus evidence for an unequivocal diagnosis was lacking.

A major problem was that the ballistocardiographic test was simple for the patients, and they treated it casually. It is easy to keep a dog without food, coffee, cigarettes, or exercise just prior to an examination, but not this type of patient. The best results by no coincidence were seen in the patients who were confined to the hospital.

Clinical Conditions

Congenital cardiac lesions. Very few characteristic ballistocardiographic recordings have been reported with congenital cardiac lesions. However, two exceptions are noteworthy. Three investigators have described an enormous H wave in the displacement and velocity ULF Bcg's in pulmonic stenosis.[83,355,389] This was felt to be caused by a back flow during atrial systole.[389]

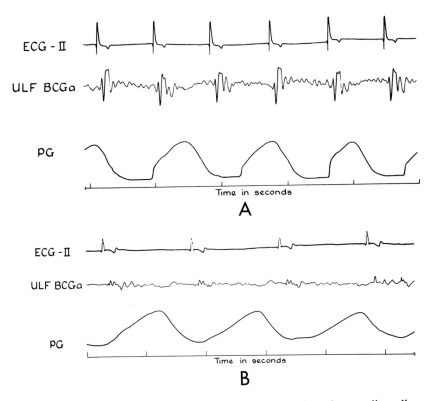

Fig. 2–27. A. The ULF acceleration Bcg from a dog after cardiac allo-transplantation (ULF Bcg$_a$, ultralow-frequency acceleration ballistocardio-gram; PG, pneumogram). Note absence of P waves in the ECG. The Bcg is remarkably close to being normal. This animal survived a year, a long survival for a dog. (From Smith NT, Angel WW: The BCG in cardiac homo-transplantation, Bibl Cardiol 20:82–93, 1968, with permission.) B. The ULF acceleration Bcg from a dog after cardiac allotransplantation (see Fig. 2–27A). This animal survived for only 4 days. It does not require an expert in ballistocardiography to see the difference between the Bcg of this animal and the one in Figure 2–27A. (From Smith NT, Angel WW: The BCG in cardiac homotransplantation, Bibl Cardiol 20:82–93, 1968, with permission.)

Elsbach and Rodrigo in 36 cases of atrial septal defect, found a characteristic pattern, in which the area of the velocity I wave was abnormally large in relation to the velocity J wave.[390] A good quadratic correlation was found between the velocity I/J ratio of the pulmonary to systemic blood flow. After closure of the defect, the abnormality tended to disappear. The authors calculated, from Noordergraaf's mathematical model, velocity Bcg curves which would result from 1 to 5 times the normal contribution to the Bcg of the pulmonary arteries and 0.5 to 2.5 times the normal cardiac contribution (Fig. 2–28).[158] Velocity (flow) curves showed the difference more conspicuously than displacement or force records.

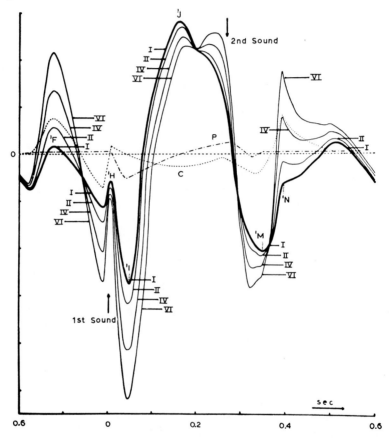

Fig. 2–28. Changes in the *velocity* Bcg predicted to accompany atrial septal defects of different magnitudes. The heavy line (I) is the velocity Bcg predicted for the normal human. The lines marked II, IV, and VI were obtained by adding to I 1, 3, and 5 times the normal contribution of the pulmonary arteries (P, light dashed-dotted line), and 0.5, 1.5, and 2.5 times the normal cardiac contribution (C, light dashed line). Thus, they are predicted curves for intraatrial septal defects of increasing size. The effect on the I wave is considerably more prominent than that on the J. (From Elsbach H, Rodrigo FA: The ultralow-frequency ballistocardiogram in atrial septal defect. A semiquantitative approach based on the analysis of the velocity curve, Am Heart J 70:186–195, with permission.)

Acquired valvular disease. Since the ejection pattern varies with the orifice size of the aortic valve, the Bcg might be expected to reflect this phenomenon. Moss and Gottovi studied 10 patients with aortic outflow disease and 12 control patients.[372] Four different acceleration ULF Bcg measurements correlated moderately well with aortic patency, with coefficients of 0.67 to 0.74. Perhaps multiple regression analysis would have improved these correlations. Deuchar[368] did not observe such good correlations, but he judged severity of stenosis by pressure gradient only, rather than by measurement of pressure gradient and flow plus angiography. The enormous amplitude of the force or acceleration Bcg is very characteristic of aortic insufficiency and has been described repeatedly* with the earliest description in 1880.[19] Retrograde flow accentuates the LMN complex in Noordergraaf's model.[395] Therefore, the physician should examine this segment to distinguish aortic insufficiency from other conditions producing increased amplitude.

One of the most striking acceleration Bcg's is seen with idiopathic hypertrophic subaortic stenosis. Many cases show an abrupt deceleration in the middle of ejection, resulting in a double I and double J wave (Fig. 2–29).[104,106,107] Verdouw has mimicked this Bcg pattern by reproducing the erratic ejection pattern using Noordergraaf's electrical model.[396] This pattern is typical of the "obstructive" type; the low-grade or nonobstructive type shows an enlarged waveform, but no splitting.[107] By using several Bcg variables and a multiple regression analytic technique, Jackson et al concluded that the acceleration ULF Bcg may be used to predict maximum dv/dt in this condition.[104]

In mitral stenosis and mitral insufficiency, several abnormal notches can be seen, particularly in the pre- and early ejection intervals.[397–398] However, they can be difficult to detect and are present in other disorders. On the other hand, if the diagnosis is already established, the Bcg can help assess the physiologic severity of the disease. Henderson plotted Brown's five classes of Bcg abnormalities against mean pulmonary arterial pressure.[399] The relation was virtually a straight line. Using a direct-body three-dimensional Bcg, Fujigaki et al noted close correlations between the anteropostero GH/IJ or JM/IJ ratios and mean pulmonary arterial pressure or pulmonary wedge pressure.[134] The coefficients ranged from 0.78 to 0.90.

Angina pectoris. Between anginal attacks, the force Bcg's of the great majority of patients are abnormal in form and/or amplitude,[394,400–402] yet the waveforms are usually easily identifiable. Further-

---

* Refs. 19, 352, 370, 392–394.

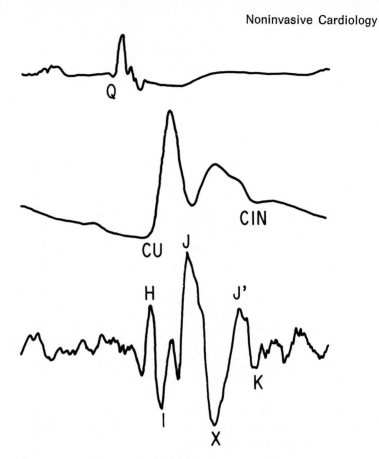

Fig. 2–29. Typical carotid pulse and Bcg tracings in idiopathic hypertrophic subaortic stenosis, with Y-lead of the Frank vectocardiograph system (CU, carotid upstroke; CIN, carotid incisura). Note in particular the deeply split J wave. (After Jackson DH et al: Ballistocardiographic and angiographic correlative study in idiopathic hypertrophic subaortic stenosis, Bibl Cardiol 27:14–19, 1972, with permission.)

more, there is nothing characteristic about these records, which can be duplicated many times during the latter half of life in patients who have never had angina. During an attack, however, ballistocardiographic confusion reigns; the cardiac contraction becomes weak and disorganized,* as if the next step were ventricular fibrillation (Fig. 2–30).

* Refs. 363, 364, 403–405.

The prodome of an attack can be detected. Kuo and Joyner[364] fed high-fat meals to susceptible patients. During the next 5 hr the Bcg steadily deteriorated until the disorganization of a full-blown attack set in.

Acute myocardial infarction. Since it usually seems unwise to move patients during the early stages of acute coronary occlusion, few studies have been conducted during this period. Recently, Winer[279,406] looked for evidence of asynergic contraction with his direct-body Bcg in 93 patients with possible acute myocardial infarction. In 71 of these patients, the diagnosis of infarction was confirmed in the early stages by characteristic enzymatic or electrocardiographic changes. However, in 22 patients, the diagnosis, unclear when the patients were first seen, was suspected solely on the basis of Bcg changes.

Almost everyone with a Bcg system has studied patients surviving more than 1 week.[407] The data have been fairly consistent. After the acute stage of infarction, the great majority of patients show force Bcg's which are abnormal in form, small in amplitude, or both. In the succeeding months, the records of many patients slowly improve, sometimes to complete normality. In other patients the record does not change; in still others it slowly deteriorates. With the newer, more sensitive ULF systems, a significant majority show specific abnormalities not seen in normal subjects or in patients affected by other types of heart disease.[404,408]

Abdominal aortic aneurysm. The K wave of the Bcg represents that portion of systole when ventricular ejection has passed its maximal acceleration phase and flow is proceeding through the systemic arterial tree prior to meeting significant resistance. With this in mind, Fischer observed that an abdominal aortic aneurysm was present in at least half of the patients with an abnormally shortened and blunted K wave.[108] Only 2 of 24 patients with a definite aneurysm did not have an abnormal K wave. The physician should therefore suspect an abdominal aneurysm in any patient with this K wave abnormality.

Hypertension. In a very recent study, Starr concluded that the presence of hypertension did not interfere with the ballistocardiographic interpretation of early systolic waveforms.[313] This finding is consistent with cadaver experiments and analog computer studies showing that the I wave is relatively insensitive to changes in systemic vascular resistance. On the other hand, the Bcg can help distinguish arteriosclerosis by

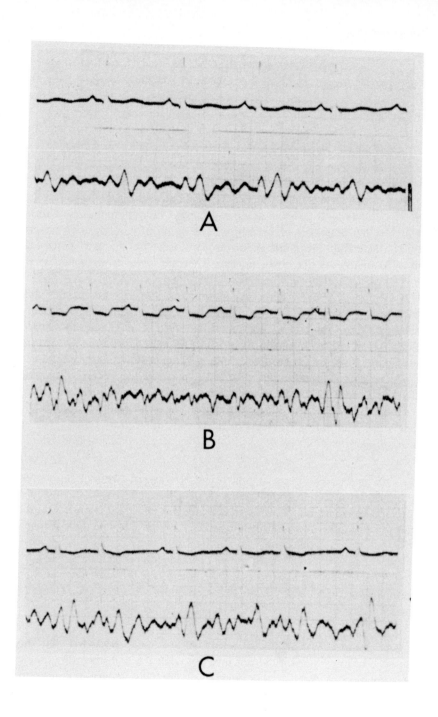

A

B

C

using information in late systole. On Noordergraaf's analog model, Verdouw showed that the IK interval decreases and the K wave becomes deeper as systemic vascular resistance or aortic wall stiffness increases.[409] In one of our baboons with an obviously increased aortic wall stiffness, as shown by a greater pulse wave velocity and pulse pressure, the K wave was much more pronounced than in the other animals.[410]

Thyroid disease. In general, Bcg's are large in amplitude in patients with hyperthyroidism,[269,325,411,412] whereas they are small in hypothyroidism.[402] Morphologically abnormal Bcg's are frequently seen with hyperthyroidism. Appropriate therapy restores most records to normal.[269,325]

BASH (BODY ACCELERATION SYNCHRONOUS WITH THE HEARTBEAT)

Ballistocardiography represents not only a noninvasive diagnostic procedure but also a potential noninvasive *therapeutic* procedure. The story of BASH is the story of a theory applied in reverse. I have repeatedly emphasized that a large portion of the early systolic Bcg arises from movement of blood in the major arteries. A Dutchman, Arntzenius,[413] in 1969 reasoned that if movements of blood could cause movements of the body, properly timed, induced movements of the body might assist the movement of blood. Accordingly, he placed piglets on a strong shake table, which delivered a 2-g footward acceleration as soon as left ventricular ejection began (Fig. 2–31). In normal piglets, flow did not change, but pressure decreased, indicating that ventricular work decreased and that energy was transferred into the circulatory system from the outside. After shock had been induced in

---

Fig. 2–30. ECG and HF (force) Bcg before, during, and after an attack of angina pectoris in a patient aged 63. This attack was a comparatively mild one, relieved promptly by one tablet of 0.6 mg nitroglycerine. Calibration is given by the bar in the top right, which indicates 275×10^3 dynes. A. Usual record when not in attack, BP, 120/80. B. During pain, BP 110/80. C. About 5 min after nitroglycerine, pain gone, BP 120/80. Note the incoordination in the middle record. (From Starr I, Noordergraaf A: Ballistocardiography in Cardiovascular Research, Philadelphia, Lippincott, 1967, p 235, with permission.)

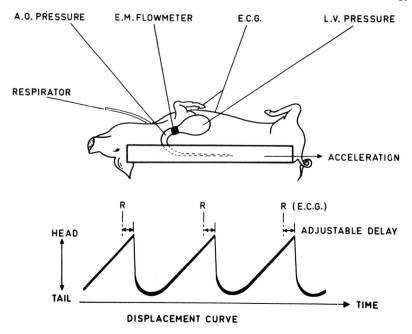

Fig. 2–31. The shake table used by Arntzenius to deliver a properly timed footward impulse (BASH) to a well-secured pig. The R wave was used to time the impulse. Since the total displacement must be equal in both directions, there is a noticeable headward acceleration. The pigs were anesthetized. For BASH to be given to conscious humans, the head must be well strapped. One BASH was given for each heart beat, but the system can be adjusted to give a BASH every second or third beat. (From Arntzenius AC, Verdouw PD: Cardiovascular responses in pigs to body acceleration applied synchronously with the heart beat, Bibl Cardiol 27:44–52, 1972, with permission.)

pigs by anoxia or by ligation of the anterior descending coronary artery, brief periods of BASH (3 to 5 min) restored the circulation for prolonged periods,[414] as demonstrated by increases in peak aortic flow, stroke volume, left ventricular pressure, and aortic pressure. The ECG showed a concomitant improvement. In animals surviving 2 weeks of ligation, a classical anterior wall infarction was demonstrated. The reason for the prolonged improvement effected by brief periods of BASH in animals in cardiogenic shock is an enigma. Preliminary studies with coronary angiograms have suggested retrograde filling after BASH, similar to that seen after ventricular assistance with the Anstadt device.[415] Arntzenius has been a paragon of caution, yet it would seem that the technique has potential as a noninvasive cardiac assist device.

For the past 2 years, careful investigations have been proceeding in patients. Two unanticipated difficulties have been to achieve proper timing and direction of the impulse. In addition, the relatively simple relation between body and table movements noted with a ULF system do not apply to BASH; that is, movements of the table are seriously distorted in transmission to the body frame.[416] The reason may be that the frequency of BASH is much higher than 0.3 Hz.

PROJECTED BALLISTOCARDIOGRAPHIC RESEARCH

This section briefly covers several areas where future investigation and development are needed. Some problems can be resolved by the practicing physician; others unfortunately still belong in the laboratory.

The vector Bcg must be thoroughly investigated. The first step is the construction of a simple, sturdy three-dimensional bed. Next, methods for analyzing data must be developed (see following item). *Then* the same procedures as those already done for single-degree Bcg's will have to be repeated, for example, model studies, correlation with standard variables, clinical studies with various disorders, and long-term prognostic studies—an overwhelming prospect.

The new computer techniques should be used to their fullest in ballistocardiography. These techniques include signal averaging, pattern recognition, adaptive systems, and parameter optimization. They go beyond human capabilities and could add new power to the Bcg. Analysis of the vector Bcg would become feasible.

The use of the Bcg to estimate regional blood flows should be investigated. Harrison has taken advantage of the fact that peripheral distribution of blood flow contributes to the Bcg.[417] Thus, the signal diminishes when the legs or neck are flexed. Harrison estimates cranial blood flow by subtracting flow calculated with the neck flexed from that calculated with the neck straight. Flows into and out of the cranium are considered. The method could be used to approximate blood flow in other regions, such as the arm, by abducting the arm from the side.

It is discouraging to be forced to begin all over with long-term studies. However, the potent new analytic techniques will make the prognostic contribution of ballistocardiography even more useful.[418]

Data should be stored on magnetic tape, so that if any new analytic techniques are developed, a fresh start in data collection will not be necessary.

The ballistocardiogram should be recorded in man simultaneously with currently accepted variables. These variables include left ventricular $(dp/dt)/KP$, V_{max}, acceleration derived from an electromagnetic flow catheter, or calculations from angiographic studies, including some index of asynergic contraction.[419] Drugs or coronary artery occlusion may be used to change these variables. All grades of disease from nearly normal to seriously ill should be studied.

A stress test compatible with the recording of the Bcg must be found. This is necessary to extract even more subtle abnormalities from the Bcg. Dinaburg* has been exploring isometric exercise and a standardized Valsalva maneuver as two possibilities. Tilting on a tilt table induces considerable stress. However, this maneuver is possible only with the new Starr HF bed.[49] Lower body negative pressure is very similar and will be useful when lighter devices are available.

Patients with acute myocardial infarction. These patients should be intermittently monitored with the Bcg from the very beginning, as Winer[278,406] has done. The Bcg will probably be useful for guiding therapy, predicting the course, and facilitating rehabilitation.

The Bcg should be studied in space, in the orbiting laboratory.[420] This laboratory should provide a unique opportunity for significantly increasing our insight into the Bcg. Furthermore, the Bcg would be useful in detecting early cardiac weakness from prolonged weightlessness, as well as in evaluating the effects of various regimens, such as exercise, on the evolution and prevention of this troublesome problem.

The Bcg should be simplified as much as possible. Winer has adhered to the direct-body system because he feels that its simplicity and applicability to a broad range of patients outweigh the obvious disadvantages.[421] He has limited himself to qualitative and descriptive analysis and has improved the system probably to its limits.

Finally, and most importantly, mass screening should be investigated thoroughly. This may prove to be the most useful service the Bcg can provide to the physician. The Bcg is a very rapid, simple test,

---

* Dinaburg AG: personal communication.

and therefore ideal for screening. The total time expended in examining an ambulatory heart transplant patient was 5 min in our series. Patients with ballistocardiographic abnormalities could undergo more complex, expensive, or even invasive tests as indicated.

PRACTICAL ADVICE FOR SETTING UP A Bcg

For those who might have been tempted to set up a clinical ballistocardiographic facility, we can offer some helpful points. The following are culled from the experience of three people in assembling ballistocardiographic systems: Dr. Aaron G. Dinaburg, for a general clinical testing facility, Dr. John Reitan, for cardiac transplant patients, and the author, for his laboratories. Thus, three different areas are represented: clinical practice, clinical research, and laboratory research. Dinaburg has set up his Bcg system as a private physician on a minimum expense basis, without benefit of outside supporting funds.

Space

The room should be 12 × 15 ft minimum floor area and 9 to 10 ft high for a pendulum bed; it can be much smaller if an air-bearing bed is used. The pendulum bed need not continuously occupy the floor space, however. We suspend ours on two coat hangers when not in use. With any bed, the room should be as quiet as possible, located in a vibration-free area far from elevators, escalators, or heavy machinery. The basement is often ideal. If vibrations are unavoidable, special isolation techniques can be used. An accelerometer with low cross-sensitivity is very useful in eliminating noise. Starr has used an 8-in. pile of nylon batting to isolate his velocity transducer.[51] For a pendulum bed, inexpensive industrial shock absorbers are available. Starr dampens the vibrating wires of his pendulum bed by loosely connecting each wire to the two adjacent wires by soft strings attached about one-quarter and one-third the distance from ceiling to bed.[51]

Equipment

Bed. Three types of beds are suggested, depending on the budget and the do-it-yourself inclination of the physician. Pendulum beds can be constructed reasonably easily. Our pendulum bed weighs only 4.5 lb and consists of a rectangular frame 78 × 28 in. constructed from aluminum tubing 2 in. in diameter and 0.045 in. in wall thickness

(Fig. 2–2). Dacron sail cloth covers the frame. Eight, 1/16-in. airplane cables 10 ft long support the bed. The wires are arranged so as to allow head-foot motion only. If the ceiling is too low, the wires can be shortened and the bed converted to a semihorizontal pendulum with two 12-in. pins, which displace the bed laterally by being set into bearings on the bed and floor frame (Fig. 2–3). Dinaburg has used this system in his office. In addition, he has added two cross members to stiffen the frame and mount the accelerometer. A wooden frame 7 × 3 ft bolted to the floor serves as a patient safety feature and as a support for the stationary bearings. Finally, the Johns Hopkins bed can be either purchased or constructed.

Accelerometer. Our variable capacitance accelerometer can be assembled for $100. However, a power supply and a special oscillator are also needed. It is recommended that a commercial accelerometer be used, such as those supplied by Endevco, SystronDonner, or Statham.* The accelerometer may be mounted at the geometric center of the bed or at the foot, provided head-foot motion only is allowed. An inexpensive oscilloscope for monitoring the signals is extremely useful, since one can verify the quality of the signals without wasting paper. A two-channel oscillograph is the minimum needed, one channel for the Bcg and one for the ECG. Such an oscillograph can be purchased for $500 to $2000. This system would include necessary amplifiers and filters. A linear frequency response of direct current to 50 Hz is needed, with paper speeds of 2.5 to 100 mm/sec.

Operation

Dinaburg† describes a procedure for clinical measurement of the Bcg and preejection period simultaneously. Initially, the patient is made comfortable in a chair, and the purpose of the procedure and the various steps of the tests are described to him. Above all, he is reassured that it is painless and that he can stop at any time he becomes uncomfortable or fearful. His name is logged in a register, along with age, height, weight, blood pressure, pulse rate, and any brief record of known diseases. He is then asked to expose his upper chest and to lie supine on the bed. Next, the various sensors are applied. The ECG

---

* All three of us have had success with the Q-flex accelerometer manufactured by Endevco. With amplifiers and filters, the cost is about $1,000. If the demand is sufficient, Endevco is prepared to manufacture an accelerometer which would cost only $50.
† Dinaburg AG: personal communication.

leads are attached one to each wrist, a pneumogram sensor is taped under the nostril, a phonocardiographic microphone is placed at the second left interspace lateral to the sternal border, and a carotid pulse transducer is placed over the right carotid artery. All wires should be connected vertically to the patient to avoid damping. The amplifiers are activated, and each channel is monitored on the oscilloscope. Of particular interest are the quality and amplitude of the carotid pulse and heart sounds. The pins are then inserted into the bearing surfaces, and the bed is checked for freedom from any restraints or interference. The patient is instructed to breathe normally without any special effort and a brief tracing at medium speed is recorded, preferably at 25 mm/sec. If this record is satisfactory, a repeat of the same passively held expiration record is taken at high speed (100 mm/sec) for timing purposes. Preferably 10 to 15 complexes are obtained. If desired, various stress tests may be done involving either respiratory maneuvers (standardized Valsalva) or isometric hand exercises. At the end of the test, the pins are removed, the sensors removed from the patient, and he is assisted off the bed.

SUMMARY

Ballistocardiography, one of the oldest noninvasive methods of cardiac evaluation, has had a stormy, controversial past. It acquired a bad reputation primarily because it was urged to do too much, too soon. However, the Bcg has emerged from its period of obscurity with excellent standards for recording, as well as extensive testing in mathematical and electrical analog models, cadaver studies, animal and human physiologic and pharmacologic experiments, and clinical studies, including prognostic investigations.

These investigations have established several important facts about the Bcg. Most older recordings, especially those from direct-body devices, were grossly inaccurate. The requirements for accurate recordings are straightforward: (1) light bed, (2) tight coupling of subject to bed, (3) minimal coupling to ground, (4) very low natural frequency, and (5) measurement of acceleration. One can list 20 conceptions about the Bcg, 15 of which are actually misconceptions.

The most useful information on myocardial performance which can be extracted from the Bcg relates to maximum aortic blood flow acceleration. Areas of usefulness include those in which an assessment of circulatory and myocardial performance is desired—pharmacologic and physiologic testing, prognosis, mass screening, evaluation of therapy,

126 Noninvasive Cardiology

detecting subclinical coronary artery disease, and evaluating the functional impact of certain diseases, such as aortic valvular disease.

Finally, areas for future research, as well as suggestions for setting up a clinical ballistocardiographic facility have been included.

ACKNOWLEDGMENTS

The efforts of many people have gone into the writing of this chapter. Organizing this help would have been impossible without the existence of the two ballistocardiographic societies—European and American. Special thanks belong to Drs. E. W. Bixby, D. M. Cunningham, A. G. Dinaburg, D. C. Fischer, E. K. Franke, W. K. Harrison, Jr., A. Noordergraaf, I. Starr, and N. J. Winer who offered constructive advice and ideas and sent copies of recent unpublished material. Dr. W. K. Harrison, Jr., provided proofs of the 1970 Proceedings of the Ballistocardiograph Research Society (American). The manuscripts and proofs have allowed this chapter to be as up-to-date as possible. Drs. A. N. Corbascio, D. M. Cunningham, A. G. Dinaburg, A. Noordergraaf, P. C. Smith, and I. Starr were kind enough to review the manuscript. Dr. Corbascio, in particular, shredded the manuscript with relish.

The invaluable aid of Mrs. Cathryn Yarnell in the preparation of the manuscript is acknowledged with particular gratitude. Mrs. Faith Murphy of the Biomedical Library of the University of California, San Diego, carefully checked the reference list.

REFERENCES

1. Scarborough WR: Ballistocardiography. A bibliography, NASA SP-7021 (FAA AM 65-15), 1965
2. Baevskiy RM: Fundamentals of practical ballisto-cardiography. Washington US Joint Publications Research Service, 1963
3. Ambrosi C, Starr I: Ballistocardiographie, in: Encyclopedie Medicochirurgicale. Paris, 1971
4. Starr I, Noordergraaf A: Ballistocardiography in Cardiovascular Research. Lippincott, Philadelphia/Montreal, 1967, 438 pp
5. Klensch H (ed): Proc 2nd European Symp Ballistocardiography, Bonn, Germany, March 27–28, 1961
6. Rochet J (ed): Proc 3rd European Symp Ballistocardiography, Brussels, Belgium, April 16–17, 1962

7. Proc 4th Congr Eur Ballistocardiographie, Lille Méd, Numéro Spécial, 1964
8. Knoop AA (ed): Proc 1st World Congress on Ballistocardiography and Cardiovascular Dynamics, Amsterdam, 1965. Baltimore, Williams and Wilkins, 1966
9. Noordergraaf A, Pollack GH: Ballistocardiography and cardiac performance. Bibl Cardiol 19:1–150, 1967
10. Scarborough WR: Ballistocardiography and circulatory function. Bibl Cardiol 20:1–171, 1968
11. Deuchar D: Ballistocardiography. Bibl Cardiol 21:1–140, 1968
12. Starr I: Ballistocardiography and cardiovascular performance. Bibl Cardiol 24:1–115, 1969
13. deFreitas F: Ballistocardiography and cardiovascular therapy. Bibl Cardiol 26:1–357, 1970
14. Harrison WK: Ballistocardiography and clinical studies. Bibl Cardiol (Basel) 27:1–82, 1971
15. Verdouw PD: Ballistics of ventricular performance. Philadelphia, Univ. Pennsylvania, 1970 (dissertation)
16. Parry CH: Collections from the unpublished medical writings of the late Caleb Hiller Parry, in: Diseases of the Heart, vol. 2. London, Underwoods, 1825, p. 111
17. Gordon JW: On certain molar movements of the human body produced by the circulation. J Anat Physiol 11:533–536, 1877
18. Trotter C: Note on Mr. Gordon's paper, On certain molar movements, etc, J Anat Physiol 11:553–559, 1877
19. Burger HC, Noordergraaf A, Verhagen AMW: Physical basis of the low-frequency ballistocardiograph. Am Heart J 46:71–83, 1953
20. Burger HC, Noordergraaf A: Physical basis of ballistocardiography. II. The quantities that can be measured with different types of ballistocardiographs and their mutual relations. Am Heart J 51:127–139, 1956
21. Burger HC, Noordergraaf A: Physical basis of ballistocardiography. III. Am Heart J 51:179–185, 1956
22. Burger HC, Noordergraaf A, Korsten JJM, et al: Physical basis of ballistocardiography. IV. The relative movement of subject and ballistocardiograph. Am Heart J 52:653–673, 1956
23. Burger HC, Noordergraaf A, Kamps HJL: Physical basis of ballistocardiography. V. The distortion of the ballistocardiogram caused by the movement of the heart inside the body. Am Heart J 53:907–921, 1957
24. Landois L: Lehrbuch der physiologie des menschen einschliesslich der histologie und mikroskopischen anatomie. Mit besonderer berucksich tigung der praktischen medicin 1 Hlft. Wien, Urban and Schwarzenberg, 1879, p 415
25. Henderson Y: The mass movements of the circulation as shown by a recoil curve. Am J Physiol 14:287–298, 1905
26. Douglas CG, Haldane JS, Henderson Y, et al: Physiological observations made on Pike's Peak, Colorado, with special reference to adaptation to low barometric pressures. Philos Trans R Soc Lond Ser B 203:351–371, 1913
27. Chignon JC, Distel R: Modifications of the ballistocardiogram in altitude. Bibl Cardiol 26:74–77, 1970
28. Satterthwaite TE: Cardiovascular Diseases. New York, Lemcke and Beuchner, 1913

29. Heald CB, Tucker WS: Recoil curves as shown by the hot-wire microphone. Proc R Soc Lond Ser B 93:281–298, 1922
30. Angenheister G, Lau E: Seismographische aufnahmen der herztatigkeit. Naturwissenschaften 16:513–515, 1928
31. Abramson E: Die ruckstosskurve des herzens (kardiodynamogramm). Skand Arch Physiol 66:191–224, 1933
32. Hamilton WF, Dow P: Cardiac and aortic contributions to the human ballistocardiogram. Am J Physiol 133:313, 1941
33. Nickerson JL, Curtis HJ: The design of the ballistocardiograph. Am J Physiol 142:1–11, 1944
34. Dock W: Recording the motions of the heart and blood for clinical purposes. Trans Assoc Am Physicians 62:148–153, 1949
35. Dock W, Taubman F: Some techniques for recording the ballistocardiogram directly from the body. Am J Med 7:751–755, 1949
36. Noordergraaf A: The role of physics in the development of ballistocardiography. 4th Eur Cong Ballistocardiography. Lille Méd 3:21–26, 1964
37. Wilson GP, Cunningham DM, Griswold HE Jr.: Experimental response of the human body to a known periodic force as a measure of ballistocardiographic fidelity. Circulation 15:280–284, 1957
38. Von Wittern WW: Ballistocardiography with elimination of the influence of the vibration properties of the body. Am Heart J 46:705–714, 1953
39. Talbot SA, Harrison WK: Dynamic comparison of current ballistocardiographic methods. Part I: Artifacts in the dynamically simple ballistocardiographic methods. Circulation 12:577–587, 1955
40. Talbot SA, Harrison WK: Dynamic comparison of current ballistocardiographic methods. Part II: Effect of a platform in ballistocardiographic dynamics. Circulation 12:845–857, 1955
41. Talbot SA, Harrison WK: Dynamic comparison of current ballistocardiographic methods. Part III: Derivation of cardiovascular force from body motions. Circulation 12:1022–1033, 1955
42. Rappaport MB: Displacement, velocity, and acceleration ballistocardiograms as registered with an undamped bed of ultra-low natural frequency. I. Theory and dynamic considerations. Am Heart J 52:483–495, 1956
43. Starr I, Braunstein JR, Dock W, et al: First report of the committee on ballistocardiographic terminology. Circulation 7:929–931, 1953
44. Braunstein JR: A proposed nomenclature and convention for recording the ballistocardiograms. Circulation 7:927–928, 1953
45. Scarborough WR, Talbot SA: Proposals for ballistocardiographic nomenclature and conventions: revised and extended Report of Committee on Ballistocardiographic Terminology. Circulation 14:453–450, 1956
46. Scarborough WR, Talbot SA, Condon JH: Technical Appendix to ref 32. Circulation 14:435–450, 1956
47. Klensch H, Noordergraaf A, Van Brummelen AGW: Preliminary proposals for ballistocardiographic methodology. Standardization and Nomenclature. Proc 2nd Eur Symp Ballistocardiog. Bonn, Germany, 1961, pp 257–261
48. Cunningham DM, Franke EK, Harrison WK Jr, et al: Specifications for the ultra-low frequency ballistocardiograph. Bibl Cardiol 26:343–353. 1970
49. Starr I, Noordergraaf A: A comparison between ultra-low frequency ballistocardiograms and those secured by an improved high-frequency technique, with studies to explain remaining differences. Am Heart J 64:79–100, 1962
50. Rappaport MB: Displacement, velocity, and acceleration ballistocardiograms

as registered with an undamped bed of ultra-low natural frequency II. Instrumental considerations. Am Heart J 52:643–652, 1956

51. Starr I: Successful methods of eliminating building vibrations in the force Bcg. Bibl Cardiol 27:76–78, 1971

52. Talbot SA, Deuchar DC, Davis FW Jr, et al: The aperiodic ballistocardiograph. Bull Johns Hopkins Hosp 94:27–33, 1954

53. Nyboer J, Sharp G: Constant mass displacement ballistocardiography. AMA Exhibit, AMA Meeting, New York, 1957

54. Martin BO: A ballistocardiograph. Astro Space Laboratories Medical Electronics Division, Huntsville, Alabama

55. Cunningham DM, Smiley PC: A hydrostatic air-bearing ballistocardiograph. J Appl Physiol 16:755–758, 1961

56. Cunningham M: Lateral acceleration fidelity on an air bearing ballistocardiograph. 4th Eur Cong Ballistocardiography, Lille Med 3:101–107, 1964

57. Cunningham DM, Saunders KV: The completely isolated air ballistocardiograph. Bibl Cardiol 19:1–6, 1967

58. Curran JT, Kerr J, MacGregor J: The foetal ballistocardiograph. Bibl Cardiol 26:230–234, 1970

59. Harrison WK, Talbot SA: Two new forms of ultra-low frequency ballistocardiograph. Bibl Cardiol 19:13–18, 1967

60. Verdouw PD, Ambrosi C, Iwazumi T, et al: The effect of a rigid support on the ultra-low frequency ballistocardiogram. Bibl Cardiol 24:45–50, 1969

61. Nyboer J, Reid KA, Gessert W: A servo counterforce ballistocardiograph: an aperiodic air-bearing system. Bibl Cardiol 19:26–32, 1968

62. Nyboer J, Gessert W, Reid KA: Counter-force ballistics in man. Biomed Sci Instrum 4:42–54, 1968

63. Tolles WE: An ultra-low frequency ballistocardiograph of simple kinematic design. Bibl Cardiol 20:99–105, 1968

64. Klensch H: The frog's ultra-low frequency ballistocardiogram, in: Proc 1st Cong Soc Ballistocardio Res, Woudschoten, Zeist, The Netherlands, 1960, pp 110–115

65. von Schwarzer F, Reetz H: Mechanisch-dynamische probleme beim ultra-niederfrequented schwingtisch, in Klensch H: Proc 2nd Eur Symp Ballistocardio, Bonn, Germany, 1961, pp 257–261

66. Smith NT: Cardiac function evaluation, in Bellville JW, Weaver CS (eds): Techniques in Clinical Physiology: A Survey of Measurements in Anesthesiology, New York, Macmillan, 1969, pp 125–176

67. Starr I, Noordergraaf A: Ballistocardiography in Cardiovascular Research, Philadelphia, Lippincott, 1967, p 385

68. Starr I: Progress towards a physiological cardiology—A second essay on the ballistocardiogram. Ann Intern Med 63:1079–1105, 1965

69. Rushmer RF: Initial ventricular impulse: a potential key to cardiac evaluation. Circulation 29:268–283, 1964

70. Noble MIM, Trenchard D, Guz A: Studies of the maximum acceleration of blood in the ascending aorta of conscious dogs, in Knoop AA (ed): Ballistocardiography Cardiovascular Dynamics. Basel, Karger, 1966, pp 243–247

71. Winter PJ, Deuchar DC, Noble MIM, et al: The ballistocardiogram and left ventricular ejection in the dog, in Knoop AA (ed): Ballistocardiography Cardiovascular Dynamics. Basel, Karger, 1966, pp 243–247

72. Winter PJ, Deuchar DC, Noble MIM, et al: Relationship between the bal-

listocardiogram and the movement of blood from the left ventricle in the dog. Cardiovasc Res 1:194–200, 1967

73. Noble MIM, Gabe IT, Trenchard D, et al: Blood pressure and flow in the ascending aorta of conscious dogs. Cardiovasc Res 1:9–20, 1967

74. Sutherland A, Haselby K, Abel FL: Comparative measurements of ventricular contractility. Fed Proc 28:327, 1969

75. Scarborough WR, Podolak E, Whitlock MB: Magnetic tape recording of ballistocardiograms and other physiologic variables from subjects with and without cardiovascular "disease." Bibl Cardiol 19:72–98, 1967

76. Talbot SA, Harrison WK Jr, Ginn WM Jr: Features of ULF-BCG pertinent to coronary heart disease, in Knoop AA (ed): Ballistocardiography Cardiovascular Dynamics. Basel, Karger, 1966, pp 55–68

77. Harrison WK, Friesinger GC, Johnson SL, et al: Relation of the ballistocardiogram to left ventricular pressure measurements in man. Am J Cardiol 23:673–678, 1969

78. Pretorius PJ: Experimental investigations on ultra-low frequency acceleration ballistocardiography (Thesis). Amsterdam, Free University, 1962

79. West JW, Corbascio AN: An experimental study of the atrial ballistocardiogram with special reference to the genesis of the H wave. Bibl Cardiol 20:110–122, 1967

80. Verdouw PD, Noordergraaf A: Left ventricular ejection as reflected in the Bcg. Bibl Cardiol 26:243–261, 1970

81. Smith NT, Van Citters RL, Verdouw PD: The relation between the ultra-low frequency ballistocardiogram, the acceleration pneumocardiogram, and ascending aortic flow acceleration in the baboon. Bibl Cardiol 26:198–205, 1970

82. Verdouw PD, Smith NT, Van Citters RL, et al: The acceleration ballistocardiogram in relation to left ventricular flow in the baboon. Bibl Cardiol 27:64–73, 1971

83. Elsbach H: Clinical investigations with the ultra-low frequency ballistocardiograph according to the method of Burger. Thesis, University of Legden, 1954 (Trans. R.D. Freeman). Baltimore, Johns Hopkins Univ. 1956

84. Noordergraaf A: Neue wege in der herz-und kreislaufforschung. Berlin Med 11:301–305, 1960

85. Starr I, Noordergraaf A: Ballistocardiography in Cardiovascular Research, Philadelphia, Lippincott, 1967, p 199

86. Strehler BL, Mildvan AS: General theory of mortality and aging. A stochastic model relates observations on aging, physiologic decline, mortality and radiation. Science 132:14–21, 1960

87. Starr I, Noordergraaf A: Ballistocardiography in cardiovascular research, Philadelphia, Lippincott, 1967, pp 140–152

88. Moss AJ: Ballistocardiographic evaluation of the cardiovascular aging process. Circulation 23:434–451, 1961

89. Smith JE: Ultra-low frequency displacement ballistocardiogram. Normal standards and clinical observations. Aerosp Med 38:1120–1129, 1967

90. Bevegard S, Holmgren A, Jonsson B: The effect of body position on the circulation at rest and during exercise, with special reference to the influence on the stroke volume. Acta Physiol Scand 49:279–298, 1960

91. Trefny Z, Wagner J: A quantitative ballistocardiograph. Bibl Cardiol 19: 19–25, 1967

92. Trefny Z: Some physiological aspects in quantitative ballistocardiography. Bibl Cardiol 26:116–118, 1970

93. Bixby W Jr: A simplified technique for obtaining the high frequency ballistocardiogram in the erect position. Bibl Cardiol 127:79–82, 1971

94. Starr I, Rawson AJ: The vertical ballistocardiograph: experiments on changes in the circulation on arising; with a further study of ballistic theory. Am J Physiol 134:403–425, 1941

95. Julius HW, Noordergraaf A: Recording of displacement and velocity ballistocardiograms during normal respiration. 4th Eur Cong Ballistocardiography, Lille Méd (special number) 3:74–76, 1964

96. Noordergraaf A, Spier DH: A new method for the elimination of the respiratory effect in ultra-low frequency displacement and velocity ballistocardiograms. Soc Ballistocardiogr Res Proc 3rd Eur Symp Ballistocardiography, Brussels, Belgium, April 16–17, pp 142–145, 1962

97. Julius HW Jr, Noordergraaf A: Progress in a study on recording displacement ballistocardiograms during normal respiration, in Knoop AA (ed): Ballistocardiography Cardiovascular Dynamics. Basel, Karger, 1966, pp. 73–77

98. Rautaharju PM, Josenhans WT: Resolution of ballistocardiographic records into cardiac and respiratory components. Can J Physiol Pharmacol 44: 691–700, 1966

99. Josenhans WT, Van Brummelen AGW: Variation of stroke volume with the phase of respiration, in Knoop AA (ed): Ballistocardiography and Cardiovascular Dynamics. Basel, Karger, 1966, pp 69–72

100. Winter DA, Lodge MA, Josenhans WT: The elimination of respiratory signals from the ultra-low-frequency ballistocardiogram. Am Heart J 71: 666–670, 1966

101. Josenhans WT: Breath holding effects on ULF displacement ballistocardiography. Bibl Cardiol 19:49–62, 1967

102. Dock W: Effects of respiration on transmission of ballistocardiographic forces from the heart to the recording system. Am Heart J 58:102–112, 1959

103. Starr I, Noordergraaf A: Ballistocardiography in Cardiovascular Research, Philadelphia, Lippincott, 1967, p 194

104. Jackson DH, Eddleman EE Jr, Bancroft WH Jr, et al: Ballistocardiographic and angiographic correlative study in idiopathic hypertrophic subaortic stenosis. Bibl Cardiol 27:14–20, 1971

105. Deuchar DC: Some further observations on the ballistocardiogram in aortic valve disease. Proc 3rd European Symp Ballistocardiography, Rochet, Brussels 225–233, 1962

106. Elsbach H, Rodrigo FA, Westerhof N: The ultralow frequency ballistocardiogram in muscular subaortic stenosis, in Knoop AA (ed): Ballistocardiography and Cardiovascular Dynamics. Basel, Karger, 1966, pp 26–30

107. Elsbach H, Rodrigo FA, Verbiest E: Further observations on the ballistocardiogram in hypertrophic cardiomyopathy. Bibl Cardiol 21:125–129, 1968

108. Fisher DC, Zobay AJ: The K wave abnormality of aneurysm of the abdominal aorta. Bibl Cardiol, in press

109. Brown HR, DeLalla V Jr, Epstein MA, et al: Clinical ballistocardiography. New York, Macmillan, 1952

110. Starr I, Noordergraaf A: Ballistocardiography in Cardiovascular Research. Philadelphia, Lippincott, 1967, p 155

111. Sherwin RW, Harrison WK, Davis FW, et al: Reproducibility of form readings of Starr and ultra-low frequency ballistocardiograms. Bibl Cardiol 24:51–56, 1969

112. von der Groeben J: ECG analysis, in Bellville JW, Weaver CG (eds.): Techniques in Clinical Physiology. A Survey of Measurements in Anesthesiology. Toronto, Macmillan, 1969, pp 53–84

113. Laverman E: Recording of the ultra-low frequency ballistocardiogram with a computer of average transients. Bibl Cardiol 21:80–85, 1968

114. Johnson STL, Johns RJ, Harrison WK: Digital computer averaging of ballistocardiograms in patients with congestive heart failure. Bibl Cardiol 24:90–95, 1968

115. Jackson DH, Molina E: The postexercise ballistocardiogram. A study method utilizing average transient computing. Bibl Cardiol 20:35–38, 1967

116. Onodera K, Sasaki K, Saito M, et al: The action of digoxin and adenosine triphosphate as demonstrated mainly by harmonic analysis of Bcg in auricular fibrillation and other cardiac diseases. Bibl Cardiol 26:24–30, 1970

117. Ozaki T, Sato K, Awazu T, et al: Some observations on minor tremors related to heart beat. Jap J Physiol 12:484–493, 1962

118. Ozaki T, Sato K, Awazu T, et al: Some observations on the effect of sensory stimulation upon minor tremors in man. Jap J Physiol 13:24–32, 1963

119. Tomonaga K: On the effect of heart beat on minor tremor. Jap J Physiol 15:560:569, 1965

120. Awazu T: Studies on human minor tremors. Jap J Physiol 15:579–595, 1965

121. Eddleman EE Jr, Bancroft WH Jr: Analysis of the ballistocardiograph by means of computer techniques. Bibl Cardiol (Abstr) 20:20, 1967

122. Harrison WK, Burton ME, Glaspell F: Computer Analysis of Ballistocardiograms. Comps Biol Med (in press)

123. Proper R: Age-related changes in professional pilots as defined by the Klensch-Schwarzer ultra-low frequency ballistocardiogram. Bibl Cardiol 20:50–56, 1967

124. Freiman AH, Steinberg CA: The analysis of simultaneously recorded cardiovascular data with the digital computer. Ann NY Acad Sci 115:1091–1105, 1964

125. Talbot SA, Harrison WK Jr, Ginn WM Jr: Features of ULF-BCG pertinent to coronary heart disease, in Knoop AA (ed): Ballistocardiography Cardiovascular Dynamics. Basel, Karger, 1966, pp 55–68

126. Harrison WK, Talbot SA: Discrimination of the quantitative ultralow-frequency ballistocardiogram in coronary heart disease. Am Heart J 74: 80–87, 1967

127. Van den Bos GC, Knoop AA, Hoitink AWJH, et al: The influence of body position and anaesthesia on the ultralow-frequency ballistocardiogram of the dog. Bibl Cardiol 21:62–68, 1968

128. Batelaan B, Knoop AA, Van den Bos GC: The configuration of the ultra-low frequency vector displacement BCG in man. Bibl Cardiol 21:12–15, 1968

129. Knoop AA, Pretorius PJ, Hoitink AWJH: Vectorballistocardiography. Proc 3rd Eur Symp Ballistocardiography, Brussels, Belgium, April 16–17, pp 121–128, 1962

130. Hoitink AWJH, Knoop AA: Physiological principles of ballistocardiography. Some aspects of the experimental ultra-low frequency ballistocardiography. 4th Eur Congr Ballistocardiography, Lille Méd 3:15–20, 1964

131. Baan J, Noordergraaf A: Some methods to control the natural frequencies in the three different modes of a 3-degree of freedom ultra-low frequency ballistocardiograph. Bibl Cardiol 20:12–19, 1968

132. Cunningham DM, Brown GW: Basis for the design of a three dimensional ballistocardiograph. Proc Soc Exper Stress Anal 13:77–84, 1954

133. Nomura Y, Fujigaki H, Fujimoto J, et al: A three-directional ballistocardiograph. Jap Circ J 30:217–223, 1966

134. Fujigaki H, Nomura Y, Fujimoto J, et al: Three directional ballistocardiogram in mitral stenosis. Ann Report Center for Adult Diseases. OSAKA. (Asaka Furitsu Seijinbye Senta. Annual Report) 4:43–59, 1964

135. Nomura Y, Fujigaki H, Fujimoto J, et al: The three directional ballistocardiogram on experimental coronary stenosis and occlusion of the dog. Jap Circ J 30:349–356, 1966

136. Fujigaki H, Nomura Y, Fujimoto J, et al: Three directional ballistocardiogram in atrial septal defect. Jap Circ J 31:601–607, 1967

137. Franke EK, Braunstein JR: Design of a three-dimensional high-frequency ballistocardiograph. Bibl Cardiol 19:7–12, 1967

138. Talbot SA: Physical Principles of Vector Ballistocardiographic Measurement. Final report on investigation of the unloaded internal ballistocardiogram: its biophysical and physiological relation to cardiac performance, Contract AF 18 (600) 1107. June, 1958, 156 p. AFOSR TR 58–72; AD-158301; PB 135626

139. Hixson WC, Beischer DE: Biotelemetry of the triaxial ballistocardiogram and electrocardiogram in a weightless environment. US Naval School of Aviation Medicine, US Naval Aerospace Medical Institute, Pensacola, Florida, 1964

140. Hixson WC, Beischer DE: Biotelemetry of the triaxial ballistocardiogram and electrocardiogram in a weightless environment, in Knopp AA (ed): Ballistocardiography and Cardiovascular Dynamics. Basel, Karger, 1966, pp 85–89

141. Baan J, Cunningham DM, Noordergraaf A: The meaning of the human lateral ballistocardiogram, in Knoop AA (ed): Ballistocardiography and Cardiovascular Dynamics. Basel, Karger, 1966, pp 198–202

142. Van de Weerd JM, Noordergraaf A: Prediction of the human lateral ballistocardiogram, in Knoop AA (ed): Ballistocardiography and Cardiovascular Dynamics. Basel, Karger, 1966, pp 281–284

143. Batelaan B, Knoop AA: The value of the displacement vector ballistocardiogram in comparison with the longitudinal BCG, in Knoop AA (ed): Ballistocardiography and Cardiovascular Dynamics. Basel, Karger, 1966, pp 198–202

144. Starr I, Rawson AJ: Role of the "static blood pressure" in abnormal increments of venous pressure especially in heart failure. I. Theoretical studies on an improved circulation schema whose pumps obey Starling's law of the heart. Am J Med Sci 199:27–39, 1940

145. Starr I: Role of the "static blood pressure" in abnormal increments of venous pressure, especially in heart failure. II. Clinical and experimental studies. Am J Med Sci 199:40–55, 1940

146. Noordergraaf A, Heynekamp CE: Genesis of displacement of the human longitudinal ballistocardiogram from the changing blood distribution. Am J Cardiol 2:748–756, 1958

147. Noordergraaf A: Further studies on a theory of the ballistocardiogram. Circulation 24:413–425, 1961

148. Noordergraaf A, Horeman HW, Holt SP: Numerical evaluation of volume pulsations in man. IV. The calculation of the human ballistocardiogram. Phys Med Biol 3:349–360, 1959

149. Noordergraaf A, Horeman HW: The prediction of the ballistocardiogram from physiological and anatomical data. Cardiolgia (Basel) 31:416–420, 1957

150. Noordergraaf A, Verdouw PD, Boom HB: The use of an analog computer in a circulation model. Prog Cardiovasc Dis 5:419–439, 1963

151. Westerhof N, Bosman F, DeVries CJ, et al: Analog studies of the human systemic arterial tree. J Biomechanics 2:121–143, 1969

152. Noordergraaf A, Verdouw PD, Van Brummelen AGW: Analog of the arterial bed, in Attinger EO (ed): Pulsatile Blood Flow. New York, Mc-Graw-Hill, 1964, pp 373–386

153. Jager GN, Westerhof N, Noordergraaf A: Oscillatory flow impedance in electrical analog of arterial system. Circ Res 16:121–133, 1965

154. Pollack GH: Electrical model of the human pulmonary circulation. Hemodynamics Internal Report H66-1, Univ. of Pa., 1966

155. Pollack GH, Reddy RV, Noordergraaf A: Input impedance, wave travel and reflections in the pulmonary arterial tree: Studies using an electrical analog. IEEE Trans Biomed Engin 15:151–164, 1968

156. Westerhof N, Scarborough WR, Noordergraaf A: Some experiments on a delay line simulating the human systemic arterial tree, with special emphasis on the ballistocardiogram. Bibl Cardiol 19:141–150, 1967

157. Verdouw PD: Ballistics of ventricular performance. Phildelphia, Univ. of Pa., pp 174–175, 1970 (Dissertation)

158. Elsbach H, Rodrigo FA: The ultralow-frequency ballistocardiogram in atrial septal defect. Am Heart J 70:186–195, 1965

159. Starr I, Noordergraaf A: Ballistocardiography in Cardiovascular Research, Philadelphia, Lippincott, 1967, p 63

160. Morse RL: A mathematical model of the ballistocardiogram. Bibl Cardiol 19:136–140, 1967

161. Baan J, Manchester JH, Shelburne JC: A quantitative relationship between the H-I slope of the head-foot BCG and the initial acceleration of flow in man. Bibl Cardiol 1972 (in press)

162. Harrison WK: Calculation of cardiovascular force from phasic regional blood flow. Bible Cardiol 26:262–268, 1970

163. Starr I, Horwitz O, Mayock RL, et al: Standardization of the ballistocardiogram by simulation of the heart's function at necropsy; with a clinical method for the estimation of cardiac strength and normal standards for it. Circulation 1:1073–1096, 1950

164. Starr I, Schnabel TG, Mayock RL: Studies made by simulating systole at necropsy. II. Experiments on the relation of cardiac and peripheral factors

to the genesis of the pulse wave and the ballistocardiogram. Circulation 8: 44–61, 1953

165. Starr I, Schnabel TG: Studies made by simulating systole at necropsy. III. On the genesis of the systolic waves of the ballistocardiogram. J Clin Invest 33:10–22, 1954

166. Starr I, Schnabel TG, Askovitz SI, et al: Studies made by simulating systole at necropsy. IV. On the relation between pulse pressure and cardiac stroke volume, leading to a clinical method of estimating cardiac output from blood pressure and age. Circulation 9:648–663, 1954

167. Starr I: Studies made by simulating systole at necropsy. VI. Estimation of cardiac stroke volume from the ballistocardiogram. J Appl Physiol 8:315–329, 1955

168. Starr I, Askovitz SI, Feder W, et al: Studies made by simulating systole at necropsy. VII. Clinical methods for estimating the work of the left ventricle, with a note on the diminution of heart work as age advances. Circulation 12:1005–1021, 1955

169. Starr I: Studies made by simulating systole at necropsy. VIII. Significance of the pulse pressure. Circulation 14:1117–1128, 1956

170. Starr I: Studies made by simulating systole at necropsy. X. State of peripheral circulation in cadaver preparations. J Appl Physiol 11:174–180, 1957

171. Starr I: Studies made by simulating systole at necropsy. XI. On the higher dynamic functions of the heart, and their reflections in the pulse wave. Circulation 17:589–600, 1958

172. Starr I: Studies made by simulating systole at necropsy. XII. Estimation of the initial cardiac forces for the ballistocardiogram. Circulation 20:74–87, 1959

173. Scarborough WR: Some circulatory effects of morphine-barbiturate anesthesia, artificial respiration, and abdominal compression based on ballistocardiographic observations on dogs, with a review of pertinent literature. Am Heart J 54:651–677, 1957

174. Corbascio AN, Smith NT: A new anesthetic technique for animal experimentation on the ULF-BCG, in Knoop AA (ed): Ballistocardiography and Cardiovascular Dynamics. Basel, Karger, 1966, pp 255–258

175. Moreira MG, de Azvedo SG: Ballistocardiographic effects of pentobarbital sodium given intravenously in the dog (in Portuguese). Med Contemp 80:29, 1962

176. Pretorius PJ, Terblanche M, Van der Walt JJ: Ballistocardiography in some domestic animals. Bibl Cardiol 21:46–52, 1968

177. Rogallo VL: Measurement of the heartbeat of bird embryos with a micrometeroite transducer. Technology Utilization Report NASA SP-5007, 1964

178. Klensch H: Ein Kleintier-Ballistokardiograph. Z Kreislaufforsch 50:350–356, 1961

179. Juznic G: The work, power, force and impulse of the heart as represented in the ULF-BCG curve of small laboratory animals. Bibl Cardiol 21:53–57, 1968

180. Juznic G: The calibration of the ULF-BCG curves (velocity and acceleration) of small laboratory animals. Bibl Cardiol 21:90–95, 1968

181. Juznic G: The ultra-low frequency ballistocardiogram of acceleration as an indicator of the force of the heart. Bibl Cardiol 20:39–43, 1967

182. Juznic G, Klensch H: Comparative investigations of cardiac stroke volume by quantitative ballistocardiography and Stewart-Hamilton dye dilution method in small laboratory animals. Proc 3rd Eur Symp Ballistocardiography, Brussels, Belgium, April 16–17, pp 199–206, 1962

183. Juznic G: The ultra-low frequency ballistocardiogram of the mouse. Bibl Cardiol 26:280–291, 1970

184. Klensch H, Alieff A: Der Kreislaug des frosches bei and rung seiner korpertemperatur. Z Kreislaufforsch 51:211–221, 1962

185. Alieff A, Klensch H: Der einfluss einiger gebrauchlicher narkotika auf den krieslauf des frosches (untersuchungen am intakten tier). Z Kreislaufforsch 51:720–729, 1962

186. Juznic G: The normal ballistocardiogram of guinea pig. Proc 2nd Eur Symp Ballistocardiography, Bonn, Germany, 1961, pp 191–194

187. Pretorius PJ, Van der Walt JJ, Rademeyer LJ: The ultra-low frequency acceleration ballistocardiogram of the albino rat, in Knoop AA (ed): Ballistocardiography and Cardiovascular Dynamics. Basel, Karger, 1966, pp 304–312

188. Rademeyer LJ: Deterioration of myocardial function in rats associated with age, as measured by the UF acceleration Bcg. Bibl Cardiol 26:188–197, 1970

189. Rademeyer LJ: The atrial wave complex in the UF Bcg aY of rats. Bibl Cardiol 26:321–326, 1970

190. Pretorius PJ, Green SCJE: The ultra-low frequency acceleration ballistocardiogram of the rabbit. Bibl Cardiol 21:37–45, 1968

191. Smith NT, Van Citters RL, Verdouw PD: Relation between the pneumocardiogram and aortic flow in the baboon. Bibl Cardiol 24:34–44, 1969

192. Smith NT, Reitan JA: The pneumocardiogram: a potential monitor for the operating room. Anesth Analg 49:781–790, 1970

193. Elzinga G, Knoop AA: The influence of ouabain on the normal heart of the dog, in Knoop AA (ed): Ballistocardiography and Cardiovascular Dynamics. Basel, Karger, 1966, pp 323–326

194. Juznic G, Klensch H: Vergleichend-physiologische untersuchungen uber das verhalten der indices fur energieaufwand und leistung des herzens. Pfluegers Arch Gesamte Physiol 280:38–45, 1964

195. West JW, Corbascio AN: Effects of intracoronary injections of drugs on the ULF Ballistocardiogram of the dog. Fed Proc (Abstr) 18:169, 1959

196. Corbascio AN, West JW: Effect of selective myocardial stimulation or depression induced by intracoronary administration of drugs or by obstruction of major vessels. Studies with the dog ultralow frequency ballistocardiogram. Am Heart J 62:785–796, 1961

197. Schennetten FPN, Laass-Rein A: Ballistocardiographic comparative examinations of the influence of different coloured light on test persons with sound hearts. Bibl Cardiol 21:141–144, 1968

198. Shenkin HA, Cheney RH, Govons SR, et al: On the diagnosis of hemorrhage in man. A study of volunteers bled large amounts. Am J Med Sci 208:421–436, 1944

199. Galdston M, Steele JM: Critique of area and height formulae for estimating cardiac output from the ballistocardiogram. J Appl Physiol 2:229–234, 1959

200. Dripps RD, Comroe JH: The effect on inhalation of high and low oxygen

concentrations on respiration, pulse rate, ballistocardiogram and arterial oxygen saturation (oximeter) of normal individuals. Am J Physiol 149: 277–291, 1947

201. Starr I, McMichael M: Oxygen transport, circulation and respiration in healthy subjects at simulated altitudes of 16,000–18,000 ft. J Appl Physiol 1:430–440, 1948

202. Moss AJ: The effect of hypoxia on the rate at which the cardiac ejection force is generated: a ballistocardiographic study. Am Heart J 59:412–427, 1960

203. Scarborough WR, Penneys R, Thomas CB, et al: The cardiovascular effect of induced controlled anoxemia. A preliminary ballistocardiographic study of normal subjects and a few patients with suspected coronary artery disease. Circulation 4:190–210, 1951

204. Otis AB, Rahn H, Brontman M, et al: Ballistocardiographic study of changes in cardiac output due to respiration. J Clin Invest 25:413–421, 1946

205. Whitehorn WV, Edelman A, Hitchcock FA: The cardiovascular responses to the breathing of 100 per cent oxygen at normal barometric pressure. Am J Physiol 146:61–65, 1946

206. Zöllner N, Lohmoller G, Schnelle K, et al: The effects of cardiac glycosides and of a β-receptor blocking agent on the ULF displacement ballistocardiogram in healthy young men. Bibl Cardiol 26:42–48, 1970

207. Smith NT, Fleischli GJ, Corbascio AN: Estimation of stroke volume by analog computer solution of the Starr ballistic formula, in Knoop AA (ed): Ballistocardiography and Cardiovascular Dynamics. Basel, Karger, 1966, pp 123–130

208. Smith NT, Whitcher CE: Monitoring of hemodynamic parameters by the BCG in conscious man. Bibl Cardiol 19:36–42, 1967

209. Smith NT, Whitcher CE: Acute hemodynamic effects of methoxamine in man. Anesthesiology 28:735–748, 1967

210. Smith NT, Whitcher CE: A comparison of the acute hemodynamic effects of methoxamine and mephentermine in man. Fed Proc 26:287, 1967

211. Hamilton WF: Measurement of the cardiac output, in Handbook of Physiology, Section 2: Circulation 1:575–578, 1962

212. Wagner HR, Gamble WJ, Albers WH, et al: Fiberoptic dye dilution method for measurement of cardiac output. Comparison with the direct Fick and the angiographic methods. Circulation 37:694–708, 1968

213. Whayne TF Jr, Smith NT, Eger EI, et al: Reflex cardiovascular responses to simulated diving: heart rate, intravascular pressure and ballistocardiographic changes. Angiology 23:500–508, 1972

214. Whayne TF Jr, Smith NT, Eger EI II, et al: The effects of halothane anesthesia on reflex cardiovascular responses to simulated diving and the Valsalva maneuver. Anesthesiology 34:262–270, 1971

215. Brick I: Circulatory responses to immersing the face in water. J Appl Physiol 21:33–36, 1966

216. Kawakami Y, Tatelson BH, DuBois AB: Cardiovascular effects of face immersion and factors affecting diving reflex in man. J Appl Physiol 23: 964–970, 1967

217. Scholander PF: The master switch of life. Sci Am 209:92–106, 1963

218. Wolf S: The bradycardia of the dive reflex; a possible mechanism of sudden death. Trans Am Clin Climatol Assoc 76:192–200, 1964

219. Olsen CR, Fanestil DD, Scholander PF: Some effects of breath holding and

apneic underwater diving on cardiac rhythm in man. J. Appl Physiol 17: 461–466, 1962

220. Smith NT, Eger EI II, Kadis LB: Analogue computers in the study of anaesthetic and ancillary agents. Prog Anaesthesiology. Amsterdam, Excerpta Medica, 1970, pp 597–605

221. Winer NJ: Observations on possible atrial contribution to ventricular dynamics as recorded by the direct body high-frequency "acceleration" BCG. Bibl Cardiol 19:116–125, 1967

222. Smith NT, Whitcher CE: A comparison of the acute hemodynamic effects of methoxamine and mephentermine in man. Fed Proc 26:287, 1967

223. Cullen BF, Eger EI II, Smith NT, et al: Cardiovascular effects of fluroxene in man. Anesthesiology 32:218–230, 1970

224. Eisele JH, Trenchard D, Stubbs J, et al: The immediate cardiac depression by anaesthetics in conscious dogs. Brit J. Anaes 41:86–93, 1969

225. Eisele JH, Smith NT: Cardiovascular effects of 40 percent nitrous oxide in man. Anesth Anal 51:956–962, 1972

226. Smith NT, Eger EI II, Stoelting RK, et al: The cardiovascular and sympathomimetic responses to the addition of nitrous oxide to halothane in man. Anesthesiology 32:410–421, 1970

227. Smith NT, Eger EI II, Gregory GA, et al: The cardiovascular responses to the addition of nitrous oxide to ether in man. Can Anaesth Soc J 19: 42–48, 1972

228. Smith NT, Eger EI II, Cullen BF, et al: The cardiovascular responses to the addition of nitrous oxide to fluroxene in man. Br J Anaesth 44:142–149, 1972

229. Starr I: History and development of ballistocardiography. Proc 3rd Eur Symp Ballistocardiography, Brussels, Belgium, April 16–17, pp 12–33, 1962

230. Starr I, Rawson AJ, Schroeder HA, et al: Studies on the estimation of cardiac output in man, and of abnormalities in cardiac function from the heart's recoil and the blood's impacts; the ballistocardiogram. Am J Physiol 127: 1–28, 1939

231. Neeley WA, Wilson FC Jr, Milnor JP, et al: Cardiac output: a clinical comparison of the direct Fick, dye and ballistocardiographic methods. Surgery 35:22–29, 1954

232. Cournand A, Ranges HA, Riley RL: Comparison of the results of the normal ballistocardiogram and a direct Fick method in measuring cardiac output in man. J Clin Invest 21:287–293, 1942

233. Cournand A, Riley RL, Bradley SE, et al: Studies of the circulation in clinical shock. Surgery 13:964–995, 1943

234. Burkhart K: Theoretical verification of Isaac Starr's formula for the calculation of stroke volume. Bibl Cardiol 24:57–62, 1969

235. Klensch H: Problems in estimation of stroke volume by ULF Bcg. 4th Eur Cong Ballistocardiography. Lille Méd 3:33–35, 1964

236. Klensch H, Caspari R: Schlag-und minutenvolumen des herzens unter dem einfluss strahlender warme. Pfluegers Arch Gesamte Physiol 267:591–599, 1958

237. Klensch H, Eger W: Die bestimmung des schlagvolumens aus dem ballistokardiogramm (vorlaufige mitteilung). Dtsch Med Wochenschr 81:1205–1206, 1956

238. Eger W, Klensch H: Qualitative und quantitative ballistographische untersuchungen am modellkreislauf. Pfluegers Arch Gesamte Physiol 262: 443–455, 1956

239. Klensch H, Eger W: Ein neues verfahren der physikalischen Schlagvolumenbestimmung. Pfleugers Arch Gesamte Physiol 263:459–475, 1956

240. Gott U, Klensch H: Kreislauf—untersuchungen unter den bedingugen von narkosen und kunstlicher blutdruckenskung. Anaesthetist 10:72–77, 1961

241. Klensch H, Hohnen HW: Bestimmung von schlag-und minutenvolumen nach arbeitsleistungmit der ballistischen methode. Pfluegers Arch Gesamte Physiol 265:207–219, 1957

242. Klensch H, Hohnen HW, Kesseler KH: Ballistische bestimmung des einzelschlagvolumens bei veranderung der atemlage und erhorung des intrapulmonalen druckes. Pfleugers Arch Gesamte Physiol 264:424–440, 1957

243. Klensch H, Schaede A, Thurn P, et al: Vergleichende untersuchung des minutenvolumens des herzens mit der ballistischen und der direkten fickschen methode. Pfleugers Arch Gesamte Physiol 269:232–239, 1959

244. Klensch H, Hohnen HW, Richter W: Das Schlagvolumen des herzens vor und nach operation traumatischer arteriovenoser fisteln der unteren extremitaten. Z Kreislaufforsch 48:153–161, 1959

245. Klensch H, Juznic G: Teststoffverfahren nach Stewart-Hamilton mit der a.v. schlinge. Pfleugers Arch Gesamte Physiol 275:574–578, 1962

246. Klensch H, Kallfelz HC: Das basale schlag-und minutenvolumen des herzens bei kindern und jugdlichen im alter von 9-22 Jahren. Verh Dtsch Kreislaufforsch 24:214–220, 1958

247. Eger W: Ballistographische untersuchungen zur frage der kreislaufwirkungen der epidural-anasthesie. Proc 2nd Eur Symp Ballistocardiography, Bonn, Germany, pp 210–215, 1961

248. Eger W, Hugin W: Ballistographische untersuchungen bei narkosen besonders zur frage der hypotonie unter halothan. Anaesthetist 10:38–48, 1961

249. Juznic G, Klensch H: Correlation between the values of cardiac output by the ULF-Ballistocardiography and Stewart-Hamilton dye dilution method in man. 4th Eur Congr Ballistocardiography, Lille Méd (Special Number) 3:56–61, 1964

250. Juznic G: Determination of cardiac stroke volume from the velocity and acceleration curve of the ULF-Ballistocardiogram. 4th Eur Cong Ballistocardiography, Lille Méd (Special Number) 3:62–64, 1964

251. Burger HC, Van Brummelen AGW: A physicist's view on the possibilities of measurement of stroke volume by means of special methods using ultra-low frequency BCG. 4th Eur Congr Ballistocardiography, Lille Méd (Special Number) 3:27–32, 1964

252. Van Brummelen AGW, Scarborough WR, Josenhans WKT: On the elimination of pulse wave velocity in stroke volume determination from the ultralow-frequency displacement ballistocardiogram. Am Heart J 67:374–378, 1964

253. Van Brummelen AGW, Josenhans WT: Elimination of the effects of variable ejection time and heart rate in ULF-Ballistocardiographic stroke volume determination, in Knoop AA (ed): Ballistocardiography and Cardiovascular Dynamics. Basel, Karger, 1966, pp 131–136

254. Rödenbeck M: Untersuchungen zur biophysik der ballistocardiographie,

M.S. thesis, Karl Marx Univ., Leipzig. (Trans. Studies on the biophysics of ballistocardiography. US Joint Publ Res Serv R-1410-D (FAA 1-6900-1) Washington, D.C. 1961, 1959

255. Nickerson JL: The low frequency, critically-damped ballistocardiograph. Fed Proc 4:201–206, 1945

256. Nickerson JL: Estimation of stroke volume by means of the ballistocardiograph. Am J Cardiol 2:642–644, 1958

257. Nickerson JL, Warren JV, Brannon ES: The cardiac output in man: studies with the low-frequency, critically-damped ballistocardiograph and the method of right atrial catheterization. J Clin Invest 26:1–10, 1947

258. Nickerson JL: Cardiac output by ballistic methods. Chicago Med Sch Quart 21:115–123, 1961

259. Nyboer J: Absolute value ULF ballistic forces as indices of pulsatile fluid pumping. Bibl Cardiol 24:7–12, 1969

260. Harrison WK: A ballistocardiographic stroke volume formula recognizing blood distribution effects. Bibl Cardiol 20:29–34, 1968

261. Starr I, Noordergraaf A: Ballistocardiography in Cardiovascular Research. Philadelphia, Lippincott, 1967, pp 98–100

262. Rushmer RF: Cardiovascular Dynamics (ed 3). Philadelphia, Saunders, 1970, p 110

263. Honig CR, Tenney SM: The relationship between the ballistocardiogram, cardiac movement and blood flow. Am Heart J 52:167–181, 1956

264. Deuchar DC: The relation of ballistocardiography to other methods of studying the cardiovascular system in man, in Knoop AA (ed): Ballisto-cardiography and Cardiovascular Dynamics. Basel, Karger, 1966, pp 225–236

265. Fox SM III, Warbasse JR, Crawford RB, et al: Studies in instantaneous ascending aortic blood velocity in intact man relative to the acceleration ballistocardiogram. Presented before the Ballistocardiographic Research Society, April 29, 1961

266. Scarborough WR: Comments on progress in ballistocardiographic research and the current state of the art. Proc 3d Eur Symp Ballistocardiography, Brussels, Belgium, April 16–17, pp 98–120, 1962

267. Darby TD, Walton RP, Gazes PC: Effects of drugs on ballistocardiographic recordings. Correlation with other cardiovascular measurements in dog and in man. Am J Cardiol 3:668–675, 1959

268. Lydtin H, Schnelle K, Lohmoller G, et al: Synchronous recordings of Bcg, ECG, carotid pulse wave, and PCG in acute pharmacological trials. Bibl Cardiol 26:36–41, 1970

269. Starr I: Further clinical studies with the ballistocardiograph on abnormal form, on digitalis action, in thyroid disease, and in coronary heart disease. Trans Assoc Am Physicians 59:180–189, 1946

270. Ambrosi C, Starr I: Incoordination of the cardiac contraction as judged by the force ballistocardiogram and the carotid pulse derivative. Am Heart J 70:761–774, 1965

271. Starr I, Ogawa S: On the aging of the heart; why is it so much more conspicuous in the ballistocardiogram than in the pulse. Am J Med Sci 242:399–410, 1961

272. Starr I, Ogawa S: On the relation between the ballistocardiogram and the

pulse; diagnostic advantages gained by simultaneous records. Proc 3rd
Eur Symp Ballistocardiography. Brussels, Belgium, pp 195–198, 1962

273. Starr I, Ogawa S: A clinical study of the first derivative of the brachial pulse.
Normal standards and abnormalities encountered in heart disease. Am
Heart J 64:482–494, 1963

274. Starr I: Progress towards a physiological cardiology: A second essay on the
ballistocardiogram. Ann Intern Med 63:1079–1105, 1965

275. Juznic G, Sketelj J, Novak Z, et al: The differential sphygmogram and lean
body mass in a group of 18 young men. Bibl Cardiol 26:94–107, 1970

276. Cunningham DM: Clinical simulation of the ballistocardiogram from pressure pulse measurements. Bibl Cardiol, in press

277. Winer NJ: The high frequency (acceleration) direct body ballistocardiogram:
I. Its interpretation in terms of the second derivative of the carotid pulse
and its own derivative. Bibl Cardiol 24:101–106, 1969

278. Winer NJ: High-frequency ('acceleration') direct body ballistocardiography:
A new concept in its application and diagnosis of early acute myocardial
infarction. Bibl Cardiol 26:52–65, 1970

279. Verdouw PD: Ballistics of ventricular performance. Philadelphia, Univ. of
Pa., 1970, p 104 (Dissertation)

280. Starr I: The place of the ballistocardiogram in a Newtonian cardiology; and
the new light it sheds on certain old clinical problems. Proc R Soc Med
60:1299–1306, 1967

281. Starr I, Mayock RL, Krumbhaar EB, et al: On the initial force of cardiac
contraction; standardization of the ballistocardiogram by physiological
experiments performed at necropsy. Trans Assoc Am Physicians 62:154–
161, 1949

282. Starr I, Noordergraaf A: Ballistocardiography in Cardiovascular Research,
Philadelphia, Lippincott, 1967, p 229

283. Smith JE: Studies of amplitude variation in the ultra-low frequency ballistocardiogram with special reference to cardiovascular reactivity. Aerosp
Med 40:258–263, 1969

284. Starr I, Noordergraaf A: Ballistocardiography in Cardiovascular Research,
Philadelphia, Lippincott, 1967, p 31

285. Starr I: The relation of the ballistocardiogram to cardiac function. Am J
Cardiol 2:737–747, 1958

286. Starr I, Ogawa S: Incoordination of the cardiac contraction in clinical conditions; as judged by the ballistocardiogram and the pulse derivative. Am
J Med Sci 244:663–680, 1962

287. Verdouw PD: Ballistics of ventricular performance, Philadelphia, University of Pennsylvania, p 272, 1970 (Dissertation)

287a. Starr I, Verdouw PD, Noordergraaf A: Clinical evidence of cardiac weakness and incoordination secured by simultaneous records of the force BCG
and carotid pulse derivative and interpreted by an electrical analogue.
Am Heart J 85:341–348, 1973

288. Osadjan CE, Randall WC: Effects of left stellate ganglion stimulation on
left ventricular synchrony in dogs. Am J Physiol 207:181–186, 1964

289. Herman MV, Heinle RA, Klein MD, et al: Localized disorders in myocardial
contraction. Asynergy and its role in congestive heart failure. N Engl J
Med 277:222–232, 1967

290. Herman MV, Gorlin R: Implications of left ventricular asynergy. Am J Cardiol 23:538–547, 1969

291. Ueda H, Ueda K, Morooka S, et al: A cineangiocardiographic study of the regional contraction sequence of the normal and diseased left ventricle in man. Jap Heart J 10:95–112, 1969

292. Segal BL, Kilpatrick DG (eds): Engineering in the Practice of Medicine. Baltimore, Williams & Wilkins, 1967

293. Franke EK, Braunstein JR: More data on the effects of the internal coupling of body segments. Bibl Cardiol 24:22–27, 1969

294. Franke EK, Braunstein JR: The effects of the internal coupling of body segments on the ballistocardiogram. Bibl Cardiol 20:21–28, 1968

295. Franke EK: Ballistocardiogram and body dynamics. Bibl Cardiol, in press

296. Tannenbaum O, Vesell H, Schack J: Relationship of the natural body damping and body frequency to the ballistocardiogram. Circulation 13:404–409, 1956

297. Weissbach GHJ: Die rolle der tischmasse und der wert einer zusätzlichen dampfung beim elongationsballistokardiographen. Pfluegers Arch Gesamte Physiol 270:529–535, 1960

298. Weissbach GHJ: Die registriertechnische eigenschaften des direkten ballistokardiographen. Z Kreislaufforsch 49:626–630, 1960

299. Tishchenko MI: Significance of natural vibrations of the human body in shaping the ballistocardiogram. Biophysics 8:311–319, 1963 (Trans)

300. Nickerson JL, Pevsner H, Johnson R, et al: Vibration transmission between heart and ballistocardiograph, in Knoop AA (ed): Ballistocardiography and Cardiovascular Dynamics. Basel, Karger, 1966, pp 49–54

301. Nickerson JL, Drazic M, Pevsner H: Further studies on transmission between heart and ballistocardiograph. Bibl Cardiol 21:74–79, 1968

302. Nickerson JL, Drazic M, Pevsner H: Further studies on transmission between heart and ballistocardiograph (Part 2). Bibl Cardiol 20:44–49, 1968

303. MacDonald DA: Hemodynamics. Ann Rev Physiol 30:525–556, 1967

304. Proper R: Correlation between age, "stroke volume index" and the "minute volume index" of Scarborough. Bibl Cardiol 24:63–65, 1969

305. Scarborough WR, Westura EE, Podolak E: Studies on a small group of normal test pilots with special reference to quantitative relationships of age with the ULF ballistocardiogram and other cardiovascular measurements. Bibl Cardiol 24:66–74, 1969

306. Starr I, Hildreth EA: The effect of aging and of the development of disease on the ballistocardiogram. A study of 80 subjects, originally healthy, followed from 10–14 years. Circulation 5:481–495, 1952

307. Scarborough WR, Folk EF III, Smith PM, et al: The nature and records from ultra-low frequency ballistocardiographic systems and their relation to circulatory events. Am J Cardiol 2:613–641, 1958

308. Rorvik K: Apexcardiography, phonocardiography and ballistocardiography— their diagnostic and prognostic significance in coronary heart disease. Acta Med Scand 404:1–77, 1963

309. Klensch H: Der informationscharakter der modernen ballistographie. Elektromedizen 6:104–118, 1961

310. Hartleb O: Forwandlungen ballistokardiographischer befund als ausdruck des alterns. Med Welt 47:2490–2493, 1960

311. Proper R, Wall F: Etiological factors associated with the diminution of

ballistocardiographic amplitudes occurring with advanced age. Bibl Cardiol 27:40–43, 1971

312. Knoop AA, Hoitink AWJH, van den Bos GC, et al: Cardiovascular effects in aging. Bibl Cardiol 21:7–11, 1968

313. Starr I: Does the presence of hypertension itself increase force BCG abnormality? Bibl Cardiol 27:36–39, 1971

314. Starr I: The physiological age of the heart. Proc 2nd Eur Symp Ballistocardiography, Bonn, Germany, 1961, pp 15–17

313. Starr I, Luchi RJ: A study of the cardiac function of extremely elderly women by the ULF force BCG and the carotid pulse derivative. Bibl Cardiol 20:94–98, 1967

316. Julius HW Jr, Van Brummelen AGW, Noordergraaf A: Distortion of the ultra-low frequency displacement ballistocardiogram for different heart rates, in Knoop AA (ed): Ballistocardiography and Cardiovascular Dynamics. Basel, Karger, 1966, pp 203–207

317. Verdouw PD, Westerhof N, Noordergraaf A: Analysis of the effect of posture on the BCG. Bibl Cardiol 24:75–84, 1969

318. Verdouw PD, Odell RH Jr, Noordergraaf A: Right ventricular forces in the ballistocardiogram. Bibl Cardiol, 1972

319. Kruger K: Metabolische aspekte der ischemischen herzkrankungen. Med Klin 62:1381, 1967

320. Kutschera-Aichbergen HV: Heuorientirung der herztherapie hach der biochemie des herzmuskul. Ther Woche 18:1935, 1968

321. Starr I, Noordergraaf A: Ballistocardiography in Cardiovascular Research. Philadelphia, Lippincott, 1967, p 43

322. Fischer DC: Use of the ballistocardiogram to assess surgical risk. Bibl Cardiol 27:21–24, 1971

323. Talakov AA: The prognostic significance of ballistocardiograms in mitral valve diseases, in Knoop AA (ed): Ballistocardiography and Cardiovascular Dynamics. Basel, Karger, 1966, pp 47–48

324. Fernandez-Garcia G: BCG and mitral valvotomy, in Knoop AA (ed): Ballistocardiography and Cardiovascular Dynamics. Basel, Karger, 1966. pp 31–35

325. Mathers JA, Nickerson JL, Fleming TC, et al: Abnormal ballistocardiographic patterns in cardiovascular disease as recorded with the low-frequency critically damped ballistocardiograph. Am Heart J 40:390–400, 1950

326. Starr I, Wood FC: Twenty year studies with the ballistocardiograph. The relation between the amplitude of the first record of "healthy" adults and eventual mortality and morbidity from heart disease. Circulation 23:714–732, 1961

327. Starr I: Prognostic value of ballistocardiograms. Studies on evaluation of the doctor's experience. JAMA 187:511–517, 1964

328. Baker BM, Scarborough WR, Davis FW Jr, et al: Ballistocardiography and ischaemic heart disease: predictive considerations and statistical evaluation. Proc R Soc Med 60:1290–1296

327. Scarborough WR, Baker BM, Davis FW Jr, et al: Ballistocardiography and coronary heart disease; prognostic evaluation based on a long-term follow-up study. Bibl Cardiol 20:57–81, 1968

330. Baker BM: Editorial, Ballistocardiography, predictor of coronary heart disease. Circulation 37:1–3, 1968

331. Smith JE: The use of ultra-low frequency ballistocardiograms in clinical practice with special reference to the causes of amplitude variations. Bibl Cardiol 26:152–155, 1970

332. S'Jongers JJ, Segers M: Differences between the ballistocardiograph of athletes and of sedentary persons. Preliminary note. Bibl Cardiol 21:145–151, 1968

333. Masini V, Venerando A, Busnengo E: Il balistocardiogramma da sforza nel soggeto normale e nello sportivo. Schweiz Z Sport-Med 2:83, 1954; in Medicino dello Sport; Sport e apparato cardiovasolare Universo Roma, 1960, pp 472–473

334. Jokl E: Heart and Sport, Charles C Thomas, Springfield, Ill., 1964, pp 27–44

335. Jokl E: Ballistocardiographic studies on athletes. Am J Cardiol 4:105–117, 1959

336. Medved R, Horvat V: Das ballistokardiogramm bei den sportlem. Dtsch Med Wochenschr 81:780–783, 1956

337. Elsbach H, Rodrigo FA, Weeda HWH, et al: The ballistocardiogram in selection for and assessment of physical conditioning in patients with ischemic heart disease. Bibl Cardiol 26:49–51, 1970

338. Holloszy JO, Skinner JS, Barry AJ: Effect of physical conditioning on cardiovascular function. Am J Cardiol 14:761–770, 1964

339. Frick MH, Katila M: Hemodynamic consequences of physical training after myocardial infarction. Circulation 37:192–202, 1968

340. Hanson JS, Tabakin BS, Levy AM, et al: Long-term physical training and cardiovascular dynamics in middle-aged men. Circulation 38:783–799, 1968

341. Starr I, Noordergraaf A: Ballistocardiography in Cardiovascular Research. Philadelphia, Lippincott, 1967, pp 203–211

342. Starr I, Noordergraaf A: Ballistocardiography in Cardiovascular Research. Philadelphia, Lippincott, 1967, pp 302–317

343. Caccese A, Schrager A: The effects of cigarette smoking on the ballistocardiogram. Am Heart J 42:589–596, 1951

344. Starr I, Noordergraaf A: Ballistocardiography in Cardiovascular Research. Lippincott, 1967, p 315

345. Chevalier RB, Krumholz RA, Ross JC: Effects of carbon monoxide inhalation on the cardiopulmonary responses of non-smokers to exercise. J Lab Clin Med (Abstr) 62:167, 1963

346. Ayres SM: Role of carbon monoxide and nicotine in circulatory effects of cigarette smoke. JAMA 219:520, 1972

347. Buchanan J: Ballistocardiographic smoking tests in thyrotoxicosis, in Knoop AA (ed): Ballistocardiography and Cardiovascular Dynamics. Basel, Karger, 1966, pp 175–179

348. Buchanan J: Ballistocardiographic smoking tests in myxoedema. Bibl Cardiol 26:89–93, 1970

349. Buchanan J, Cameron AJV: Ballistocardiographic smoking tests in young patients with diabetes mellitus. Proc 2nd Eur Symp Ballistocardiography, Bonn, Germany, pp 27–28, 1961

350. Starr I, Noordergraaf A: Ballistocardiography in Cardiovascular Research, Philadelphia, Lippincott, 1967, pp 318–355

351. Van Lingen B, Gear JH, Whidborne JC, et al: Some effects of digitalis on the circulation in congestive cardiac failure. S Afr J Clin Sci 1:336–346, 1950

352. Dock W, Mandelbaum H, Mandelbaum R: Ballistocardiography; the application of the direct ballistocardiograph to clinical medicine. St. Louis, Mosby, 1953

353. Wendhut G, Reichel H: Zur frage der reproduzierbarkeit direkter ballistokardiogramme im hinblick auf ihre verwendung zu verlaufskontrollen. Z Kreislaufforsch 46:399–406, 1957

354. Arbeit SR, Moret P: A biologic test for digitalis effect. Am Heart J 53: 293–300, 1957

355. Jonnart L: Le ballistocardiogramme d'ultra-basse frequence. Acta Cardiol Suppl 9:1–75, 1960

356. Bedrova NN: The effect of glycosides on myocardial contraction ballistocardiographic studies (in Russian). Klin Med (Moskva) 41:35–38, 1963

357. Winer NJ: The effect of certain drugs on myocardial dynamics as recorded with the high-frequency (acceleration) direct body ballistocardiograph. Bibl Cardiol 26:160–173, 1970

358. Winer NJ: The BCG reflections of the pathophysiology of the heart beat as recorded with the high frequency ('acceleration') direct body BCG. Bibl Cardiol 21:102–115, 1968

359. Starr I, Luchi RJ: Blind study on the action of digitoxin on elderly women. Am Heart J 78:740–751, 1961

360. Warembourg H, Merlen JF, Flament G, et al: Ballistocardiographic study of amyl nitrite effects in normal and in ischaemic heart disease. Bibl Cardiol 26:156–159, 1970

361. Starr I, Pedersen E, Corbascio AN: The effect of nitroglycerine on the ballistocardiogram of persons with and without clinical evidence of coronary heart disease. Circulation 12:588–603, 1955

362. Moreira MG: L'interet du ballistocardiogramme en pharmacodynamie, 4th Eur Congr Ballistocardiography, Lille Méd 3:97–100, 1964

363. Scarborough WR: Ballistocardiogram in the diagnosis of coronary atherosclerosis. Minn Med 38:880–887, 1955

364. Kuo PT, Joyner CR: Angina pectoris induced by fat ingestion in patients with coronary artery disease, ballistocardiographic and electrocardiographic findings. JAMA 158:1008–1013, 1955

365. Klensch H, Juznic G: Untersuchungen uber die hamodynamisch bedingte sauerstoff-einsparung des herzen durch nitroglyzerin. Z Kreislaufforsch 53: 117–130, 1964

366. Urbach F, Hildreth EA, Wackerman MT: The therapeutic uses of low fat, low cholesterol diets. J Clin Nutr 1:52–65, 1952–53

367. Scarborough WR: Current status of ballistocardiography. Prog Cardiovasc Dis 2:263–291, 1959

368. Kuo PT, Whereat AF, Horwitz O: The effect of lipemia upon coronary and peripheral arterial circulation in patients with essential hyperlipemia. Am J Med 26:68–75, 1959

369. Davis FW Jr: The role of the ballistocardiograph in the diagnosis and man-

agement of patients with coronary heart disease, stress tests and the cigarette test. Am J Cardiol 3:103–110, 1959

370. Deuchar DC: Some further observations on the ballistocardiogram in aortic valve disease. Proc 3rd Eur Symp Ballistocardiography, Brussels, Belgium, April 16–17, pp 225–233, 1962

371. Hugin W: Das ballistographische Bild vor und nach der operation von aorten-isthmusstenosen. Thoraxchirurgie 8:563–566, 1961

372. Moss AJ, Gottovi D: Correlation of the acceleration ballistocardiogram with cardiovascular dynamics in aortic outflow disease, in Knoop AA (ed): Ballistocardiography Cardiovascular Dynamics. Basel, 1966, pp 21–25

373. Henderson CB: The ballistocardiogram in congenital heart disease. Am J Cardiol 3:799–810, 1959

374. Cossio P, Berreta A, Mosso HE, et al: El balistocardiograma en la estrechez mitral. Medicina (Buenos Aires) 15:368–376, 1955

375. Ming-Hsin H, Kuo-Juei Y: Ballistocardiographic changes in rheumatic mitral valvular disease. China Med J 75:693–701, 1957

376. Talakov A: Prae- und postoperative veranderungen im ballistokardiogramm bei der mitralstenose. Bull Int Soc Surgery 19:46–52, 1960

377. Starr I, Noordergraaf A: Ballistocardiography in Cardiovascular Research. Philadelphia, Lippincott, 1967, p 343

378. Black A, Delmonico JE Jr: An evaluation of three revascularization pro-cedures in the rehabilitation of the coronary patient. Am J Cardiol 3:68–73, 1959

379. Starr I, Noordergraaf A: Ballistocardiography in Cardiovascular Research, Philadelphia, Lippincott, 1967, p 347

380. Brofman BL, Arbeit SR, Adicoff A: Coronary heart disease. Ballistocardio-graphic evaluation of surgical treatment. Am J Cardiol 3:54–60, 1956

381. Starr I, Joyner CR, MacVaugh H III: Preliminary report of studies made in cases of severe angina pectoris before and after the Vineberg operation. Bibl Cardiol 24:96–100, 1968

382. Starr I, Joyner CR, MacVaugh H III: Further studies of the effect of the Vineberg operation on patients with severe angina pectoris. Bibl Cardiol 26:31–35, 1970

383. Lower RR: Cardiac transplantation in proper perspective. Surg Gynecol Obstet 126:838–839, 1968

384. Nora JJ, Cooley DA, Fernbach DJ, et al: Rejection of the transplanted hu-man heart. Index of recognition and problems in prevention. N Engl J Med 280:1079–1086, 1969

385. Smith NT, Hurley EJ, Corbascio AN: The ultra-low frequency ballisto-cardiogram in dogs after autotransplantation of the heart, in Knoop AA (ed): Ballistocardiography and Cardiovascular Dynamics. Basel, Karger, 1966, pp 298–303

386. Smith NT, Angell WW: The BCG in cardiac homotransplantation. Bibl Cardiol 20:82–93, 1968

387. Shakespeare T, Reitan JA, Smith NT, et al: ULF ballistocardiography in hu-man cardiac transplantation. Bibl Cardiol 27:1–9, 1971

388. Stinson EB, Griepp R, Clark DA: Cardiac transplantation in man. VIII. Survival and function. J Thorac Cardiovasc Surg 60:303–321, 1970

389. Jonnart L: Auricular activity from the ballistocardiogram. Proc 2nd Eur Symp Ballistocardiography. Bonn, Germany, March 27–28, pp 33–43, 1961

390. Elsbach H, Rodrigo FA: The ultralow-frequency ballistocardiogram in atrial septal defect. A semiquantitative approach based on the analysis of the velocity curve. Am Heart J 70:186–195, 1965

391. Starr I, Schroeder HA: Ballistocardiogram: II. Normal standards, abnormalities commonly found in diseases of the heart and circulation and their significance. J Clin Invest 19:437–450, 1940

392. Debenedetti V: Il balistocardiogramma; limiti della sua applicazione practica. Minerva Cardioangiol 2:176–188, 1954

393. Smith JE, Rosenbaum R, Ostrich R: Studies with the displacement velocity, and acceleration ballistocardiograph in aortic insufficiency. Am Heart J 48:847–863, 1954

394. Scarborough WR, Mason RE, Davis FW Jr, et al: A ballistocardiographic and electrocardiographic study of 328 patients with coronary artery disease; comparison with results from a similar study of apparently normal persons. Am Heart J 44:645–670, 1952

395. Verdouw PD: Ballistics of ventricular performance. Philadelphia, Univ. of Pa., 1970 (Dissertation), p 171

396. Starr I, Verdouw PD: Physiological interpretation of the abnormal ballistocardiograms (Bcg) and pulse waves found in the clinic by their simulation in an electrical model of the circulation. Fed Proc (Abstr) 29:797, 1970

397. Tuveri A, Pitzus F: La morfologia del balistocardiogramma nelle valvulopatie reumatiche. Minerva Med 2:332–340, 1954

398. Starr I, Noordergraaf A: Ballistocardiography in Cardiovascular Research, Philadelphia, Lippincott, 1967, pp 247–252

399. Henderson CB: The abnormal ballistocardiogram in mitral stenosis. The relationship of the abnormal waves to right ventricular ejection and to the mean pulmonary artery pressure. Circulation 12:858–868, 1955

400. Starr I, Wood FC: Studies with the ballistocardiograph in acute cardiac infarction and chronic angina pectoris. Am Heart J 25:81–101, 1943

401. Masini V, Martini G, Rossi P: Ricerche ballistocardiografiche II-II ballistocardiogramma nei cardiopatici. Riforma Med 66:477–480, 1952

402. Brown H, Rinzler SH, Benton JG: Correlation of ballistocardiogram with work performance and energy cost for guidance in rehabilitation of cardiac patients. Circulation 7:740–746, 1953

403. Davis FW Jr, Scarborough WR, Mason RE, et al: The effects of exercise and smoking on the electrocardiograms and ballistocardiograms of normal subjects and patients with coronary artery disease. Am Heart J 46: 529–542, 1953

404. Isaacs JX, Wilburne M, Gunther L: Ultra-low frequency acceleration (force) ballistocardiogram in myocardial infarction. Am J Cardiol 1:323–333, 1958

405. Rosenblatt WH, Harbour JH: The value of the ballistocardiograph in the diagnosis of the prodromal stage of acute myocardial infarction; case report. Mississippi Doctor 33:309–313, 1956

406. Winer NJ: The high frequency (acceleration) direct body ballistocardiogram: II. The diagnosis of early acute myocardial infarctions in terms of the second derivative of the carotid pulse and its own next derivative. Bibl Cardiol 24:107–112, 1969

407. Starr I, Noordergraaf A: Ballistocardiography in Cardiovascular Research, Philadelphia, Lippincott, 1967, pp 247–252

408. Moss AJ: Ischemic heart disease and accelerated cardiovascular aging. A ballistocardiographic study. Circulation 25:369–375, 1962

409. Verdouw PD: Ballistics of ventricular performance. Philadelphia, Univ of Pa., 1970 (Dissertation), p 111

410. Verdouw PD: Ballistics of ventricular performance. Philadelphia, Univ. of Pa., 1970 (Dissertation), p 192

411. Frankel AL, Rothermich NO: Clinical experiences in ballistocardiography. Ann Intern Med 36:1385–1412, 1952

412. Starr I, Noordergraaf A: Ballistocardiography in Cardiovascular Research, Philadelphia, Lippincott, 1967, pp 285–286

413. Arntzenius AC, Koops J, Rodrigo FA, et al: Circulatory effects of body acceleration given synchronously with the heart beat (BASH). Bibl Cardiol 26:180–187, 1970

414. Arntzenius AC, Verdouw PD: Cardiovascular responses in pigs to body acceleration applied synchronously with the heartbeat. Bibl Cardiol 27:44–52, 1971

415. Hoffer RE, Almond CH, Elefson EE, et al: Acute anterior descending coronary artery ligation, ventricular fibrillation and ventricular assistance. Arch Surg 98:703–708, 1969

416. Verdouw PD, Noordergraaf A, Arntzenius AC, et al: Relative movement between subject and support in body acceleration applied synchronously with the heartbeat (BASH). Bibl Cardiol 1973 (in press)

417. Harrison WK: Measurements of cranial blood flow using ballistocardiography. Bibl Cardiol 27:53–58, 1971

418. Talbot SA, Harrison WK Jr: Computer evaluation of graphical physiologic data for diagnosis of coronary heart disease. Meth Inform Med 5:81–85, 1966

419. Ingels NB, Daughters GT II, Smith NT, et al: A comparison of directly measured and hemodynamically inferred indices of myocardial performance. Proc Biomed Eng Soc, 1972

420. Niess OK, Sparks BW: Use of the orbital space laboratory for research in biology and medicine. Dis of Chest 51:384–391, 1967

Richard L. Popp
Donald C. Harrison

3
Echocardiography

INTRODUCTION AND HISTORICAL BACKGROUND

The application of ultrasound technology for a study of medical problems has occurred only in the past two decades. In 1953 Drs. Inge Edler and Helmuth Hertz conceived of using the ultrasonic ocean floor detectors developed during World War II for visualizing cardiac structures. Dr. Hertz borrowed such a sonar apparatus from a local shipyard and was able to record echoes from his own heart. These investigators were able to interest a medical electronics company in developing an "ultrasonic reflectoscope," based on their design. Over the next few years, extensive studies were done on the genesis of the echographic patterns they observed.[1-3] Initially, Drs. Edler and Hertz thought that they were recording echoes from the left atrial wall, which allowed them to differentiate normal patients from those with mitral stenosis.[3] They later discovered that this echo was arising from the anterior leaflet of the mitral valve. Anatomic and physiologic studies led to labeling of the various echo patterns observed.[4,5] That the identity of the origin of these echoes has been confirmed repeatedly over the subsequent two decades is a tribute to the care and thorough-

This work was supported in part by NIH Grants (HE-5709, HE-5866 and HE-5107), a grant from the National Aeronautics and Space Administration (NGR-05-020-305) and grants from the American Heart Association and the Bay Area Heart Association. Dr. Popp is a recipient of a Research and Career Development Award, No. 1-K04-HL704-39.

ness of the original investigations. In the 1950s, Edler and Hertz popularized the echographic technique for cardiac use in Europe, with subsequent extensive basic studies by Dr. Sven Effert in Germany.[6,7] In the early 1960s, these investigators visited the United States, and the interest they generated in Dr. Claude Joyner's laboratory in Philadelphia, and in other laboratories, served as the impetus for the development of ultrasound in the United States. Until approximately 7 years ago, the clinical use of ultrasound had been limited to the assessment of mitral valve stenosis and rare cases of ball valve thrombus or atrial tumor. A great deal of experience with mitral and tricupsid valve lesions had accrued in Europe and the United States. However, during the last few years, the use of ultrasound for the diagnosis of pericardial effusion, mitral valve prolapse, hypertrophic subaortic stenosis, and as a noninvasive means to assess ventricular function has generated considerable enthusiasm in many centers around the country. This enthusiasm has brought unusually rapid growth of the understanding of the technique and its level of application. The current high quality of ultrasonic studies performed in academic institutions is due, in large part, to the skill and hospitality of Dr. Harvey Feigenbaum in allowing physicians and interested investigators to visit and to work in his laboratory. This laboratory at Indiana University has been quite active in the development and assessment of ultrasound techniques.

Part of the excitement in the use of ultrasound in cardiology is because this is a young field which is still in its developmental stages. As more centers begin to use this technique, more applications will be developed. The limitations of ultrasound for cardiac diagnosis are not yet known, since intriguing new patterns continue to emerge as experience expands. There has been some slow but gradual improvement in the quality of the ultrasonic equipment commercially available during the last 10 years. As factors limiting the usefulness of specific procedures have been recognized, new types of transducer designs and display techniques have been devised. It is encouraging to see that new research and development appears to be occurring among commercial firms and engineering laboratories, giving rise to the expectation of new and better equipment for specific applications of ultrasonics in diagnosis.

BASIC PRINCIPLES

Engineering and Physics

Sound waves with a frequency above 20,000 Hz (cps) are defined as ultrasound. Medical ultrasound uses piezoelectric material to generate and detect these high-frequency waves. The application of an electric field to such crystals causes a compression and expansion of the crystal, thereby converting the electrical energy to mechanical energy. Short bursts of high-frequency waves formed in this manner may be directed into biological tissue and are transmitted within this tissue. The physical principles of sound and the similar principles of light waves are generally quite familiar. If a packet of sound waves traveling through a medium encounters an interface of materials of different acoustic impedance (density times sound velocity), then part of the sound will be transmitted into the new media, and part will be reflected by the interface. If the interface is nearly perpendicular to the path of the sound beam, then the reflected sound will travel back to the transducer, and the piezoelectric property of the transducer will reconvert the sound waves into electrical energy. It is possible to calculate the distance between the transducer and the echo source if the speed of sound through the material and the time elapsed from transmission of the sound to reception of the echo are known. The velocity of sound transmission in human tissue varies from 1,450 meters per sec in fat to 1,585 meters per sec in muscle, and 1,620 meters per sec in the optic lens.[8] An average value of 1,540 meters per sec is used in most ultrasonic equipment to calculate the location of an echo source. Timing circuits are a basic part of the ultrasonoscope's electronic circuitry. In practice, the ultrasonic transducer is pulsed for a very short period of time, usually 1 μsec or less, with the transducer acting as its own receiver for the remaining 99 μsec until the next pulse. Thus, 1,000 distance readings are made per second, and variations in the distance between the transducer and echo sources may be observed with a sampling rate equal to this repetition rate. Most commercially available instruments have a repetition rate of 500 to 1,000 pulses per sec.

The most usual method of display for the ultrasonic signals is by the use of a cathode-ray tube. The A-mode, or amplitude modulated display, presents time from sound transmission to echo return, as a measurement of distance, along the X axis, and the amplitude of the returning sound, or intensity of the echo, on the Y axis (Fig. 3–1). Time of transmission, or zero distance, is displayed on the left side

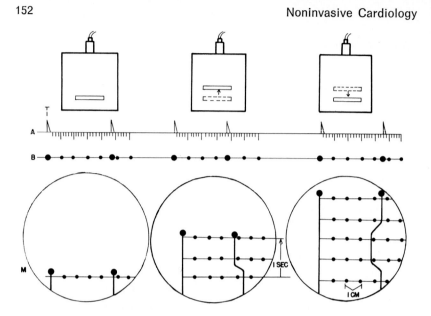

Fig. 3–1. Echo display techniques. A transducer directed toward a reflecting surface, with movement toward the transducer in the middle panel, and movement away from the transducer in the right-hand panel (A, A mode display of the motion of the reflecting surface with respect to the transducer. T, transducer artifact; B, B mode display of the signal; M, motion mode showing the basis of time and distance measurements from the oscilloscopic display). In M mode records, the B mode presentation is swept from the bottom to the top of the oscilloscope.

of the oscilloscope. Elapsed time from transmission to reception of an echo is represented by horizontal distance from left to right. A series of calibrated electronic spikes representing tissue depth is usually generated along the X axis and appears on the A-mode trace. These calibration markers allow precise measurement of the distance between intracardiac interfaces. There is a large amount of electronic circuitry needed for signal processing, in order to transform the raw signal form, which is generated in the transducer by returning echoes, into the spikes seen on the cathode-ray tube. A single returning echo is made up of a series of high-frequency oscillations with increasing and then decreasing amplitude. The basic external outline, or envelope, that encloses this packet of oscillations is detected and transformed, by subsequent signal processing, into a triangular voltage spike. Generally, it is this triangular spike, representing the outline of the returning echo, which is displayed on the cathode-ray tube. The great variation and the appearance of echographic signals from one ultrasonoscope to another is mainly because of the differences in signal processing techniques. As an example, an instrument that uses a very narrow envelope detecting technique may neglect the low-frequency oscillations on either side of a central high-amplitude area which contains higher frequency components, whereas another instrument may display echo return envelopes which enclose low-frequency oscillations as well as the central, high-frequency oscillations. As a result of these two types of processing, the signal will appear broader in the latter case. Such broad signals allow echoes from two interfaces which are close together to be blended, so that one is unable to recognize the difference between these signals. If two interfaces are close together and the echoes from these interfaces are processed so that they present narrow signals, it is possible to separate the two returning echoes and recognize that there are two interfaces present. In the past, some instruments have used circuitry that sensed the returning echoes as just described, but instead of displaying these directly on the oscilloscope, these ultrasonoscopes generated a square-wave marker in place of the envelope of the sound. Most modern instruments differentiate the rectified signal, and a thin, sharply defined electronic spike results.

As one watches the cathode-ray tube of an ultrasonoscope, using the A-mode display, the motion of the echo source can be observed as the electronic representation of the structure moves along the X axis. In cardiac echography, it is the pattern of motion that is recognized as identifying certain intracardiac structures. In order to record this pattern of motion, a M-mode, or time-motion display, is recorded (Fig. 3–1). In this presentation, the ultrasonoscope converts each echo spike into a dot on the oscilloscope screen, with distance again represented on the X axis. In this mode, however, we have an intensity-modulated display wherein the stronger, or high-amplitude, echoes are represented by a bright dot, and the weak echoes by a less intense dot. The oscilloscope is allowed to drift from the bottom to the top of the tube face, so that time is represented along the Y axis. As a consequence of this electronic manipulation, the moving dots trace out their patterns as they move from the bottom to the top of the oscilloscope. In this method of operation, distance calibration marks are flashed on the oscilloscope at specific time intervals, so that a calibration grid of distance against time is generated. Most ultrasonoscopes contain an electrocardiographic amplifier, which permits a display of the electrocardiogram simultaneously with the echoes for timing. Such echograms are generally photographed from the oscilloscope face using a Polaroid, or other rapid-process camera. The hard-copy records are usually viewed by rotating the original orientation of the record 90° clockwise. This allows one to view the electrocardiogram in the conventional manner. It is also possible to use a tape recorder or oscilloscopic strip chart recorder to display the data. Strip chart records may be made using an analog output device, which allows one to record the motion of only one echo-producing structure on the strip chart recorder (Fig. 3–2). Alternately, the whole echographic display may be recorded by strip chart, in order to display other physiologic parameters simultaneously (Fig. 3–3, see also Fig. 3–17).

The transducers which are used in medical-pulsed ultrasound are usually made of lead zirconate titanate with electrodes tightly bound to this crystal, and various backing materials used to control the ringing of the crystal. The whole apparatus is put in an insulating case, which should be comfortable to hold during the examination, and small enough to fit into an intercostal space on the chest. The active face of the transducer may be flat, or acoustic lenses may be placed on the transducer, in order to focus the sound beam. Although there are no good data concerning the form of the sound beam within the chest, we assume that a strong central beam of sound is preferable to a diffuse beam for the purposes of localization of structures and producing returning echoes of sufficient intensity to be displayed. We know that the ability to penetrate biological tissue is inversely proportional to the frequency of the ultrasound used. However, the resolution of two structures which are very close to each other improves directly with the frequency of the ultrasound used. For example, since deep-tissue penetration is not critical in opthalmologic uses of ultrasound, very high-frequency transducers (10 to 20 mHz) are used for this application. In techniques requiring penetration of the abdomen with ultrasound, low frequencies such as 1 mHz are used. In cardiac work, a compromise between penetration and resolution has resulted in the general use of transducers in the 1 to 5 mHz range, with 2 or 2.25 mHz being the standard frequency used in most laboratories.

As sound penetrates tissue, part of the energy is reflected from each succeeding interface, and the sound beam has diminishing energy as it penetrates deeper into the tissue. In order to compensate for this attenuation, most ultrasonoscopes have the capability of changing the gain of their receiving amplifiers as a function of time, and thus as a function of tissue depth, so that the weaker signals returning from the more distant interfaces are amplified to a greater degree than the strong signals returning from near structures. These devices for the time-compensated gain adjustments are used routinely in cardiac work.

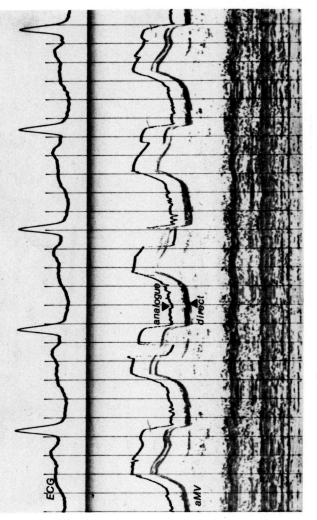

Fig. 3–2. Analog record. Simultaneous analog and direct presentations of a mitral valve echogram demonstrates the variation in analog presentation owing to alterations in the character and strength of the direct signal. The patient has mitral stenosis (aMV, anterior mitral valve leaflet).

155

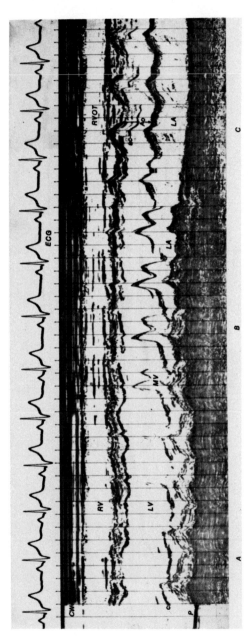

Fig. 3–3. Standard echographic patterns. The transducer on the chest wall is rocked from a caudal and lateral direction, recorded on the left portion of this tracing, toward a cephalad and medial direction, recorded on the right (see Fig. 3–4). A. The body of the right and left ventricle and the echoes from the chordae tendineae (c) within the left ventricle are shown. B. The patterns of the mitral valve are displayed. The echoes from the chordae tendineae are seen to join the mitral valve, and both anterior and posterior mitral leaflets are seen. The amplitude of anterior mitral leaflet motion decreases as the beam records areas nearer the mitral annulus. The patterns of left ven- tricle and left atrium are contrasted during this continu- ous sweep. Note the altered pattern of interventricular septal motion in area B compared with that in area A. C. The pattern of the aortic root and left atrium are shown. The aortic cusps are seen between the two aortic walls. The altered pattern of left atrial motion from the lateral to the posterior aspect of the left atrium is apparent (CW, chest wall; **RV**, right ventricle; LV, left ventricle; P, pericardium; c, chordae tendineae; MV, mitral valve; LA, left atrium; RVOT, right ventricular outflow tract; Ao, aorta; ac, aortic cusp).

The energy levels used in diagnostic ultrasound are quite small. The average power output of ultrasonic therapy devices used for generating heat in muscle tissue is 1 watt per cm^2. The average output of most diagnostic ultrasonic instruments is 0.02 watt per cm^2 or less.[9] Peak intensity appears to be in the range of 20 watts per cm^2, but the duration of this intensity level is extremely short. Studies on the biological effect of ultrasound show no evidence for tissue damage at these power levels,[4,10] and such levels are used in monitoring the fetus without demonstrable effect.[11,12] Effect of ultrasound on cells in tissue culture using chromosomal studies as the end-point shows no significant difference between the cultures which had been insonated and the controls.[13] In addition, investigators such as Dr. Edler have not noted any untoward effects of ultrasound in their long-term experience.[4] Thus, it would appear that diagnostic ultrasound is not only relatively simple to perform in a noninvasive manner without discomfort to the patient but also it is safe.

Terminology

As a result of confusion in the terminology used in early ultrasonic literature, the American Institute of Ultrasonics in Medicine has suggested terminology for the various display techniques, in order to avoid this confusion (Fig. 3–1). A-mode presentation is the amplitude-modulated display, and this is a method of data presentation in which the coordinate along the trace of the oscilloscope represents time, whereas the amplitude of the echo is displayed along the other co-ordinate. B-mode is the brightness or intensity-modulated display, and is a method of data presentation in which the coordinate along the trace of the oscilloscope represents time, whereas the amplitude of the echo is represented as brightness, or intensity of the appropriate portion of the tracing. M-mode is a method of data presentation generally used in the intensity-modulated display, but in which the trace is moved along the oscilloscope to display the pattern of movement of echoes while the transducer is kept stationary. As opposed to these modes of presentation, echographic techniques which are described as *scans* are techniques in which the transducer is moved while making the trace follow and indicate motion of the transducer. The type of two-dimensional imaging which is used in abdominal work, using a storage oscilloscope and intensity modulated display, is called a *B-scan*.

TECHNIQUES

Anatomical Considerations

There is a large area of the anterior chest of the normal adult human which permits the waves from an ultrasonic transducer to enter the soft tissues without encountering bone or air-containing lung. This "ultrasonic window" is in the shape of the letter "L" with the base of the window extending from the cardiac apex to the left sternal border, and the vertical portion of the window extending from the fifth to the second intercostal space along the left sternal border. In infants, the noncalcified ribs neither reflect nor absorb enough sound to be an obstacle to transmission and reception, which is in contrast to the situation in the adult. Adult patients with significant pulmonary hyperinflation often have a very small ultrasonic window on the anterior chest, as a result of pulmonary tissue being interposed between the heart and the anterior chest wall. We should appreciate that the ultrasonic beam passing through the window on the anterior chest is analogous to a flashlight beam passing through the window of a room in a darkened house. In both cases, only a small area can be visualized at a time, and the structures on the other side of the window must be recognized either by their unique characteristics seen with one beam orientation or by the integration of information gained by illuminating various parts of the structure in sequence.

Structures within the heart are recognized by *patterns of motion* which are characteristic of the structure, and by the *anatomic relationship* between structures showing various specific patterns of motion. The classic anatomic work of Edler and Hertz in delineating the motion patterns of various cardiac structures[4] has been confirmed and extended by investigators using intracardiac ultrasonic indicators.[14-16] Substances such as indocyanine green or ordinary saline produce microbubbles within the cardiac chamber when these substances are injected at high pressure through a catheter. There is evidence that this microbubble formation is a cavitation phenomenon, rather than the presence of dissolved or carried particulate matter.[17,18] However, the high-pressure injection of these substances within a specific chamber produces very strong ultrasonic reflections which define the cavity. Studies using this technique have delineated the patterns seen in the great vessels of the heart, as well as the atrial and ventricular chambers. Such indicator studies have allowed one to recognize left atrial from left ventricular wall motion, and endocardium from epicardium, for example.

Observation of the sequence of the structures encountered allows the reconstruction of the path of the sound beam through the heart. That is, one can tell if the sound beam passes through the aorta on the way to the left atrium, or through the mitral valve on the way to the left atrium. Then, assuming an adequate knowledge of the three-dimensional anatomy of the heart, the examiner may identify the structures encountered by the sound beam from any transducer location, and either angulate the transducer or move it to a new position on the chest wall, and aim the transducer from this new point to obtain any desired path of the ultrasonic beam to intersect the specific cardiac structures that are sought (Fig. 3–4). Figure 3–4 illustrates a sound path, A, through the chest wall, right ventricular wall, interventricular septum, chordae tendineae, posterior left ventricular wall, pericardium, and lung. If the pattern so produced is recognized, then the transducer need only be directed in a cephalad and medial direction to encounter the mitral valve with its characteristic motion (path B, Fig. 3–4). Continued movement of the transducer in a cephalad and medial direction will demonstrate a smooth progression to the pattern characteristic of the aortic root, with the left atrium posterior to it (path C, Fig. 3–4). It is important to emphasize the anatomic continuity of the posterior left ventricular wall with the atrioventricular ring and left atrium; the

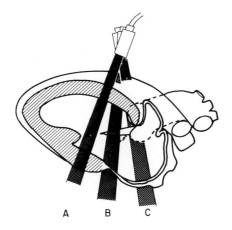

A   B   C

Fig. 3–4. Standard sound beam orientations. From one position on the chest wall, the beam can be directed in position A to encounter the body of the left ventricle below the mitral valve, and above the papillary muscle. Position B: the sound beam encounters the mitral valve. Position C: the sound beam traverses the aortic root and proceeds through the left atrium.

continuity of the anterior mitral valve leaflet with the posterior wall
of the aorta, and the continuity of the interventricular septum with
the anterior aortic wall (Fig. 3–3). These continuities are anatomic
facts which permit the examiner to imagine the path of the sound beam
through the heart in any specific case. The practice of sweeping the
sound beam along the left ventricular outflow tract while observing
the transition from one area to the contiguous area has clarified the
origin of most echoes. This coupling of ultrasonic patterns with anatomic relations is especially important for standardization of studies
among patients and reproducibility of studies in a single patient. The
currently used method of sweeping the sound beam is based on
Gramiak's rediscovery[14–15] of the patterns identified by Edler and
Hertz, and by Effert. This method of transducer direction has taken the
mystery out of the ultrasonic examination. A practical example of this
approach is in the diagnosis of atrial masses. Authors show echoes
of an atrial mass as the mass protrudes down through the mitral
orifice and appears behind the echoes from the anterior leaflet of the
mitral valve. Of course, if the transducer is quite superior to the level
of the mitral valve, the sound beam will pass from this cephalad
position on the chest wall in an inferior direction through the anterior
mitral leaflet and strike the left ventricular wall (Fig. 3–5, path A).

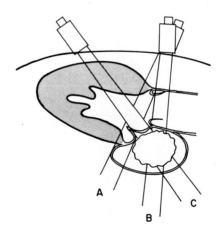

A   C
B

Fig. 3–5. Transducer positions to encounter a left atrial
mass. Position A records the mitral valve, but may not
intersect a mass that remains in the atrium throughout
the cardiac cycle. Position B permits the sound beam to
enter the left atrium and encounter an atrial mass. Position C allows the transducer to record the mitral valve and
proceed into the left atrium to evaluate the presence of an
atrial mass.

Then, if one wishes to send the sound beam into the left atrium, one may rotate the transducer in a cephalad and medial direction, in which case the aorta and left atrium will be visualized (Fig. 3–5, path B). Alternately, one may replace the transducer one or two interspaces lower on the chest wall, and direct the sound beam from this more caudal position up through the anterior leaflet and into the left atrium (Fig. 3–5, path C). In this way, even a mass which does not really protrude through the mitral orifice might be seen.

Physiological Considerations

Because of the anatomy of the heart, there are several characteristic patterns which have been defined by echographers and have been alluded to above. The generation of these patterns is most easily explained and visualized using a lateral projection of the heart (Fig. 3–4). We will assume a single transducer position on the chest wall at the level of the mitral valve. From this position, the transducer may be rocked to inscribe a plane parallel with the left ventricular outflow tract. The exact plane is oriented differently in space from one patient to another, but the proper plane is found by sweeping the transducer from a cephalad and medial direction to a caudal and lateral direction at varying angles with the vertical. When this plane is found, four specific patterns can be observed. The first pattern is that recorded as the sound beam passes through, in order, the chest wall, anterior right ventricular wall, right ventricular outflow tract, anterior aortic wall, posterior aortic wall, left atrium, posterior left atrial wall, and mediastinum or lung (Fig. 3–3 and 3–6). This pattern is most easily recognized by the synchronous movement of the two aortic walls.[14] The aorta is seen to move toward the transducer during systole and away from the transducer during diastole. The left atrial posterior wall shows virtually no motion and is recorded behind the moving aortic echoes. That the left atrial wall does not move in this area is accounted for by the attachment of this posterior portion of the atrial wall to the mediastinum at the level of the pulmonary veins. The area of the aorta that is recorded is the sinuses of Valsalva, and it is necessary to direct the transducer slightly more cephalad than this level, in order to record the movement of the aortic valve leaflets. The leaflets are recognized by their position midway between the two aortic walls during diastole, and their abrupt opening motion at the onset of ejection (Fig. 3–7). One of the recorded leaflets moves toward the anterior wall, and the other leaflet toward the posterior aortic wall, so that a boxlike pattern is inscribed with opening and reclosure of the valve leaflets during each cardiac cycle. The pattern of aortic motion is one of the most easily

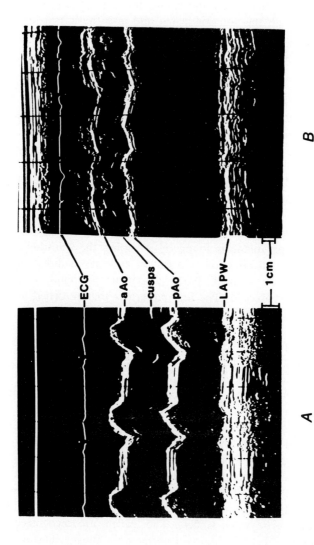

Fig. 3–6. Echographic patterns of the aorta and left atrium. A. Echogram of a normal patient showing anterior displacement of the aortic root during ventricular systole. Portions of the aortic valve cusps are seen; structures near the chest wall have not been displayed. B. Echogram from a patient with an enlarged left atrium and atrial fibrillation (aAo, anterior aortic wall; pAo, posterior aortic wall; LAPW, left atrial posterior wall; cusps, aortic valve cusps).

162

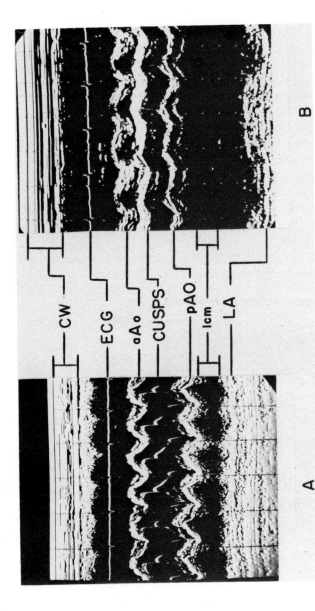

Fig. 3–7. Aortic valve patterns. A. Echogram of a normal aorta with the valve cusps displayed. The leaflets can be seen to separate during systole and join to form a thin, relatively low-intensity echo during diastole. B. Echogram from a patient with calcific, aortic stenosis. Note the multiple echoes of high intensity arising from the area of the valve cusps. These echoes are of greater intensity than the echoes of the anterior or posterior aortic walls.

163

recognized patterns and often serves as the landmark for subsequent localization of other structures. The anatomy of the semilunar valves allows recording of echoes from a maximum of two of the three leaflets during systole in optimal records.[19,20]

A second characteristic echo pattern is produced as the sound beam traverses the chest wall, anterior right ventricular wall, right ventricle, interventricular septum, anterior leaflet of the mitral valve, posterior heart wall, and lung (Fig. 3–8). It is quite useful to remember that the interventricular septum is continuous above this level with the anterior aortic wall, just as the anterior leaflet of the mitral valve is continuous above this level with the posterior aortic wall. Thus, as one rotates the transducer in a caudal and lateral direction, from the position that produced the pattern of aortic motion, the interventricular septum will replace the anterior aortic wall, and the mitral valve will replace the posterior aortic wall, on the oscilloscope (Fig. 3–3). If the transducer is on the anterior chest wall caudal to the level of the mitral valve, then the left atrium will be seen behind the valve (Fig. 3–9, see also Fig. 3–11). If the transducer is placed on the chest wall at a level cephalad to the level of the valve, then the left ventricle will be seen behind the mitral valve. The pattern of motion

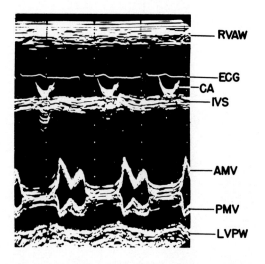

Fig. 3–8. Mitral valve leaflets. The anterior mitral valve leaflet and posterior mitral valve leaflet show mirror image configuration (RVAW, right ventricular anterior wall; CA, catheter in right ventricle; IVS, interventricular septum; AMV, anterior mitral valve leaflet; PMV, posterior mitral valve leaflet; LVPW, left ventricular posterior wall).

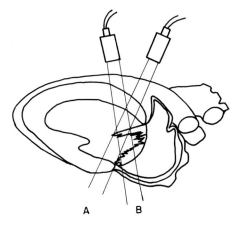

A   B

Fig. 3–9. Transducer positions in recording the mitral valve. Beam orientation A will show the left ventricular posterior wall behind the mitral valve. Beam orientation B will show the left atrial posterior wall behind the mitral valve.

of the anterior mitral leaflet is so characteristic[5,21] that it is recognized immediately. To understand fully the echographic pattern inscribed by the anterior leaflet, one must appreciate that mitral valve motion is being judged relative to a fixed point on the anterior chest wall (Fig. 3–10). It is this fixed point of reference that accounts for the systolic motion of the anterior leaflet that is normally observed. Of course, the mitral valve is in the closed position in the mitral orifice at the level of the annulus. The systolic motion that is recorded echographically is caused by movement of the total mitral valve apparatus, including the mitral annulus, forward toward the chest wall, as the volume of blood in the ventricles decreases.[22,23] The mitral valve motion is recorded through the right and left ventricles and, since the ventricular volume decreases during systole, the valve structures are closer to the transducer at end-systole than at end-diastole. The normal echogram shows a gradual and rather smooth anterior motion during systole. The anterior leaflet of the mitral valve then moves toward the transducer abruptly as the valve opens, and diastolic filling of the ventricle is initiated. The end-systolic point of the mitral valve tracing has been called the *D-point*, and the maximum opening of the valve at the onset of diastole has been termed the *E-point* (Fig. 3–10).[21] There are four phases to diastolic filling which can be observed in the normal mitral echogram after the E-point. During the earliest phase of diastole, there is a rather smooth motion of the open mitral leaflet away

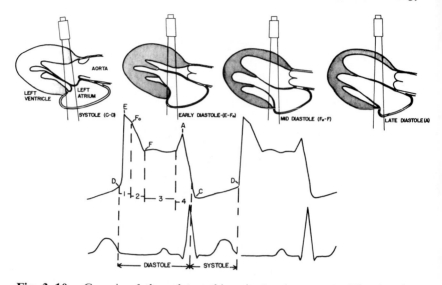

Fig. 3–10. Genesis of the echographic mitral valve pattern. The drawing of the echographic mitral valve pattern in the center section is labeled with letters corresponding to the phases of the cardiac cycle, and with numbers corresponding to phases of motion during diastole described in the text. See text for full discussion.

from the transducer ($E-F_o$) that represents motion of the total mitral valve apparatus away from the chest wall as ventricular filling begins.[22] At the end of rapid filling, there is an accelerated posterior motion of the anterior leaflet (F_o-F), as the anterior and posterior mitral leaflets actually approach each other to come to a semiclosed position. The third diastolic phase is seen only if there is sufficient time between the end of rapid filling and atrial systole to permit its appreciation. This third phase is represented by low-frequency oscillations of the anterior mitral leaflet, as blood continued to flow through the valve during slow ventricular filling. The fourth phase is related to atrial systole, and is a rapid motion of the anterior leaflet towards the chest wall, as the valve is completely reopened (A-point).[21] Studies have shown that the mitral valve is closing as a result of atrial systole before ventricular systole completes this closure.[24,25] As mentioned above, the peak of the atrial wave is termed the *A-point*, and the point of complete closure of the valve is termed the *C-point*. It is common to see a notch of varying amplitude in this A–C slope, and this notch is termed the *B-point*. The B-point may be related to atrial preclosure of the valve before completion of closure by ventricular systole, or a temporary hesitation in the closure motion caused by reversal of the ventricular-atrial gradient.* The C-point normally should be the most posterior point in the valve record. The valve apparatus moves toward the transducer on the anterior chest wall again, from point C to point D during systole. It is the early diastolic opening motion to the E-point and the late diastolic reopening motion, to the A-point, which give the characteristic "M-shaped" configuration to the mitral valve echogram. If the posterior mitral leaflet is also recorded, one will see a reciprocal "W-shaped" mirror-image pattern (Fig. 3–8). The area of the left atrium that may be recorded behind the mitral valve is a rather lateral portion of this chamber, and the lateral free wall of the atrium can be recognized by its own characteristic pattern (Fig. 3–3).[4,26] Basically, the left atrial pattern reflects volume changes suggested by mitral valve motion. The posterior left atrial wall moves toward the transducer during diastole, as the atrium empties and the space between the mitral valve and the left atrium decreases; during systole, the left atrial wall moves away from the transducer and mitral echo, as the atrial volume increases owing to pulmonary venous inflow (Fig. 3–11).

The third basic echographic pattern that is easily recognized is that seen as the sound beam passes through the chest wall, anterior right ventricular wall, ventricle, interventricular septum, chordae tendineae, posterior left ventricular wall, pericardium, and lung (Fig. 3–12). This third pattern is seen to emerge as the transducer is rocked from the mitral valve orientation in a caudal and lateral direction. When this is done, the high-amplitude "M-shaped" mitral valve pattern markedly decreases in amplitude as the sound beam passes from the free edge of the valve and into the chordae tendineae with their reflections of valve motion (Fig. 3–3). It is usual to record two sets of chordae tendineae near the posterior left ventricular endocardium. These two sets of echoes appear to be produced by the sets of chordae which attach the posterior medial papillary muscle to both the anterior leaflet and the posterior leaflet. The recognition of the origin of these chordal echoes is based on their continuity with the mitral valve echoes when the transducer is directed toward the valve once again. The echoes from the chordae tendineae near the papillary muscle have a pattern similar to the ventricular motion, but of lower amplitude. It is common to see the myocardial echoes approach the posterior chordal echo during systole and move away during diastole. The pattern of the posterior ventricular myocardium shows motion toward the transducer during systole and away from it during diastole, resulting from ventricular

* Feigenbaum, H. Personal communication.

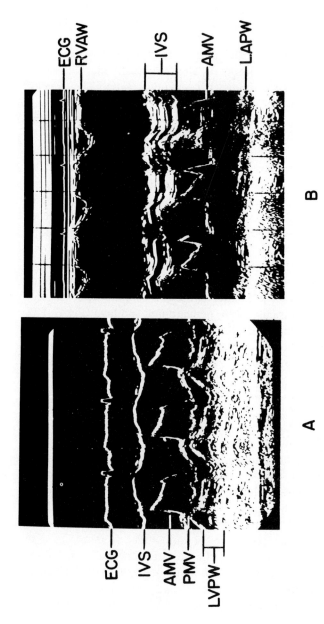

Fig. 3–11. Reduced mitral valve diastolic slopes seen in patients with aortic stenosis. A. Posterior mitral valve leaflet moves in direction opposite the anterior mitral valve leaflet during diastole. This is not seen in mitral valvular stenosis. The left ventricular posterior wall (LVPW) is recorded behind the mitral leaflets. B. The prominent atrial wave shows evidence against mitral valvular stenosis. The left atrial posterior wall (LAPW) is recorded behind the anterior mitral valve leaflet (IVS, interventricular septum; RVAW, right ventricular anterior wall).

volume changes.[26] The endocardial echo characteristically has a higher amplitude of motion than the epicardial portion of the wall. As a result, the myocardium appears thicker at end-systole than at end-diastole. It is appropriate to note here that the epicardial-pericardial-pleural area is an extremely fine sound reflector. This high-reflectivity may be the result of the interface between the dense connective tissue of the pericardium and pleura and the air-containing lung. However, it is noted consistently that the strongest posterior echo is that arising from the pericardial area.[4] Thus, if the gain setting of the instrument is reduced, the pericardial echo will be the last to disappear, and it will be the first to be redisplayed as the gain is increased (Fig. 3–12).

The last basic echographic pattern from the left ventricular outflow tract is obtained if the transducer is rotated still further in a caudal and lateral direction from its last orientation through the body of the left ventricle. During this maneuver, the chordal echoes will merge with a thick posterior band of echoes which are thought to represent the ventricular myocardium at the level of the posterior medial papillary muscle (Fig. 3–13). With this sound beam orientation, the

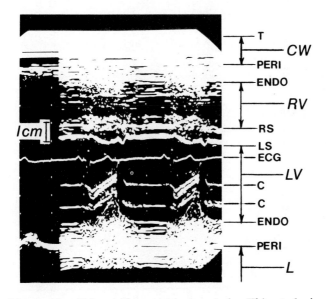

Fig. 3–12. Echographic ventricular study. This study is from a normal patient (T, transducer; CW, chest wall; PERI, pericardium; ENDO, endocardium; RV, right ventricle; RS, right-side interventricular septum; LS, left-side interventricular septum; LV, left ventricle; C, chordae tendineae; L, lung).

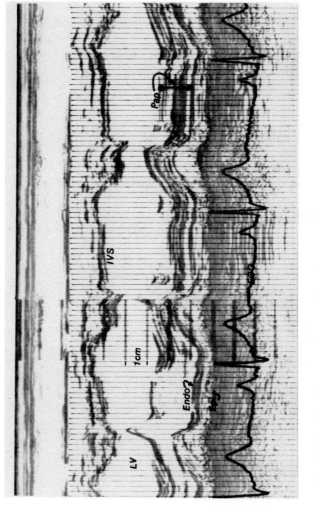

Fig. 3–13. Papillary muscle. During the recording of this echogram, the transducer is directed first through the body of the left ventricle and then toward the apex, in order to encounter the papillary muscle. The left ventricular posterior wall in the left part of the tracing shows a clear endocardial echo, and the posterior wall thickness is 0.8 cm. To the right of the calibration, the left ventricular posterior wall is recorded at the posterior papillary muscle. At this point, the papillary muscle echoes are apparently superimposed on the previous endocardial echoes (LV, left ventricle; IVS, interventricular septum; Endo, endocardium; Epi, epicardium; Pap, papillary muscle).

structures encountered are chest wall, anterior right ventricular wall, right ventricle, interventricular septum, posterior left ventricular myocardium, pericardium, and lung. The patterns of motion are similar to those just described, but the left ventricular cavity is of smaller size. If one recognizes the patterns established for the various areas of the outflow tract described above, it is possible to produce the same beam orientation from patient to patient, regardless of the relationship between the heart and the interspaces on the chest wall. Observations of the transducer orientation which produces a specific pattern permits the examiner to visualize the relationship between the heart and the transducer. Fig. 3–14 shows that a specific area of the posterior ventricular myocardium may be recorded from several interspaces. However, recognition of the transducer orientation needed to record this area from each position allows the examiner to choose the interspace that is appropriate for the purpose. Obviously, the patterns of the outflow tract may be optimally recorded from the third interspace in one patient and from the fifth interspace in another. In addition, it is the deviation from these established normal patterns which allows ultra-

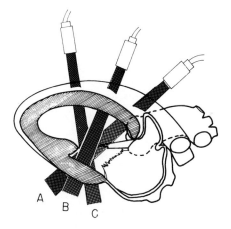

Fig. 3–14. Transducer positions. A single portion of the left ventricular posterior wall may be recorded from various transducer positions on the chest wall. Position A is being used if the transducer is still directed in a caudad direction as the mitral valve is encountered. Position C is being used if the transducer is pointed cephalad when the left ventricular posterior wall is recorded. Beam orientation B is the desired standard position for left ventricular studies.

sound records to be used for the diagnosis of pathologic cardiac conditions.

ULTRASONIC METHODS FOR DIAGNOSIS IN CARDIOLOGY

Cardiologic conditions in which ultrasound is of proved diagnostic value will be discussed separately from those conditions for which ultrasound must still be considered investigational.

Mitral Stenosis

Valve movement. Ultrasonic techniques have been used for the analysis of mitral valve motion for 19 years, and consequently mitral valve motion in health and disease has been studied extensively.* The characteristic "M-shaped" normal pattern of the anterior mitral valve leaflet (Fig. 3–15) is replaced by a square-wave pattern in the presence of mitral stenosis (Fig. 3–16). The genesis of this typical pattern is directly related to the hemodynamics of the disease. Mitral valve opening is somewhat delayed compared to normal valve motion[21,27] but occurs abruptly, with the maximal opening of the valve (E-point) coincident with the opening snap recorded by phonocardiography (Fig. 3–17).[43] Since there is no rapid ventricular filling phase, and since the atrioventricular pressure gradient maintains the valve in an open position,[22] the normal middiastolic oscillations of the valve are not seen.[21] The valve motion away from the transducer during diastole is caused by an increase in volume of the ventricles, with displacement of the whole mitral valve apparatus away from the anterior chest wall.[22,23] Again, since the valve is maintained in a completely open position because of the pressure gradient between atrium and ventricle and continued blood flow, there is no further reopening as a result of atrial systole, and the A-point is not seen. In mild mitral stenosis, a small A wave may be visible on the mitral valve recordings (Fig. 3–16c). At end-diastole the mitral valve tracing makes a rapid-closing motion with the most posterior point (C-point) being coincident with the mitral component of the first heart sound.[4,5,21]

Determining severity. There are two quantitative points that can be gleaned from measurements taken from such ultrasound tracings. The

* Refs. 1–7, 15, 16, 21, 22, 24, 25, 27–50.

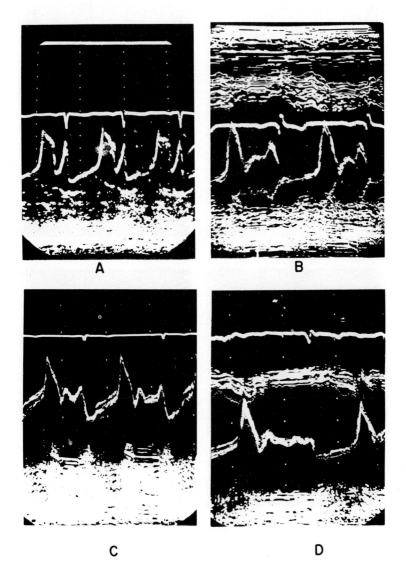

Fig. 3–15. Examples of nonstenotic mitral valve motion. A. A clear E-F_0 slope is noted prior to the F_0-F slope in diastole (see text). B. Normal anterior and posterior leaflet motion. C. middiastolic oscillations observed with a slow heart rate. D. Pattern of atrial fibrillation with lack of a terminal atrial (A) wave.

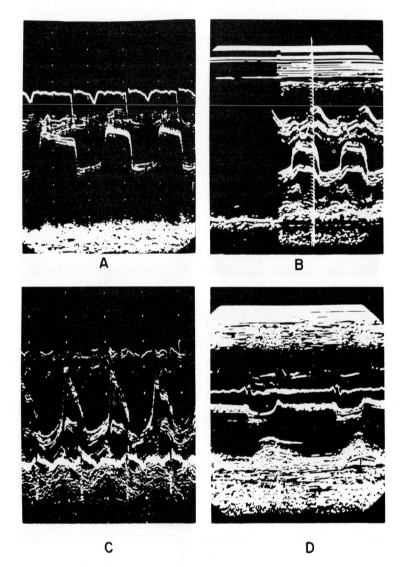

Fig. 3–16. Examples of stenotic mitral valve patterns. A. Atrial fibrillation, severe stenosis with a mobile anterior leaflet. B. Abnormal motion of the posterior leaflet seen with mitral stenosis. The posterior leaflet moves in the same direction as the anterior leaflet throughout diastole. C. Mild mitral stenosis; mitral diastolic slope 70 mm/sec; however, the posterior leaflet moves in an abnormal fashion typical of mitral stenosis. D. Severely scarred, immobile mitral valve. This patient had predominant mitral regurgitation at hemodynamic study and surgery.

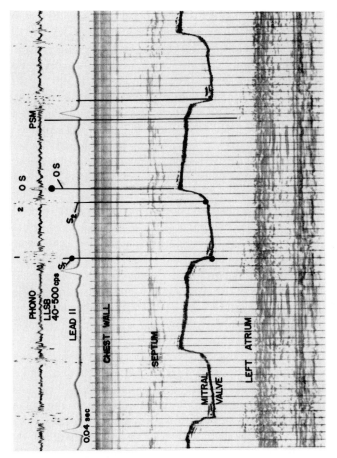

Fig. 3–17. Strip chart recording in mitral stenosis. Stenotic mitral valve pattern shows the correlation of maximal mitral valve opening with the opening snap recorded on the phonocardiogram. The closing motion of the mitral valve during the presystolic murmur (PSM) is recorded. Complete closure of the mitral valve occurs as the high frequency components of the first sound are recorded (S_1 and 1, first heart sound; S_2 and 2, second heart sound; OS, opening snap; PSM, presystolic murmur; LLSB, lower left sternal border).

175

first point is a rough quantitation of the severity of the stenosis. Several studies have shown a correlation between mitral orifice size and the slope of posterior valve motion during diastole.* If one measures the normal initial diastolic slope, the vast majority of normal patients will show posterior motion at the rate of 80 mm/sec, or greater.[7,21,27] A diastolic slope of less than 40 mm/sec generally is recorded when patients with mitral stenosis are studied. If the posterior diastolic slope is measured in large groups of patients with mitral stenosis, the small valve orifices are seen in those patients with diastolic slopes of 10 mm/sec or less, and the larger orifices are seen in patients in the 30 to 40 mm/sec range. Patients with mitral stenosis of very mild degree rarely have been seen with diastolic slopes up to 60 to 70 mm/sec (Fig. 3–16c). It is reasonable to expect the posterior motion of the mitral valve to indicate the severity of stenosis if one assumes that the most limiting factor for ventricular filling is the stenotic mitral orifice. Then the rate of ventricular filling, as measured by the posterior diastolic slope, would be expected to correlate with the mitral valve area. This is only a rough measurement, however, since the rate of ventricular filling should be affected by many factors, including atrioventricular gradient, total diastolic flow, ventricular filling period related to heart rate, ventricular compliance, and the presence of aortic valve disease. It is important for those interpreting cardiac echograms to recognize that in order to make a valid measurement of diastolic posterior slope, the most initial portion of the diastolic tracing should be measured. Of course, this requires a clear and present diastolic posterior slope on the record. Studies have shown the mean maximum diastolic descent rate or slope to be virtually constant in a single patient during repeated examinations at one period of time.[27] The mean maximum descent rate varied less than 5 mm per sec comparing two recording sites in individual patients.[27] The slope was virtually independent of R-R interval in atrial fibrillation (Fig. 3–16a), and the mean slope in both sinus rhythm and atrial fibrillation in the same patients was not different statistically.[27] Valve area correlates with diastolic slope better in sinus rhythm than in atrial fibrillation.[28] A group of patients with very low diastolic slopes and a group with relatively high diastolic slopes showed similar mean cardiac outputs.[27] However, the group with low diastolic slopes showed an increased mean pulmonary artery pressure compared with the group with high diastolic slopes.[27]

Many patients with rapid heart rates show mitral valve echograms

* Refs. 7, 21, 27–36, 43, 44.

which can only be interpreted as showing the mitral valve opening and closing, without sufficient time between these two motions to allow measurement of the true posterior diastolic slope.[45] In these patients, either one must somehow slow the patient's heart rate to permit proper assessment of the diastolic mitral phase, or reserve comment (Fig. 3–18). In such patients, one additional diagnostic clue has proved helpful. As previously stated, the normal motion of the posterior mitral leaflet is a mirror image of the anterior leaflet. However, Duchak et al noted that in mitral stenosis the posterior leaflet appears to move toward the chest wall when opening, with a pattern similar to that of the anterior leaflet but with a much reduced amplitude (Fig. 3–16B and C).[50] This may be related to the fusion of the two leaflets at their commisures and the large area of the anterior leaflet mechanically pulling the smaller leaflet in a predominantly anterior direction.[7,27,50] Whatever the true explanation for this phenomenon, finding motion of the posterior leaflet in this abnormal manner is quite useful in evaluating patients with a very rapid heart rate and patients with very mild mitral stenosis, or both. In this latter group, it may be necessary to decide whether a 70 mm/sec slope represents mild stenosis or a low normal slope owing to nonvalvular causes (Fig. 3–11). Edler[21] and others* have shown that the diastolic slope in patients with mitral stenosis increases after mitral commissurotomy, and the slope may decrease again in the presence of mitral restenosis, with a second increase in diastolic slope after reoperation.[30] Thus, echocardiography provides a means for quantitatively following the course of mitral valve disease. Diastolic slope is often below the normal range after commissurotomy, and serial studies are necessary for adequate postoperative evaluation. The two patients that we have seen displaying virtually no posterior motion or slope during diastole were patients with true silent mitral stenosis, with an extremely low cardiac output. In these two patients who were thought to have primary myocardial disease, mitral stenosis was discovered by cardiac echography.

Leaflet pathology. The second point of important information that can be inferred from the mitral valve tracing is related to the pliability of the valve leaflets. It appears that the D-E amplitude, i.e., opening amplitude, is related to the amount of motion of which the anterior leaflet is capable. If one envisions a stenotic mitral valve attached superiorly to the mitral annulus and inferiorly to the fibrotic subvalvar apparatus, the maximum amplitude of motion would be in

* Refs. 7, 27, 29, 39, 44.

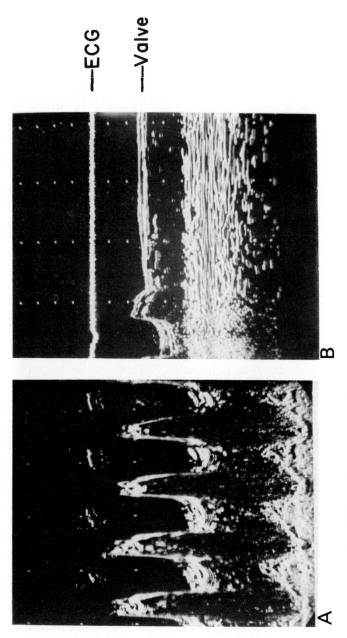

ECG

Valve

Fig. 3–18. Mitral valve motion with rapid heart rate. A. During the baseline record, the rapid heart rate produced a pattern which precluded evaluation of mitral valve motion. B. With carotid sinus massage, the heart rate was slowed to evaluate the mitral valve pattern.

the midportion of the valve. This is confirmed by sweeping the sound beam from the mitral annulus toward the area of the papillary muscle and observing the maximum amplitude of the valve in the midportion (Fig. 3–3; see also Fig. 3–23). Parenthetically, it is obvious that the midportion of the valve must be recorded if one wishes to assess mobility of the anterior leaflet properly. In most patients with mitral stenosis of significant degree, the D-E amplitude (opening amplitude), and A-C amplitude (closing amplitude) are equal.[21] That is, if a pandiastolic gradient is present, the valve is maximally opened from the onset of diastole to the onset of systole. The normal excursion or amplitude is 20 mm or greater. In a broad sense, a high-amplitude motion represents the type of pliable leaflet that is amenable to commissurotomy without the production of severe mitral insufficiency (Fig. 3–16A, B, C). If there is a low-amplitude motion, less than 12 mm, then one may expect to find a fibrotic, relatively immobile anterior leaflet. Such a highly fibrotic leaflet is often calcified, and in our experience, valve replacement is usually required. In addition, we have noted that with low-amplitude valve excursion, it is difficult or impossible to tell whether the valve is scarred with a fixed, very small orifice or with a fixed, large orifice.[7,27,39,43] In the latter case, a large degree of mitral insufficiency rather than stenosis may be present as the end-stage of rheumatic disease (Fig. 3–16D).[40] Mitral orifice size cannot be measured from the distance between the anterior and posterior leaflets, as seen on echogram. This fact may be expected since the shape of the mitral valve is similar to a funnel. With such a configuration, the distance between the anterior and posterior leaflets will vary, depending on the level of the funnel traversed. The echoes returning from the leaflets of a stenotic mitral valve will be abnormally intense if the leaflet is severely scarred, thickened and calcified, or both. This appears to be the basis of the correlation between the thickness of the mitral echo signal and the thickness of the valve tissue, using early instruments.[34] Segal noted the "ski-slope" echographic configuration suggestive of mitral stenosis, combined with significant mitral regurgitation (Fig. 3–19).[36] Small degrees of mitral regurgitation have little effect on either the diastolic slope or the pattern.[28]

Reliability of measurements. False-negative tests for mitral stenosis are extremely rare, and we are not aware of such a condition in our experience. A false-negative test may be simulated by some records in which only the opening motion (D-E) and a portion of the closing motion (A-C) are seen, but in which the diastolic position of the

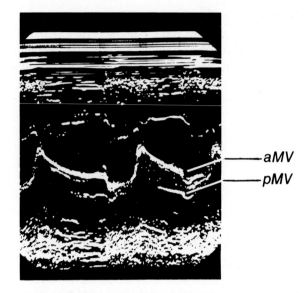

Fig. 3–19. Combined mitral stenosis and regurgitation.
The curved "ski-slope" appearance of the anterior mitral
leaflet suggests a combination of regurgitation and stenosis.
Note the abnormal posterior mitral valve leaflet showing
diastolic motion similar to that of the anterior leaflet.

valve is not well recorded. One should not infer diastolic motion of
the valve from the opening and closing portions, but should require a
solid continuous echo during diastole for the diagnosis of mitral stenosis. False positive diagnoses of mitral stenosis could be made on the
echogram in several conditions. The pattern of mitral stenosis may be
seen in the presence of atrial masses resulting in obstruction of the
mitral orifice (Fig. 3–20). This will be discussed subsequently. In
addition, any condition resulting in an extremely slow ventricular filling
rate may simulate mitral stenosis. Patients with ventricular hypertrophy,
such as is routinely seen in patients with aortic stenosis (Fig. 3–11)[51]
or hypertrophic subaortic stenosis (see Fig. 3–23), may present a
problem in echographic interpretation, as the initial diastolic slope may
be between 40 and 80 mm/sec.[52] In these cases, there are generally
two clues that the delayed initial slope is of nonvalvular cause. These
clues are the presence of a sharp and relatively normal atrial wave of
the mitral tracing, and the presence of a mirror image posterior leaflet
in these patients. In addition, it is common to find patients with
severe aortic insufficiency, in whom a diastolic murmur of true mitral

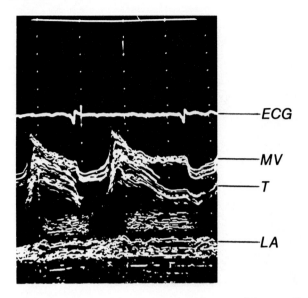

Fig. 3–20. Mitral valve echogram with an atrial mass. In the first complex, tumor echoes are seen behind the mitral valve echoes during diastole. In the second complex, the tumor apparently floats away from the mitral leaflet during a prolonged diastolic period (MV, anterior mitral valve leaflet; T, atrial tumor; LA, left atrium).

stenosis must be differentiated from the Austin-Flint murmur. In these patients, an interesting and sometimes troublesome phenomenon is seen (Fig. 3–21). Patients with aortic insufficiency show high-frequency vibrations of the anterior leaflet of the mitral valve which is not seen in other conditions.[41,53] The oscillations are of much greater frequency than the diastolic oscillations seen in atrial flutter or fibrillation (Fig. 3–15D).[45] The oscillations in aortic insufficiency give the appearance of short vertical lines in place of the usual solid diastolic tracing. This may be troublesome in that the peaks of these lines may coalesce to simulate a low diastolic slope. It is important to recognize that these high-frequency oscillations are present and this recognition can only occur with a well-focused oscilloscope. As in the previous conditions presenting possible false-positive tests, an atrial wave is usually seen on the mitral tracing, the posterior leaflet has its normal motion, and in addition, measurement of multiple diastolic intervals will show that the slope varies grossly from cycle to cycle. This pattern may be seen in aortic regurgitation without the Austin-Flint murmur.[54]

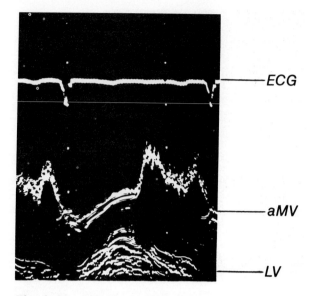

Fig. 3–21. Mitral valve pattern in aortic regurgitation. High-frequency oscillations of the anterior mitral leaflet occur during diastole (aMV, anterior mitral valve leaflet; LV, left ventricle).

Atrial Masses

The presence of any type of mass acting as a ball valve in the mitral orifice may produce a picture similar to that seen with mitral stenosis. A great many atrial masses have been detected using the ultrasound technique, and of course, most of these have been myxomatous tumors.[55–63] However, true ball valve thrombi were the first such masses reported,[2,64] and we have had experience with another pathologic type of intracardiac tumor.* As would be expected, the echoes produced by such a mass are not related to its histology. In most cases, left atrial masses are diagnosed by the appearance of a dense set of echoes behind the anterior mitral leaflet during diastole (Fig. 3–20). Any mass that prolapses through the valve during diastole will encounter the sound beam and appear on the echogram during diastole. Since most of these masses return to the atrium during systole and no longer intersect the sound beam, the appearance of cyclic motion is seen on the echogram. In many patients without atrial masses, it is possible to see multiple echoes during diastole in the area behind the

* Popp RL and Levine RB. In preparation.

anterior mitral leaflet (Fig. 3–16; see also Fig. 3–25). However, the high intensity of the echoes, the multiple bands of echoes moving in parallel, and the cyclic motion of these echoes are the distinguishing features that are seen with true atrial masses. In addition, many of the reported masses show a very short interval between the opening motion of the valve and the appearance of the tumor echoes. That is, there is a very short but definite period in early diastole in which no echoes are seen behind the open valve (Fig. 3–20). This period represents the interval between opening of the valve and the prolapse of the tumor into the orifice. If there is question as to the presence or absence of an atrial mass, we recommend two procedures. The first is to rotate the transducer up toward the left atrium using the standard technique by which one records the aorta and left atrium (Fig. 3–5B). In this manner, one may confirm that a mass is residing in the atrium during systole and prolapsing into the ventricle during diastole by recording a high-intensity echo pattern with cyclic motion seen in this atrial chamber (Fig. 3–22). In addition, or alternately, the transducer may be placed near the cardiac apex in order to direct the sound beam along the long axis of the ventricle through the mitral orifice and up into the left atrium to intersect a nonprolapsing atrial mass (Fig. 3–5C). There

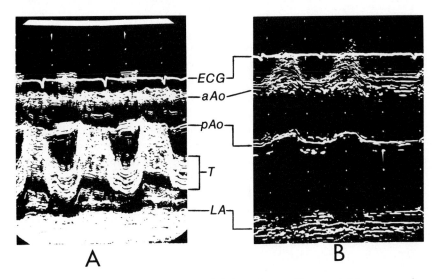

Fig. 3–22. Echogram of aorta and left atrium with an atrial mass.   A. Preoperative echogram showing the motion of the left atrial mass during the cardiac cycle. B. Postoperative echogram showing absence of the tumor echoes (T, tumor; LA, left atrial wall; the scale of the records is not identical).

have been two types of atrial masses, or atrial structures, which we have not been able to recognize adequately and consistently with the echogram. We have not appreciated a specific consistent pattern for the common type of atrial thrombus which is layered on the left atrial wall, and does not move as a free body within the atrium. Dr. Raymond Gramiak has suggested that a patient with mitral stenosis showing an echographically measured left atrium, which is quite small rather than the expected large size, should be suspected of having intraatrial thrombus.* The second inapparent type of atrial clot is a very thin layer of thrombotic material which may develop across the mitral orifice after implantation of a prosthetic valve. This layer of material acts as a flap valve and leads to the left atrial hypertension. We have not been able to recognize this material using the echogram.

Hypertrophic Subaortic Stenosis

There are two conditions for which we shift our attention to the systolic phase of mitral valve motion. Shah and Gramiak first described an abrupt systolic anterior motion of the anterior mitral valve leaflet during systole in patients with hypertrophic subaortic stenosis (Fig. 3–23).[65] This abnormal motion of the anterior leaflet is well demonstrated in angiographic studies[66,67] and appears to be a significant factor in the left ventricular outflow tract obstruction. The systolic anterior motion may be quite striking in some patients and, if one is able to record the free edge of the valve, the juxtaposition of the anterior mitral leaflet and the interventricular septum may be recorded (Fig. 3–24). From a diagnostic and therapeutic standpoint, it is interesting to note that the presence of this systolic anterior motion correlates with a left ventricular outflow tract gradient, whereas a normal pattern may be observed during systole in the same patient if no gradient is present.[52] Of course there are various forms of this disease, and the presence of an outflow tract obstruction may be variable from beat to beat.[68] From the foregoing discussion, two points emerge. The first is that in screening for hypertrophic subaortic stenosis the patient should have some type of provocative maneuver during the echogram, such as the Valsalva maneuver or amyl nitrite inhalation, before the test can be considered adequate. The second point is that one must record the mitral leaflet near its free edge in order to make a reliable assessment of the presence or absence of systolic anterior motion. As previously noted, there is a greater excursion of the leaflet

---

* Gramiak R. Personal communication.

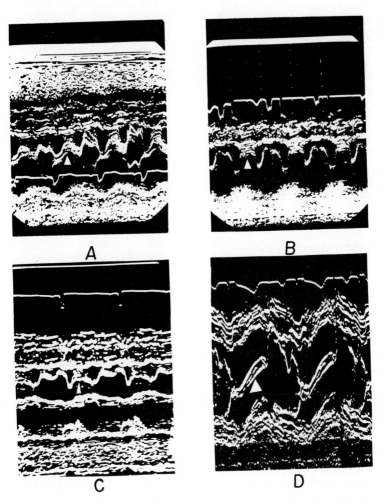

Fig. 3–23. Mitral valve patterns and pseudopattern of idiopathic hypertrophic subaortic stenosis. A, B, and C. Systolic anterior motion characteristic of IHSS. The early abrupt anterior motion and posterior return of the mitral valve echo in late systole is a characteristic feature. D. A patient with atrial septal defect and no evidence of hypertrophic subaortic stenosis. Note the later and more gradual systolic anterior motion, with very little return in the posterior direction prior to opening of the valve. The mitral valve echo meets the interventricular septal echo in diastole.

185

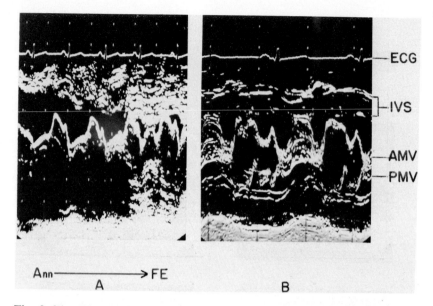

Fig. 3–24. Transducer direction in IHSS. A. The sound beam is swept from the point of attachment of the mitral annulus to the free edge of the mitral valve, from left to right. It is apparent that near the mitral annulus the systolic anterior motion characteristic of IHSS is not seen. Near the free edge of the valve, however, there is a clear systolic anterior motion. B. A high-speed recording of the mitral valve pattern at the free edge of the same patient as in A. Note the abrupt systolic anterior motion, which touches the echoes from the interventricular septum (Ann, annulus; FE, free edge; IVS, interventricular septum; AMV, anterior mitral valve leaflet; PMV, posterior mitral valve leaflet).

along a continuum from the annulus to the free edge, owing to the attachment of the mitral leaflet to the annulus. If one records the leaflet too close to the annulus, only truncated motion will be seen and the systolic anterior motion, which is the abnormal finding, may be completely missed (Fig. 3–25 and 3–23). Another hallmark of true hypertrophic subaortic stenosis is the presence of a low initial diastolic slope of mitral valve motion.[52] The exact cause of this is not known; however, it is our personal opinion that this low slope is related to the ventricular hypertrophy seen in these patients. Some of our patients with hypertrophic subaortic stenosis have such a low diastolic valve slope as to be confused with patients with mitral stenosis (Fig. 3–23B,C). Confusing or frankly false-positive diagnoses of hypertrophic subaortic stenosis have been suggested from the echograms of patients with atrial or ventricular septal defect and in some

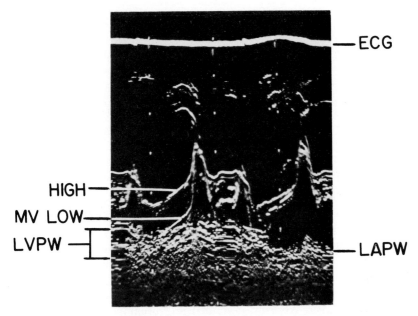

Fig. 3–25. Mitral valve echogram. During this recording the transducer is rocked from the free edge of the valve, with left ventricular posterior wall displayed behind the valve echoes toward the mitral annulus area, and the left atrial posterior wall displayed behind the valve echoes. It is thought that the low-amplitude portion marked "high" arises from the mitral valve leaflet near the annulus, and the part of the tracing marked "MV low" arises from a lower portion of the valve closer to the free edge. Such multiple patterns as seen here are commonly observed and are thought to result from the width of the sound beam.

patients with tachycardia and high cardiac output. Apparently, the problem arises from a high-amplitude convex systolic motion of the mitral annulus, which is, in turn, related to large volume changes during systole. The critical point between these false-positive records and the records from patients with true hypertrophic subaortic stenosis is that the systolic anterior motion in the latter case begins early, peaks in midsystole, and returns away from the transducer before the mitral valve opens (Fig. 3–23A,B,C). In the false–positive cases, there is a rather more gradual systolic anterior motion, which accelerates in mid-systole and ends in late systole with little or no posterior motion before the valve opens (Fig. 3–23D). Moreyra et al described impingement of the interventricular septum on the anterior mitral leaflet during early diastole as the typical finding in patients with idiopathic hypertrophic subaortic stenosis.[69] Other studies have failed to confirm this finding as specific for hypertrophic subaortic stenosis, whereas the systolic anterior motion is a consistent finding in other series.[70,71]

Recent studies have emphasized another abnormality of left ventricular anatomy which can be identified echocardiographically, namely, the presence of asymmetric septal hypertrophy. According to Henry, Clark, and Epstein the finding of a mean septal-free wall ratio of 1.3 or greater lends highly specific and sensitive diagnostic evidence for the presence of IHSS.[71a]

Mitral Valve Prolapse Syndromes

A systolic abnormality is also seen in the mitral valve pattern recorded in patients with the midsystolic click–late systolic murmur syndrome of nonrheumatic mitral regurgitation. There are a group of syndromes and the abnormality seen on echocardiogram may be anywhere in the spectrum of abnormalities. Since the definition of this click-murmur pattern by echocardiogram by Shah and Gramiak,[46] most echographers have recognized many cases in their files and continued prospective studies. Kerber[47] described an abrupt posterior motion of the mitral leaflets, especially the posterior leaflet, in midsystole coincident with the midsystolic click (Fig. 3–26A,B). The continued posterior motion of these leaflets coincided with the generation of a late systolic murmur. Dillon et al[48] demonstrated the temporal displacement of this pattern using pharmacologic agents to alter the timing of the click and murmur during systole. It would seem, from our personal experience, that this click and murmur sequence correlates with a systolic pattern which resembles a question mark rotated 90 degrees (Fig. 3–26A,B), whereas nonrheumatic mitral insufficiency of holosystolic variety correlates with a "U-shaped" systolic configuration (Fig. 3–26C,D). The C-point normally should be the most posterior point of the mitral valve echogram. Continued posterior movement from the C-point during systole suggests leaflet prolapse toward the atrium. Judging from our own experience again, it is not necessary to record the posterior leaflet to find these abnormalities, since the anterior and posterior leaflets rest against each other during systole. Segal et al have proposed that an exaggerated diastolic slope suggests mitral regurgitation of any cause.[37] However, there is overlap between the mean slope of groups with mitral regurgitation and the mean slope of normal groups. In addition, the measurement of the initial diastolic slope ($E-F_o$) rather than the hybrid E-F slope, shows even less striking separation of the patients with mitral regurgitation from the normals (Fig. 3–10). The $F_o - F$ motion occurs as the leaflets move to the

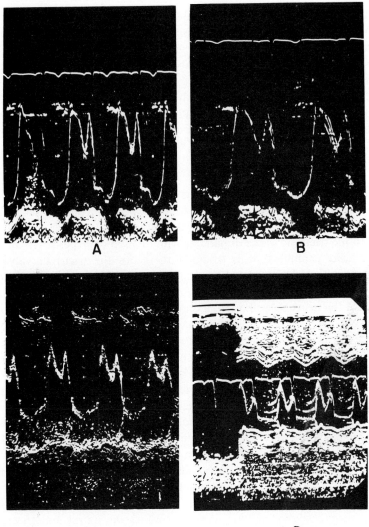

Fig. 3–26. Mitral valve prolapse syndromes. A. and B. Patient with the midsystolic click–late systolic murmur syndrome of mitral valve prolapse. Note the flat, initial systolic portion and late systolic posterior motion. C. Echogram from a patient with a holosystolic murmur and mitral valve prolapse, showing continuous posterior motion from the onset of systole. D. The pattern of mitral valve prolapse in a patient with Marfan's syndrome. There is continued posterior motion during systole, which is abnormal.

semiclosed middiastolic position, and the slope criteria should not be applied to this portion of the tracing (Fig. 3–8). Early diastolic ventricular filling is rapid in those patients with mitral regurgitation, but we have not been able to make a reliable echographic separation of these patients from normal patients and those with other types of heart disease. The high amplitude of valve excursion (D-E, A-C) seen in some patients with mitral regurgitation is probably the result of complete diastolic opening after systolic prolapse toward the atrium.[42]

Tricuspid Stenosis

The basic echographic patterns of the mitral and tricuspid valves are identical.[72] Of course, this is to be expected from the anatomic and physiologic similarity of the valve positions. It is not difficult to record the tricuspid valve in patients with dilation or hypertrophy of the right heart chambers. It is common to record the tricuspid valve in patients with right atrial enlargement. A complete record of tricuspid valve motion is quite difficult to obtain in normal patients. Displacement of the heart as well as rotation seems to play a role in moving the tricuspid valve into a position that can easily be intercepted by the ultrasonic beam. Rotation produces tricuspid leaflet motion along a path perpendicular with the axis of the sound beam. Such motion results in an echo signal which is continuous and traces out the pattern of leaflet motion. The tricuspid valve is most consistently intercepted using a technique which uses the aortic root echoes as the reference point.[15,73] The transducer is placed on the chest wall and angulated in the standard manner to record the aorta and left atrium as described above. From this position the transducer is directed in a ventral and slightly caudal direction. The anterior leaflet of the tricuspid valve then appears in the position of the anterior aortic wall (Fig. 3–27A). This is a convenient method of locating the tricuspid valve, since it is easy to confuse the mitral and tricuspid patterns. The tricuspid valve is located in the position of the anterior aortic wall, whereas the mitral valve appears in the position of the posterior aortic wall (Fig. 3-27B). Thus, if there is any question in the examiner's mind, he need only shift the transducer to intercept the aorta and differentiate which atrioventricular valve has been recorded. In cases with extreme rotation of the heart, caused by right ventricular enlargement, occasionally it is possible to record both the tricuspid and mitral valves with a single sound beam orientation (Fig. 3–28). In such cases, the intraventricular septum is seen between the tricuspid and mitral valves.

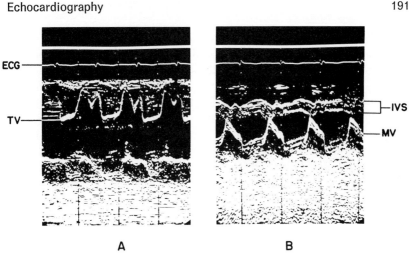

A   B

Fig. 3–27. Relative positions of the tricuspid and mitral valves. A. The tricuspid valve recorded in the position taken by the interventricular septum as the transducer is rocked to record the mitral valve in B. That is, both records are taken from one transducer position on the chest wall without change in scale.

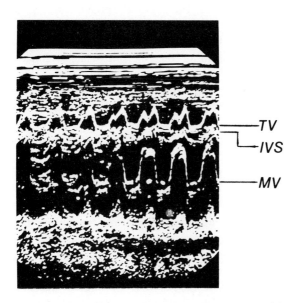

Fig. 3–28. Simultaneous recording of the tricuspid and mitral valve echoes in a patient with mitral stenosis. This pattern is only seen in patients with right ventricular dilation.

Joyner studied tricuspid valve motion in 37 patients with mitral stenosis.[74] The early diastolic tricuspid valve slope was between 60 and 120 mm/sec in the 31 patients with normal tricuspid valve function by hemodynamic and surgical criteria. The six patients with evidence of tricuspid stenosis had early diastolic tricuspid valve slopes between 8 and 30 mm/sec. Two of these latter patients had combined tricuspid stenosis and insufficiency. The diastolic slope ranged from 4 to 22 mm/sec in three patients with tricuspid stenosis reported by Effert.[30] Edler[72] and Bleifeld and Effert[73] place the normal range of tricuspid valve slope at 47 to 173 mm/sec. A recent review of ultrasound experience with congenital heart disease noted a tricuspid valve slope of less than 25 mm/sec in patients with Ebstein's anomaly.[51]

At least one case of right atrial tumor has been found using the echographic technique described for recording the tricuspid valve.[56] The echographic appearance is analogous to the appearance of such a mass on the left side of the heart.

Pericardial Effusion

The impetus for the current widespread interest in diagnostic ultrasound in the United States stems directly from the discovery and use of ultrasound for the diagnosis of pericardial effusion. Edler made mention of the separation of the anterior heart wall from the chest wall in a patient with pericardial effusion in 1955.[2] Likewise, Effert mentioned separation of the anterior heart from the chest wall in articles prior to 1964.[6,7] However, the use of ultrasound in this condition stems from the work of Feigenbaum in the experimental and clinical situation with his results published in a series of articles.[75–80]

Principles. The principle underlying the use of ultrasound for the diagnosis of pericardial effusion is the ability to visualize the separation of the anterior myocardium from the chest wall and the posterior myocardium from the lung, resulting from the accumulation of fluid (Fig. 3–29). Since most pericardial fluid is relatively clear, such an effusion is recorded as an echo-free space separating the structures usually in contact. Because of the anatomy of the pulmonary veins and the pericardium, it is not possible for fluid to accumulate directly behind the left atrium (Fig. 3–30). Therefore, in order to avoid false-negative tests on this basis, studies for pericardial effusion require the operator to direct the ultrasonic beam toward the area of the left ventricle. Even in the presence of effusion, one can usually locate the

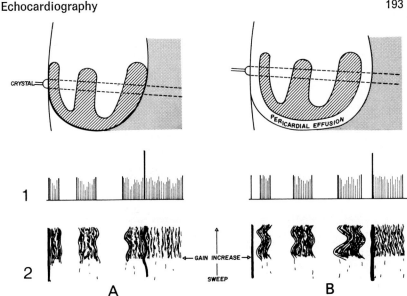

Fig. 3–29. Genesis of the echographic pattern of pericardial effusion. A. Normal position of the chest wall relative to the right ventricular anterior wall, and the posterior pericardium relative to the left ventricular posterior wall. Section 1 shows a diagram of the A mode presentation. Section 2 shows a diagram of the M mode presentation. B. Separation of the right ventricular anterior wall from the chest wall and the left ventricular posterior wall from the pericardium in the presence of pericardial effusion. In section 2, with low-gain settings, only the posterior pericardial echo is recorded, but a gain increase in the middle of the recording permits the myocardial echoes to be seen.

mitral valve echoes as a reference point from which to direct the transducer in a caudal and lateral orientation to insure recording of the left ventricle. When this is done in a normal patient, as previously described, the echogram shows the nonmoving echoes from the chest wall in contact with the low-amplitude oscillations of the anterior myocardial wall. The strong posterior pericardial-lung interface mimics left ventricular myocardial motion and is in contact with the myocardial echoes (Fig. 3–12). In the presence of pericardial effusion, however, the strong posterior pericardial-lung interface is separated from the myocardial echoes (Fig. 3–31). The fluid acts to insulate the posterior pericardial echo and decrease its amplitude of motion, as a rule. Some of the older ultrasonic instruments were apparently very insensitive to, or incapable of, presenting the pattern of a small pericardial effusion owing to signal processing techniques used. That is, echoes from structures which were separated by a small distance could not be dis-

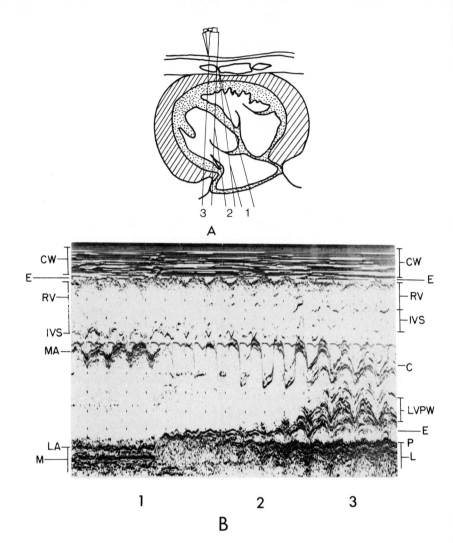

Fig. 3–30. Transducer position in recording pericardial effusion. A. Transducer positions and beam orientations corresponding to the echogram in B. B. Strip chart recording of a patient with pericardial effusion, taken while the transducer is rocked from a medial to a lateral direction on the chest wall. In portion 1, the transducer is intersecting the interventricular septum and mitral annulus near the aorta, and is recording the left atrium. In portion 2, the transducer is recording the mitral valve and the lateral portion of the left atrium. In portion 3, the transducer has been pointed laterally and is now recording the left ventricular echoes. Note the appearance of posterior effusion as one turns the transducer laterally, and the absence of effusion behind the posterior area of the left atrium (CW, chest wall; E, effusion; RV, right ventricle; IVS, interventricular septum; MA, mitral annulus; LA, left atrium; M, mediastinum; C, chordae tendineae; LVPW, left ventricular posterior wall; P, pericardium; L, lung).

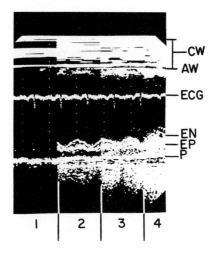

Fig. 3–31. Gain settings for recording pericardial effusion. Four separate increasing gain settings are used in the sections of the record marked 1, 2, 3 and 4. In section 1, only the pericardium is recorded, and very little motion is seen. In section 2, the myocardium is seen and is separated from the pericardium by a space. Section 3 also shows the presence of an epicardial and endocardial echo, separated from the pericardium, but recognizable separation is more difficult because of echoes from within the effusion space. Section 4, with excessive gain, does not allow separation of the epicardium and pericardium. Note the lack of anterior effusion (CW, chest wall; AW, anterior wall; EN, endocardium; EP, epicardium, P, pericardium).

tinguished as separate structures. This may still present a problem in current instruments if the oscilloscope beam is not properly focused. In this case, the myocardial and pericardial echoes each are broad and blur together to obliterate the clear pericardial space between them. In addition, even in a modern instrument which is properly focused, it is possible to obliterate the echo-free space of pericardial effusion by using excessively high-gain settings during the examination (Fig. 3–31). In this case, back-scattered sound or weak echoes appearing from within the pericardial fluid may be overly amplified and fill the pericardial space with echoes. Most experienced operators take the precaution of making ultrasound records at several different gain settings in order to obviate this problem.

Reported experiences. It has been shown that most patients have less than 5 cc of pericardial fluid at surgery, in the absence of congestive heart failure. Experimental studies show that 25 cc of fluid can be detected in the dog pericardium using echographic techniques.[75,82] It would appear that 50 cc of fluid can be reliably detected in the adult human.[81,83] Indeed, it may have been the sensitivity of the ultrasound technique that led Goldschlager[84] to cite a high incidence of false-positive results, since he was using a less sensitive isotope scanning technique as the standard for comparison. The ability to quantitate the volume of pericardial fluid by echocardiography has been both suggested[76,85] and denied[83,86] in the past. Quantitation of the amount of fluid present is complicated because pericardiocentesis seldom removes all the fluid visualized by the echogram. Our own opinion is that the quantity of fluid can be estimated in a very gross way from the appearance of the echogram.

Also, there is controversy concerning the sequence of appearance of anterior versus posterior fluid in the echogram. If one notes that in the echogram performed in the proper manner to evaluate pericardial effusion and that the transducer is pointed so as to record the posterior and *lateral* recesses of the pericardium, then some of the controversy arising from prior angiographic data[87-89] may be resolved. The weight of evidence from the studies of Feigenbaum[76,78,80] and those of Klein[83] suggest that the posterolateral space appears on the echogram first with the anterior pericardial space separating the anterior structures secondarily. In addition, when pericardial fluid is removed, the anterior space usually disappears first, with the posterior and lateral space resolving later.[83] In our experience, only small quantities of fluid are present when only a posterior space is seen (Fig. 32a). In most moderate or large effusions the anterior pericardial space is visualized in addition to the posterior and lateral space, and both spaces should be used as criteria for pericardial effusion (Fig. 3–32B). On the other hand, it is common to find a small separation of the anterior heart wall from the chest wall without evidence of posterior and lateral effusion in patients in whom no fluid is present. Anterior separation is seen in normal patients occasionally and results from the possibility that material such as adipose tissue, pulmonary tissue or loose connective tissue may be present in sufficient quantity to allow separation of the anterior myocardium from the chest wall (Fig. 3–11B). We have observed one patient with very striking separation of the anterior heart wall from the chest wall, with no separation of the posterior pericardium from the myocardium (Fig. 3–33). This patient had a foramen of Morgagni hernia with the stomach lying anterior to the right ventricle. Thus, anything that allows separation of the chest wall and myocardium may give a false-positive anterior effusion pattern.

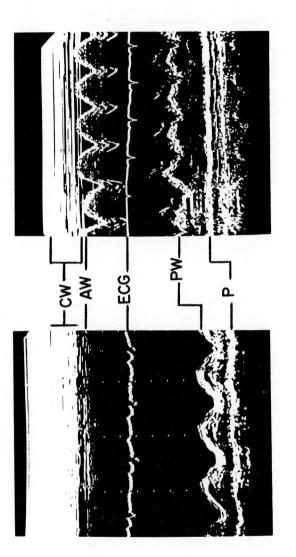

A

B

Fig. 3-32. Pericardial effusion. A. Echogram from a patient with small volume pericardial effusion. A separation of the pericardium and posterior wall is seen only posterior to the heart, with no effusion seen near the anterior wall. Note the small separation of pericardium and posterior wall and the damped pericardial motion. B. Echogram from a patient with moderate volume pericardial effusion. Separation of the anterior wall from the chest wall is seen, as well as separation of the posterior heart wall from the pericardium. The predominant posterior wall echo is from the epicardium, and faint endocardial echoes are seen. Note the damped pericardial motion in contrast to the synchronous movement of the anterior and posterior wall (CW, chest wall; AW, anterior wall; PW, posterior wall; P, pericardium).

197

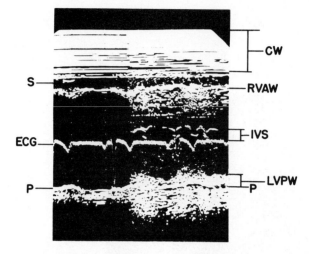

Fig. 3–33. False-positive anterior pericardial effusion. Echogram from a patient with a foramen of Morgagni hernia represented by the space separating the right ventricular anterior wall and chest wall. There is no evidence of posterior pericardial effusion. The gain is increased midway through the record (CW, chest wall; S, echo-free space; RVAW, right ventricular anterior wall; IVS, interventricular septum; LVPW, left ventricular posterior wall; P, pericardium).

Technique emphasis. For emphasis we restate that studies for effusion should be done with relatively low-gain settings and with the transducer oriented in an inferior and lateral direction from the left sternal border. Our current practice is to find the posterior pericardial echo first by its characteristic high intensity. The pericardial lung interface is the last echo to disappear as one reduces the sensitivity of the instrument, and it is possible to adjust the sensitivity to record this strong pericardial echo alone. If one observes this pericardial echo and abruptly increases the gain setting to various degrees on repeated occasions, it is possible to record the pericardial echo for reference and observe the position of the weaker myocardial echoes in relation to the strong echo (Fig. 3–31). Of course, if there is no separation, then effusion is not present. Generally speaking, one sees a small posterior separation and decreased pericardial motion with small pericardial effusion (Fig. 3–31 and 3–32A). With effusions of moderate size, the anterior myocardium separates from the anterior chest wall, in addition to a significant (greater than 1 cm) distance between the myocardium and pericardium, posteriorly. With moderate-sized effusions, in the range of 100 to 500 cc, it is common to record the anterior myocardium quite well while having difficulty in finding strong echoes from the posterior myocardium (Fig. 3–32B). In these cases, it is the presence of anterior fluid and the absence of a normal posterior pattern which causes immediate recognition of the true situation. In very large effusions, it is common to see synchronous oscillation of both the anterior and posterior heart walls of such amplitude that the opposing motion of these walls is overshadowed (Fig. 3–34). That is, the whole heart appears to swing like a pendulum within the pericardial sac in the presence of a large effusion. In such cases with very large effusion and a very striking cardiac motion, it is often impossible to identify the individual intracardiac structures giving rise to the echoes. In these cases, the extremely high-amplitude oscillation with the same frequency as the heart rate is a pathognomonic sign of large pericardial effusion.[77] It is interesting to note in this context that patients with large volume pericardial effusion and cardiac tamponade show electrical alternation of the electrocardiogram, which correlates with cardiac oscillations within the pericardial sac at one-half the heart rate (Fig. 3–35). This was originally described by Feigenbaum[77] and has

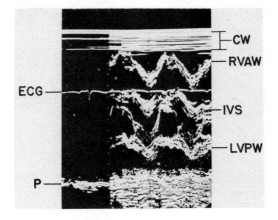

Fig. 3–34. Large pericardial effusion. The left section of the echogram shows the strong posterior pericardial echo displayed with low-gain setting of the instrument. The right area of the record shows the cardiac echoes with congruous motion of the right ventricular anterior wall and left ventricular posterior wall within the pericardial sac. The frequency of oscillation is the same as the heart rate (CW, chest wall; RVAW, right ventricular anterior wall; IVS, interventricular septum; LVPW, left ventricular posterior wall; P, pericardium).

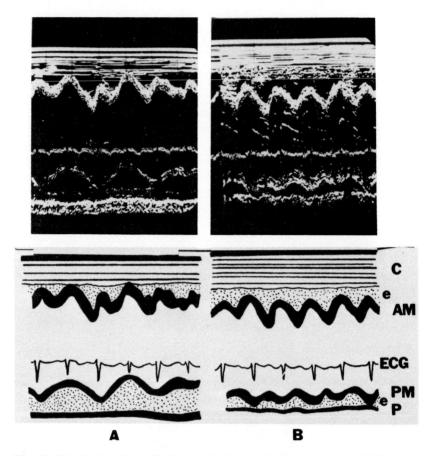

Fig. 3–35. Pericardial effusion with electrical alternans. A. Echogram from a patient with a large pericardial effusion and pericardial tamponade, displaying electrical alternans. Note that the oscillations of the heart within the pericardium occur at a frequency one-half that of the heart rate. B. Echogram from the same patient as in A, after the removal of pericardial fluid. Though pericardial effusion persists after the relief of tamponade, the oscillations of the heart within the pericardial sac are now at the same frequency as the heart rate (C, chest wall; e, effusion; AM, anterior myocardium; PM, posterior myocardium; P, pericardium). (From Usher B, Popp RL: Electrical alternans: Mechanism in pericardial effusion, Am Heart J, *83*:459, 1972, with permission.)

subsequently been confirmed by others.[90,91] To our knowledge, this finding has been seen only in the presence of pericardial tamponade. It is possible to have pericardial tamponade without this finding however, and authors have described markedly diminished myocardial motion in the presence of very small effusions in acute cardiac tamponade of traumatic nature.[76,92]

From a practical standpoint, we have found it most useful to approach the patient with the assumption that pericardial effusion is not present. With this assumption the echographic examination is performed in the usual manner, first locating the aortic echoes, then the mitral echo, and turning the transducer caudal and lateral from the mitral valve to observe the posterior left ventricular echoes (Fig. 3–30). If the normal pattern cannot be found, care is taken to keep the transducer oriented in a caudal and lateral direction, and the gain of the instrument is reduced to identify the pericardial lung interface. In the presence of effusion, this strong echo will have an abnormal or diminished pulsation and will be separated from the myocardial echoes by a space.[75,76] When this is observed, then care is taken to adjust the instrument so that the anterior chest wall and anterior myocardium can be visualized optimally. If a separation between these structures is observed, and even if a separation is not observed, then records are taken at several gain settings to avoid technical errors. It may be useful to go through this procedure using more than one intercostal space and having the patient's chest elevated at a 20–45° angle. Experience has taught us that lack of separation of the anterior myocardium from the chest wall signifies a low yield in apical or subxiphoid pericardiocentesis. On the other hand, if the patient can be turned into a position which shows separation of the anterior myocardium from the chest wall, fluid will be more easily obtained in this position.

Reliability of diagnosis. As mentioned previously, the lateral direction of the transducer is important to avoid false-negative results. Medial direction of the transducer may give false-positive results if the echoes from the aortic root or the mitral annulus are mistaken for myocardial echoes (Fig. 3–6 and 3–30). In addition, with a medial transducer position it is possible to obtain echoes from the descending aorta and vertebral column, which may be confusing. Several authors have pointed this out in the past, but transducer direction bears emphasis as the single source of most confusion in the diagnosis of pericardial effusion from the echogram.* Real false-positive results may occur

* Refs. 76, 80, 83, 93, 94.

when a separation of pericardium and myocardium is the result of material other than pericardial fluid. Pate has reported that he was unable to tell fibrous pericardial material from fluid,[81] and he cited one case in which 100 cc of clotted blood simulated anterior pericardial effusion in a case of stab would to the chest. Other types of material that may allow anterior separation have been noted above. It is common to record a distinct echo from the posterior left ventricular endocardium separated from the epicardial or pericardial echo by a nearly echo-free space (Fig. 3–36). This occurs with careful gain adjustments and therefore, the area between the endocardium and pericardium is filled with echoes if the gain adjustment is increased slightly. Familiarity with this pattern will avoid improper interpretation of such records as (false) positive studies. The identification of the endocardial echo in addition to the pericardial or epicardial echoes, or both, in each study

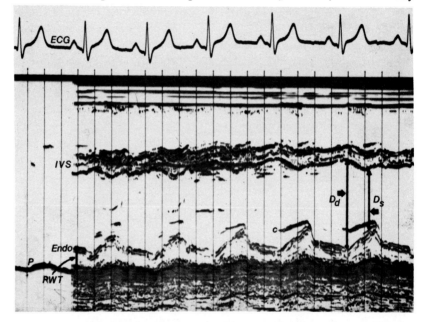

Fig. 3–36. Left ventricular echogram. This echogram is made by the direct strip-chart recording technique. The intensity of the instrument has been adjusted to display a discrete endocardial echo. With this adjustment, the myocardium appears echo-free. The appearance of the chordal echoes in contact with the endocardium at end-systole, and the ability to fill in the myocardium with echoes with slight gain adjustment, make this pattern recognizable. At low-gain setting, note the good motion of the pericardial echo (IVS, interventricular septum; Endo, endocardium; P, pericardium; PWT, posterior wall thickness; c, chordae tendineae; Dd, end-diastolic ventricular dimension; Ds, end-systolic ventricular dimension).

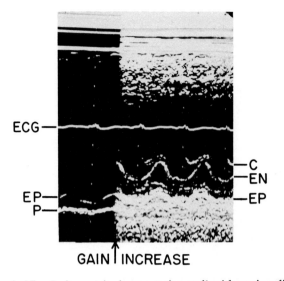

Fig. 3–37. Left ventricular posterior wall with pericardial effusion. The left portion of the record at low-gain setting shows the damped pericardial echo, and the epicardial echo is seen. With a gain increase, the endocardial echo and chordal echoes are displayed. This technique allows one to recognize a small, echo-free space between the pericardium and epicardium, representative of pericardial effusion (C, chordae tendineae; EN, endocardium; EP, epicardium; P, pericardium).

avoids this problem (Fig. 3–37).[16] That is, separation of epicardium from pericardium signifies pericardial effusion, whereas separation of endocardium from the properly moving pericardium-epicardium signifies specific gain setting of the instrument (see sections on wall thickness and ventricular volume).

Theoretically, left pleural effusion could simulate pericardial effusion, however, we agree with the findings of others [82,92,94] that pleural effusion can be recognized in the presence or absence of coexisting pericardial effusion (Fig. 3–38). In the cases of combined effusion, the parietal pericardium and pleura usually remain the dominant or the highest intensity echo. Thus, the relationship between the myocardium and pericardium may still be assessed reliably. In addition, in the presence of pleural effusion, there is separation of the pericardium and pleura from the lung by an echo-free space which appears to increase and decrease in size as the result of respiratory variation. In this way, the pattern of pleural effusion is different from that of pericardial effusion, and the frequency of oscillation in the space between the

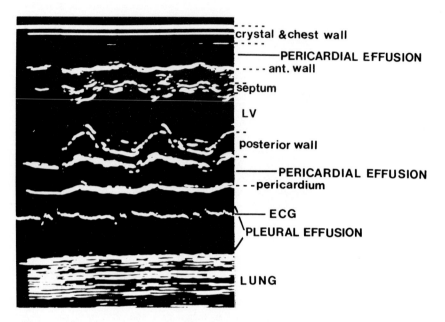

crystal &chest wall

————PERICARDIAL EFFUSION

- - - - ant. wall

septum

LV

posterior wall

————PERICARDIAL EFFUSION

- - -pericardium

—— ECG

PLEURAL EFFUSION

LUNG

Fig. 3–38. Pericardial and pleural effusions. Separation of the chest wall and anterior wall define the anterior pericardial effusion. The detail of the posterior wall shows endocardial and epicardial echoes separated from the damped pericardial motion by posterior pericardial effusion. The electrocardiogram is displayed in the echo-free space between the pericardium and the lung, representing pleural effusion.

nonmoving pericardial and pleural echo and the next echo relates to heart rate less than respiratory rate in pericardial effusion. When present, left pleural effusion is not always noted in echographic studies for pericardial effusion.

False-negative results are obtained only if fluid is loculated in an area of the pericardium which is not encountered by the ultrasonic beam. Casarella and Schneider have reported a case of loculated effusion caused by tuberculous pericarditis, in which the posterior pericardium was adherent to the myocardium and the anterior space was very large owing to loculation of the fluid.[93] They point out that recognition of the true mitral valve pattern during their study might have led them to the correct diagnosis, since they mistakenly labeled the anterior myocardium as the mitral valve. It is easy to imagine the presence of fluid loculated in the right lateral pericardial recess with no evidence of this by echogram using the standard technique, though we have not encountered such a case.

There are few false-negative and few false-positive diagnoses of pericardial effusion when there is moderate experience in the performance and interpretation of echograms. This fact, coupled with the sensitivity of the technique and the ability to perform the test in a short period of time at the patient's bedside has made echocardiography the method of choice for the diagnosis of pericardial effusion in those institutions in which it is used.

Myocardial Thickness

The ability to display separate pericardial and endocardial echoes by varying the sensitivity of the ultrasonoscope has allowed quantitative measurement of myocardial thickness (Fig. 3–39). The standardization of the procedure requires that the posterior left ventricular myocardium be recorded between the free edge of the mitral valve and the papillary muscle, with the transducer directed caudally and laterally from the left sternal border. The thickness of this area is assumed to have a constant relation to the rest of the myocardium in all patients. Twenty-five normal patients showed myocardial wall thicknesses of 0.8 to 1.3 cm in the original studies by Feigenbaum et al.[95] In this study, echographically determined myocardial thickness was within 5 mm of the thickness measured by needle insertion at surgery, and was within 3 mm of the thickness measured at autopsy. Sjogren et al reported less accuracy using different equipment, but noted "almost identical values" on repeated studies of the same patient.[96] We have compared echographic thickness measurements in the preterminal period with autopsy measurements the same day in six cardiac transplantation patients who died in rejection.[97] The echographic measurements were within 1 mm of the autopsy data in these edematous, stiff hearts, which may have been less affected by postmortem changes than the normal. In another study, echographic myocardial thickness showed a standard error of 1 mm, compared with angiographic measurements.[98] In this study, there was close agreement of the data obtained and measured by two observers. The thickness of the interventricular septum can be measured accurately in a similar manner.[99]

INVESTIGATIONAL USES OF ECHOCARDIOGRAPHY

The last area for discussion in this section is on the borderline between those techniques considered of established use and those which must still be considered investigational in nature. The use of echo-

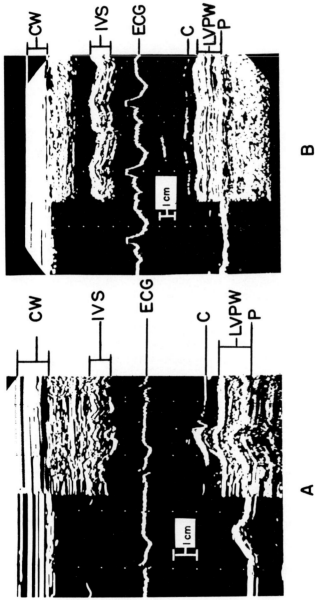

Fig. 3–39. Patterns of left ventricular wall motion. A. Echogram of a normal patient showing brisk posterior wall motion and myocardial thickness of 1 cm. B. Echogram of a patient with cardiomyopathy in heart failure. Note the sluggish left ventricular wall motion and posterior wall thickness of 1.6 cm. The chordal echoes are seen in both panels (CW, chest wall; IVS, interventricular septum; C, chordae tendineae; LVPW, left ventricular posterior wall; P, pericardium).

graphic techniques for the diagnosis of congenital heart disease is in this gray area.

Congenital Heart Disease

Left-to-right shunts. The first studies of qualitative measurement of right and left ventricular size by ultrasound were performed on normal subjects, patients with proved atrial septal defect and consequent right ventricular dilation, and patients with mitral and/or aortic regurgitation and consequent left ventricular dilation.[100] In this study and a subsequent confirmatory study,[101] the dimension of the right ventricle recorded by the standard echographic ventricular technique was increased in patients with atrial septal defect and left-to-right shunt. The increased right ventricular dimension appears to correlate with a dilated right ventricle, and this finding occurs in ventricular septal defect with large left-to-right shunt, or with severe right ventricular hypertension. Patients with patent ductus arteriosus do not show an increased right ventricular dimension.[101] An intriguing finding from both of these studies concerns the motion of the interventricular septem during ventricular systole. The typical normal motion of the interventricular septum shows a small amplitude motion toward the transducer at the time of atrial systole, with reversal of this motion near the peak of the QRS complex and the onset of ventricular systole. During ventricular systole the septum undergoes a posterior motion in an arc, concave to the transducer or convex to the left ventricular posterior wall. At the end of ventricular ejection, the septum reaches its most posterior point. A notch characteristic of septal motion is seen after this point, and this notch initiates ventricular diastole, with subsequent motion of the interventricular septum toward the transducer in a rather smooth arc terminating in the next presystolic atrial wave. This motion of the interventricular septum is essentially the reciprocal of the posterior left ventricular wall motion, with the exception of the notch at the end of ventricular systole (Fig. 3–12). It appears that, at the end of ventricular ejection, the left ventricular cavity is isovolumic for a short period, during which the whole left ventricular chamber rotates toward the chest wall.* It is this rotation which causes the notch in the interventricular septum and continued anterior motion of the posterior ventricular wall at this point. Basically, the septum and posterior wall separate between the P wave and QRS of the electrocardiogram, and approach each other between the QRS and the end

---

* Ian McDonald, personal communication.

of the T wave. This normal pattern is not found in patients with diastolic volume overload of the right ventricle (Fig. 3–40).

Abnormal interventricular septal motion and right ventricular dilation. Patients with left-to-right shunt caused by atrial septal defect or anomalous pulmonary venous return fail to show the usual posterior motion of the interventricular septum during systole. In some patients, there is reversal of the interventricular septum motion, with net anterior motion during systole. In most patients, there is only flattening of the septal motion, so that only small amplitude oscillations are seen during systole. In either of these two cases, however, net decrease in left ventricular cavity size can be measured, since there is an apparent increase in amplitude of the systolic motion in the ventricular free wall. This abnormal septal pattern has been found in tricuspid regurgitation[101] and Ebstein's anomaly of the tricuspid valve[102] as well as in atrial septal defect. This abnormal pattern is not found in patients with ventricular septal defect or atrial septal defect with pulmonary hypertension which causes balancing of the shunt.[101] Normal septal motion is seen in pulmonary hypertension not related to atrial septal defect and with pressure or volume overload, or both, of the left ventricle.[101] The combination of increased right ventricular dimension and abnormal septal motion has been a reliable indicator of atrial septal defect in the institutions where it has been used. Normalization for body surface area by the use of a right ventricular dimension index yields figures of 0.3 to 1.1 cm/m^2 as the normal range, with no significant difference between men and women.[101] Abnormal right ventricular dimension indices were found in patients with atrial septal defect, regardless of the volume of the shunt, patients with anomalous pulmonary venous return, and patients with tricuspid insufficiency. Abnormally large right ventricular dimension indices were found only in those patients with very large volume left-to-right shunt with ventricular septal defect, and only in those patients with extreme primary pulmonary hypertension.[101]

The increase in right ventricular dimension measured echographically is a true reflection of right ventricular dilation and rotation of the heart. However, satisfactory explanation of the abnormal septal motion described above has not yet been developed.

False-positive diagnoses of right ventricular diastolic volume overload may be avoided if both an increase in right ventricular volume index and abnormal septal motion are required for this diagnosis. If abnormal septal motion is the only criterion used, false-positives may arise from recording the interventricular septum high in the left ventricular outflow tract. Near the membraneous portion, the interven-

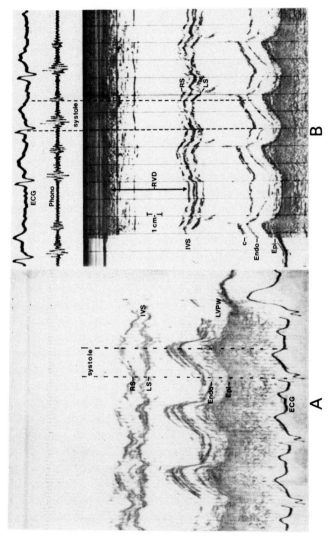

Fig. 3–40. Patterns of septal motion in right ventricular diastolic volume overload. A. and B. Both examples demonstrate lack of normal systolic posterior motion of the left side of the interventricular septum. During systole, either there is no net septal motion (A) or net anterior motion (B). An enlarged right ventricular dimension is characteristic of these patients' records. The right ventricle is not recorded in A. (RS, right side, interventricular septum; LS, left side, interventricular septum; IVS, interventricular septum; Endo, endocardium; Epi, epicardium; LVPW, left ventricular posterior wall; RVD, right ventricular dimension; c, chordae tendineae).

tricular septum has a motion pattern intermediate between the described normal ventricular pattern and the pattern of aortic motion (Fig. 3–3). Therefore, one cannot use the area of the septum below the aortic root in order to evaluate septal motion by these criteria. We have seen one false-positive diagnosis in a 20-year-old girl with pectus excavatum deformity of the chest, in which atrial septal defect was part of the differential diagnosis. False-negative results occur, and we have seen one patient with the echogram negative for abnormal septal motion, although the right ventricular volume index was abnormally large, and in this patient, large volume anomalous pulmonary venous return was found at cardiac catheterization and surgery.

More complex lesions. A group of investigators in South Africa have applied echocardography to the diagnosis of more complex congenital anomalies in the pediatric age group.[103,104] In the presence of a single ventricle, they have found absence of the interventricular septal echoes, and have been able to differentiate a single common AV valve from separated tricuspid and mitral valves.[103] Excessive mitral valve motion has been seen in cases of hypoplasia of the right heart chambers, whereas excessive tricuspid motion was seen with hypoplasia of the left heart chambers.[103] The simple presence of the tricuspid valve allowed these authors to rule out the diagnosis of tricuspid atresia. Similar studies have been done in this country.[105,106] In another study, the normal continuity of the aortic root and mitral valve was used to differentiate patients with double-outlet right ventricle from physiologically similar conditions, since there is discontinuity between the aorta and mitral valve in double-outlet right ventricle.[104] Lundstrom and Edler[51] have reported the echographic patterns present in congenital mitral stenosis to be similar to the patterns of acquired mitral stenosis. They were able to record the mitral valve echoes in all infants except those with mitral atresia. Likewise, the tricuspid valve could not be recorded in cases of tricuspid atresia. These authors note that the tricuspid valve is most easily recorded in children with right ventricular dilation caused by congenital anomalies, and report the normal tricuspid slope during diastole to be 55 to 160 mm/sec. In Ebstein's anomaly of the tricuspid valve, these authors noted an abnormally high amplitude of valve motion and a diastolic slope of less than 25 mm/sec. Three adult cases of this condition of the tricuspid valve were reported by Kotler,[102] in which the diastolic tricuspid valve slope was reduced, and the tricuspid valve amplitude was greater than the mitral valve amplitude in each case. Lundstrom and Edler[51] noted an echo in the left ventricular outflow tract just below the aortic root echoes in cases of membraneous subaortic stenosis. However, they could find no abnormality of the aortic valve in patients with aortic stenosis. One other group reported finding a subaortic diaphragm.[107]

Aortic Valve Disease

The ultrasonic patterns of aortic valve motion have been studied extensively.[14,15,19,20] Echocardiography appears to be useful only in cases of calcific aortic stenosis. In the normal situation, a maximum of three cusp echoes are seen in diastole; when there is severe calcific disease of the aortic valves, more than three echoes from the area of the aortic cusps are seen.[19] Cases of restrictive aortic valve motion have been noted in patients with aortic stenosis, but this has not been a consistent finding. The intensity of the aortic cusp echoes is normally less than the intensity of the aortic wall echoes, but in one study, 14 of 16 cases in which the cusp echoes were of greater intensity than the wall echoes showed the presence of calcific aortic stenosis. (Fig. 3–7).[19]

Although many of the techniques we have just described have been discovered recently, the new techniques that are clearly investigational will now be described.

Assessment of Ventricular Dimensions and Stroke Volume

The qualitative assessment of left ventricular size, in connection with studies of right ventricular volume overload, has already been mentioned.[100] Prior to the discovery of techniques for reliably recording the echoes of the interventricular septum, attempts were made to quantitate left ventricular size, using the distance from the chest wall to the posterior left ventricular wall as a measure of left ventricular diameter. Feigenbaum reported a good correlation of this overall heart size with the left ventricular end-diastolic volume in 52 patients in whom there was some reason for left ventricular cineangiogram.[108] An empiric combination of overall heart size and mitral ring amplitude was then used to estimate stroke volume.[109] Subsequent experience showed that this correlation did not hold if a significant degree of right ventricular dilation or hypertrophy was present. However, since the discovery of the interventricular septal echoes, and the ability to measure the left ventricular internal dimension in a standard manner, echocardiography has been used again to quantitate left ventricular volume. As expected, left ventricular volume correlates most directly with the cube of the left ventricular diameter. This relationship holds at end-diastole and end-systole as well.[110] The ability to calculate left ventricular stroke volume follows this correlation, since the stroke volume represents the difference between the diastolic and systolic volumes. In our laboratory, we have used the assumptions from the angiocardiographic method of left ventricular volume calculation, and we have assumed the left ventricle to be represented by a prolate ellipse.[111] We have assumed that the long axis of this ellipse is nearly twice the diameter measured by echocardiogram, and that this relationship remains relatively constant from end-diastole to end-systole. Using these assumptions, drawn from angiographic data,[112,113] we found an excellent correlation between the stroke volume calculated by echocardiography and the simultaneously determined output calculated by the Fick method. Subsequent studies have confirmed these findings.[114-118] Since echographic stroke volume is the total volume ejected from the ventricle, patients with aortic or mitral regurgitation, or both, show a smaller stroke volume calculated by the Fick method than by the echographic method. The difference of the echographic and Fick values is an estimate of the regurgitant volume and the severity of the lesion judged angiographically.[118] This technique relies on a full understanding of the anatomic principles of transducer direction in order to standardize the path of the sound beam through each ventricle. It is not difficult to locate the area of the left ventricular posterior wall between the free edge of the mitral valve and the tip of the papillary muscle. However, one must recognize that this spot may be found from a transducer position near the base of the heart or near the apex (Fig. 3–14). Since the goal is to measure a diameter of the ventricle, one would ideally like to have the transducer and sound beam perpendicular to the long axis of the ventricle. In practice, we try to obtain this goal by using the intercostal space which allows us to record the mitral valve when the transducer is almost perpendicular to the chest wall. From this position, a slight lateral and caudal rocking of the transducer brings the desired area of the ventricle into view. If we are above the desired interspace, we will observe a significant caudal direction of the transducer to record the mitral valve. If we are below the desired interspace, the transducer will still be directed in a cephalad direction when the desired area of the ventricle is recorded. In fact, it is difficult to record the interventricular septum and posterior left ventricular walls simultaneously from the interspace below the standard one described. It is possible to record the interventricular septum and posterior wall from the interspaces cephalad to the standard one. A difficulty with this procedure is most obvious in patients with hyperinflation of the lung. In such patients, the ultrasonic window on the chest wall is small and may be located in interspaces which are not optimal for recording ventricular studies as described above. In such patients, at least, one should be aware that standard studies are not being obtained.

In addition to these limitations, the assumptions on which the geometric calculation is based become less valid at some point as the heart dilates and begins to approximate the shape of a sphere rather than the shape of an elongated prolate ellipse.[113,117] With these reservations, we feel that the echocardiographic determination of stroke volume, ejection fraction, and the time course of these events may be used in the future as an accepted routine method for the calculation of these values. It is premature to advocate a single method of handling the data or even a single method of obtaining studies. This area of echocardiography is a very exciting one, but is still in the developmental stages.

For those involved in echocardiography, it is always striking to see the dynamic echographic display of normal brisk cardiac motion, contrasted with the sluggish motion of patients with severe myocardial disease (Fig. 3–39).

Monitoring Wall Motion

In our own experience in monitoring patients following cardiac transplantation using echographic techniques, we have been intrigued to see normal brisk myocardial wall motion progress to sluggish motion during episodes of cardiac rejection.[97] The use of isoproterenol or other inotropic agents may bring myocardial motion toward normal temporarily, whereas reversal of the rejection process will convert the sluggish motion back to a brisk normal motion within a few days time (Fig. 3–41). Studies of this type make us quite optimistic that echocardiography may be used for monitoring of cardiac function in the future. Already there have been attempts at monitoring cardiac function by quantitation of left ventricular posterior wall motion using the pericardial or epicardial echo as the basis for measurement.[119–122] In these studies, a normal range can be defined at rest, with increasing mean velocity of wall motion with exercise or other inotropic stimuli, and decreased mean velocity of posterior wall motion with myocardial infarction or other types of left ventricular failure. As stated earlier, the endocardium shows a greater amplitude of motion than the epicardium, and it would seem that this former echo would be superior to the latter as an indicator of myocardial function. Fortuin has proposed

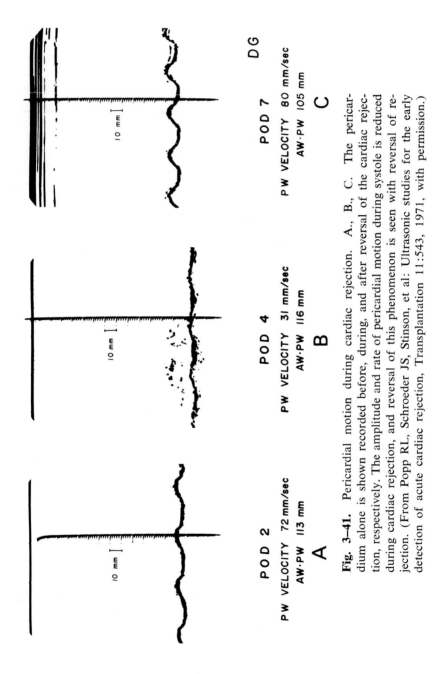

Fig. 3–41. Pericardial motion during cardiac rejection. A., B., C. The pericardium alone is shown recorded before, during, and after reversal of the cardiac rejection, respectively. The amplitude and rate of pericardial motion during systole is reduced during cardiac rejection, and reversal of this phenomenon is seen with reversal of rejection. (From Popp RL, Schroeder JS, Stinson, et al: Ultrasonic studies for the early detection of acute cardiac rejection, Transplantation 11:543, 1971, with permission.)

the use of the echographically determined left ventricular diameters in diastole and in systole to calculate left ventricular circumference and measure velocity of circumferential fiber shortening.[117,123] In this study, patients with either congestive heart failure or hypertrophic subaortic stenosis could be separated from the normal group. This work was confirmed by Paraskos et al[124] and Cooper et al.[124a] Frequently, it is possible to record echograms of sufficient quality to allow calculation of *maximum* velocity of circumferential shortening rate, which requires measurement of diameter at many points during each cycle. The drawback in all of these studies of ventricular function has been the inability to record technically adequate studies in every patient. Studies sufficient for calculation of stroke volume ejection fraction, and other parameters of ventricular function, are obtained in from 60 to 85 percent of patients, depending on the experience of the investigator.[111,114-117] In the older age group, the yield is approximately 60 to 70 percent even in the most experienced hands because of the inability to obtain good studies on older men with significant degrees of hyperinflation of the lungs. Consequently, the lowest yield is obtained in those patients with coronary disease, in whom one would be most anxious to use this non-invasive technique for the assessment of ventricular function. We believe that technical advancements in the design and production of echographic equipment, transducers, and display techniques may reduce this problem.

The use of ultrasound for studies of ventricular function requires an extensive understanding of the basic three-dimensional cardiac anatomy and transducer positioning which is required to standardize studies among patients. Even if the posterior ventricular wall motion is to be analyzed alone, it is critical to know what portion of the myocardium is being recorded. If the intracardiac structures neighboring the portion of myocardium recorded are not noted as landmarks, then varying portions of the myocardium may be analyzed from time to time in the same patient and among different patients. All motion recorded with the ultrasonoscope is recorded relative to the transducer. Consequently, motion of one portion of the myocardium toward a transducer near the cardiac apex should not be compared with motion of a similar area of the myocardium toward a transducer near the cardiac base. It is possible that a similar area of myocardium can be recorded consistently from a similar relative transducer position in most patients. However, this takes a good deal of time and experience. Experience is needed in learning to visualize the path of the sound beam through the various intracardiac structures, whereas time is needed on each patient to go through the procedure of carefully placing the transducer in various interspaces, noting the structures encountered with specific transducer angles, and finding the correct transducer position for an individual patient.

Detecting Rejection after Cardiac Transplantation

We have already mentioned our experience with monitoring of patients after cardiac transplantation using the echocardiogram,[97] and we continue to use this technique in the human cardiac transplantation program at Stanford. We have found that during cardiac rejection, the classical finding of decreased voltage on the surface electrocardiogram correlates with the echographic finding of an increase in posterior wall thickness, which may be related to the histologic findings of myocardial edema and cellular infiltration. The finding of right axis deviation on the electrocardiogram correlates with an increase in right ventricular dimension recorded by echocardiogram, whereas myocardial decompensation is seen in those patients with a decreasing velocity of posterior wall motion. All of these findings may be reversed after treatment of cardiac rejection.

Left Atrial Dimensions

Left atrial dimensions have been assessed echographically using two approaches. The original studies by Hirata[125] used standard echograms of the aortic root and left atrium, as described earlier (Fig. 3–6) (see Techniques section). The echographic dimension of the left atrium, measured at end-ventricular systole, showed very good correlation with the angiographic calculation of left atrial size. The echogram was superior to the chest radiograph and cardiac fluoroscopic study using barium, in the assessment of left atrial enlargement. The normal left atrial dimension in this study was divided by body surface area to give a normal index of 1.0 to 2.0 cm/m^2. Mild atrial enlargement was represented by 2.0 to 3.0 cm/m^2; moderate enlargement was 3.0 to 4.0 cm/m^2; and marked enlargement was over 4.0 cm/m^2. In this study, the dimension was measured approximately in the anteroposterior direction through the atrium. The cephalocaudal dimension has been estimated by placing the ultrasonic transducer in the suprasternal notch and directing the sound beam through the left atrium.[126] Patient groups expected to have left atrial enlargement showed an increase in this atrial dimension also.

Prosthetic Valve Motion

Metallic, plastic, and silastic materials used in the construction of prosthetic valves are very strong sound reflectors. The motion of both aortic and mitral valve prostheses have been studied by several authors.[23,127-131] Such studies have explained the sounds which are heard from such prostheses and have provided important information regarding the factors involved in normal mitral valve motion. As would be expected, the poppet of such a valve is against the sewing ring when the valve is in the closed position. Any motion of the closed valve during this period reflects motion of the whole prosthesis and the valvular ring to which it is attached (Fig. 3–42). When opening, the

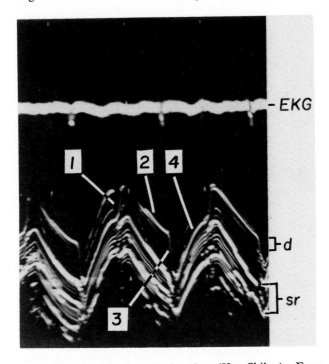

Fig. 3–42. Prosthetic mitral valve (Kay-Shiley). Four phases of disc motion are recorded: (1) Disc motion from the sewing ring to the top of the cage during opening of the mitral valve; (2) posterior motion of the open mitral valve caused by movement of the mitral annulus; (3) closure of the valve as the disc moves from the top of the cage to the sewing ring; (4) systolic motion of the closed valve caused by movement of the mitral annulus (d, disc; sr, sewing ring).

poppet abruptly moves from the sewing ring to the apex of the cage
and may bounce in the apex of the cage after opening. However, the
poppet remains in the apex of the cage in most cases of normal motion,
and motion of the cage and poppet is an indicator of motion of the
valve ring during this phase of the cardiac cycle. Such valves close
abruptly as the poppet moves back toward the sewing ring and the
pattern is repeated. In one series of patients with Kay-Shiley valves in
the mitral position, malfunction of the valve was diagnosed on serial
studies of the patients.[130] That is, the diastolic slope of prosthetic valve
motion became reduced when thrombus formed on the valve causing a
reduced orifice size. In one patient, such thrombotic material was surgi-

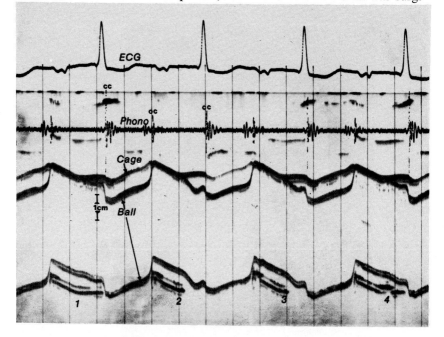

Fig. 3–43. Starr-Edwards mitral valve. Echoes are obtained from the apex
of the cage and the two surfaces of the ball. The sewing ring is not recorded.
The ball is seen to move toward the transducer and the apex of the cage
with opening, and away from the cage toward the sewing ring with closing.
In cycle 2, the ball floats toward a closed position prior to ventricular systole. The amplitude of the closing click is reduced in comparison with cycle
1, during which the ball is at the apex of the cage at the onset of ventricular
systole. In cycles 3 and 4 the ball separates slightly from the cage at end-
diastole. The dimensions of the ball are artifactually large, owing to the
slow speed of sound within the ball (see text).

cally removed, without valve replacement, and the diastolic slope recorded by echogram was stable for over a year after this procedure. This suggests that serial studies on a single patient may give some clue to mitral valve malfunction of this type. We would suppose that valves which stick in an open or closed position, or valves which show impaired poppet motion, could be found using the echographic technique. Such studies must await further confirmation. Echograms of Starr-Edwards prosthetic valves show artifactually large poppet dimensions caused by the altered sound velocity through the silastic material. The effect causes the distal edge of the poppet to appear detached from the cage (Fig. 3–43).

SUMMARY

Although ultrasound is a relatively new area of medical diagnosis, it has been expanding rapidly. The basic principles of physics on which the technique is based are familiar to most physicians and scientists. However, the anatomic and physiologic variables that must be considered in using an external probe to localize internal structures make mastering of the technique more difficult than most other noninvasive techniques. Three-dimensional anatomy of the heart, the basic echographic patterns emanating from the intracardiac structures, and the use of this information to guide the transducer's direction, all must be mastered in order to get consistent, high-quality echographic studies. Once such high-quality studies are obtained, the technique is extremely useful in the diagnosis of mitral stenosis and the evaluation of the severity of the lesion, as well as the condition of the leaflets themselves. The echographic disgnoses of atrial masses, hypertrophic subaortic stenosis, and the mitral valve prolapse syndromes have certainly been established. We believe that the method of choice for evaluation of pericardial effusion is echocardiography. The ability to perform studies in acutely ill patients at the bedside in a short period, as well as the ability to do repeated examinations and the sensitivity of the technique, have been factors which outweigh all other methods for the diagnosis of this condition.

The two most exciting areas for the advancement of echocardiography are in the diagnosis of congenital heart disease and the assessment of ventricular function. Advances in the diagnosis of prosthetic valve malfunction should be developed using echocardiography.

ACKNOWLEDGMENTS

The authors wish to acknowledge the assistance of Mr. O.R. Brown, Mr. F. LaManna, and Miss M.E. Stone in the accumulation of the data included in this chapter, and the secretarial assistance of Mrs. S. McCain.

REFERENCES

1. Edler I, Hertz CH: The use of ultrasonic reflectoscope for the continuous recording of the movements of heart walls. Kungl Fysiogr Sällsk i Lund Förhandl 24:5, 1954
2. Edler I: The diagnostic use of ultrasound in heart disease. Acta Med Scand Suppl 308:32, 1955
3. Edler I, Hertz CH: Ultrasound cardiogram in mitral valvular diseases. Acta Chir Scandinav 111:230, 1956
4. Edler I: The use of ultrasound as a diagnostic aid and its effects on biological tissues. Continuous recording of the movements of various heart structures using an ultrasound echo method. Acta Med Scand Suppl 370:7, 1961
5. Edler I, Gustafson A, Karlefors T, et al: Mitral and aortic valve movements recorded by an ultrasonic echo method—An experimental study. Acta Med Scand Suppl 370:68, 1961
6. Effert S, Erkerus H, Grosse-Brockhoff F: Ueber die Anwendung des Ultrashall echoverfahrens in der Herzdiagnostik. Dtsch Med Wochenschr 82: 1253, 1957
7. Effert S, Bleifeld W, Deapmann FJ, et al: Diagnostic value of ultrasonic cardiography. Br J Radiol 37:920, 1964
8. Wells PNT: Physical Principles of Ultrasonic Diagnosis. New York, Academic, 1969, p 6
9. Smith-Kline Instruments, Inc. Technical Data, Ekoline Twenty Ultrasonoscope
10. Posakony GJ, VanValkenburg HE: Diagnostic Ultrasound. Boulder, Colorado, Automation Industries, 1966, p 12
11. Woodward B, Pond J, Warwick R: A study of the hazards of diagnostic ultrasonography using mice. Proc Am Inst Ultrasound Med, 1970
12. Abdulla U, Campbell S, Dewhurst CJ, et al: Effect of diagnostic ultrasound on maternal and fetal chromosomes. Lancet 2:830, 1971
13. Franco J, Rydquist R, Kovaleski B: Chromosome abberations and Doppler ultrasound. Proc Am Inst Ultrasound Med, 1971
14. Gramiak R, Shah PM: Echocardiography of the aortic root. Invest Radiol 3:356, 1968
15. Gramiak R, Shah PM, Kramer DH: Ultrasound cardiology: Contrast studies in anatomy and function. Radiology 92:939, 1969
16. Feigenbaum H, Stone JM, Lee DA, et al: Identification of ultrasound echoes from the left ventricle by use of intracardiac injections of indocyanine green. Circulation 41:615, 1970

17. Bove AA, Ziskin MC, Mulchin WH: Ultrasonic detection of in vivo cavitation and pressure effects of high-speed injections through catheters. Invest Radiol 4:236, 1969

18. Kremkau FW, Gramiak R, Carstensen EL, et al: Ultrasonic detection of cavitation at catheter tips. Am J Roentgenol 110:177, 1970

19. Gramiak R, Shah PM: Echocardiography of the normal and diseased aortic valve. Radiology 96:1, 1970

20. Hernberg J, Weiss B, Keegan A: The ultrasonic recording of aortic valve motion. Radiology 94:361, 1970

21. Edler I: Atrioventricular valve motility in the living human heart recorded by ultrasound. Acta Med Scand Suppl 370:83, 1961

22. Zaky A, Nasser WK, Feigenbaum H: A study of mitral valve action recorded by reflected ultrasound and its application in the diagnosis of mitral stenosis. Circulation 37:789, 1968

23. Winters WL Jr, Gimenez J, Soloff LA: Clinical application of ultrasound in the analysis of prosthetic ball valve function. Am J Cardiol 19:97, 1967

24. Zaky A, Steinmetz E, Feigenbaum H: Role of atrium in closure of mitral valve in man. Am J Physiol 217:1652, 1969

25. Shah PM, Kramer DH, Gramiak R: Influence of the timing of atrial systole on mitral valve closure and on the first heart sound in man. Am J Cardiol 26:231, 1970

26. Winsberg F, Goldman HS: Echo patterns of cardiac posterior wall. Invest Radiol 4:173, 1969

27. Gustafson A: Ultrasound cardiography in mitral stenosis. Acta Med Scand Suppl 461, 1966

28. Gustafson A: Correlation between ultrasound cardiography hemodynamic and surgical findings in mitral stenosis. Am J Cardiol 19:32, 1967

29. Effert S, Deupmann FJ, Karytsiotis J: Registration of movement of cardiac walls using the ultrasonic reflection procedure, in Kelly E (ed): Ultrasonic Energy. Chicago, Univ. of Illinois, 1965, p 327

30. Effert S: Pre- and postoperative evaluation of mitral stenosis by ultrasound. Am J Cardiol 19:59, 1967

31. Edler I: Ultrasoundcardiography in mitral valve stenosis. Am J Cardiol 19:18, 1967

32. Joyner CR, Reid JM, Bond JP: Reflected ultrasound in the assessment of mitral valve disease. Circulation 27:503, 1963

33. Joyner CR, Reid JM: Applications of ultrasound in cardiology and cardiovascular physiology. Prog Cardiovasc Dis 5:482, 1963

34. Joyner CR, Dyrda I, Barrett JS, et al: Preoperative determination of the function anatomy of the mitral valve. Circulation 31 and 32 (Suppl II): 120, 1965

35. Segal BL, Likoff W, Kingsley B: Echocardiography. Clinical application in mitral stenosis. JAMA 195:99, 1966

36. Segal BL, Likoff W, Kingsley B: Echocardiography. Clinical application in combined mitral stenosis and mitral regurgitation. Am J Cardiol 19:42, 1967

37. Segal BL, Likoff W, Kingsley B: Echocardiography: Clinical application in mitral regurgitation. Am J Cardiol 19:50, 1967

38. Winters WL: Ultrasound cardiology. Pa Med 70:53, 1967

39. Winters WL, Riccetto A, Gimenez J, et al: Reflected ultrasound as a diagnostic instrument in study of mitral valve disease. Br Heart J 29:788, 1967

40. Winters WL, Hafer J, Soloff LA: Abnormal mitral valve motion as demonstrated by the ultrasound technique in apparent pure mitral insufficiency. Am Heart J 77:196, 1969

41. Pridie RB, Benham R, Oakley CA: Echocardiography of the mitral valve in aortic valve disease. Br Heart J 33:296, 1971

42. Wharton CFP: Reflected ultrasound patterns in mitral valve disease. Guys Hosp Rep 118:187, 1969

43. Wharton CFP, Bescos LL: Mitral valve movement: A study using an ultrasound technique. Br Heart J 32:344, 1970

44. Silver W, Rodriguez-Torres R, Newfeld E: The echocardiogram in a case of mitral stenosis before and after surgery. Am Heart J 78:811, 1969

45. Gabor GE, Winsberg F: Motion of mitral valves in cardiac arrhythmias: Ultrasonic cardiographic study. Invest Radiol 5:355, 1970

46. Shah PM, Gramiak R: Echocardiography recognition of mitral valve prolapse. Circulation 42 (Suppl III):45, 1970

47. Kerber RE, Isaeff DM, Hancock EW: Echocardiographic patterns in patients with the syndrome of systolic click and late systolic murmur. N Engl J Med 284:691, 1971

48. Dillon JC, Haine CL, Chang S, et al: Use of echocardiography in patients with prolapsed mitral valve. Circulation 43:503, 1971

49. Friedman NJ: Echocardiographic studies of mitral valve motion. Genesis of opening snap in mitral stenosis. Am Heart J 80:177, 1970

50. Duchak JM, Chang SJ, Feigenbaum H: The posterior mitral valve echo and the echocardiographic diagnosis of mitral stenosis. Proc Am Inst Ultrasound Med, 1971

51. Lundström N, Edler I: Ultrasound in infants and children. Acta Paediatr Scand 60:117, 1971

52. Popp RL, Harrison DC: Ultrasound in the diagnosis and evaluation of therapy of idiopathic hypertrophic subaortic stenosis. Circulation 40:905, 1969

53. Winsberg F, Gabor GE, Hernberg JG, et al: Fluttering of mitral valve in aortic insufficiency. Circulation 41:225, 1970

54. Craige E, Fortuin NJ: Studies of mitral valve motion with the Austin-Flint murmur. Circulation 44 (Suppl II):33, 1971

55. Schattenberg TT: Echocardiographic diagnosis of left atrial myoxom. Mayo Clin Proc 43:620, 1968

56. Wolfe SB, Popp RL, Feigenbaum H: Diagnosis of atrial tumors by ultrasound. Circulation 39:615, 1969

57. Popp RL, Harrison DC: Ultrasound for the diagnosis of atrial tumor. Ann Intern Med 71:785, 1969

58. Finegan RE, Harrison, DC: Diagnosis of left atrial myxoma by echocardiography. N Engl J Med 282:1022, 1970

59. MacVaugh H, Joyner CR: Mitral insufficiency due to calcified myxoma. J Thorac Cardiovasc Surg 61:287, 1971

60. Trinkle JK, Edelstein SG, Yoshonis KF: Left atrial myxoma. Diagnosis and excision. J Thorac Cardiovasc Surg 61:765, 1971

61. Spencer WH, Peter RH, Orgain ES: Detection of a left atrial myxoma by echocardiography. Arch Intern Med 128:787, 1971

62. Glasser SP, Bedynek JL, Hall RJ, et al: Left atrial myxoma, Am J Med 50: 113, 1971

63. Kraus R: Ultrasound evaluation of left atrial myxoma. Report of a case and differential diagnosis. Proc Am Inst Ultrasound Med 1971

64. Effert S and Domanig E: Diagnostik intrasurikularer Tumoren und grosser Thromben mit den Ultraschallechoverfahren. Dtsch Med Wochenschr 84:6, 1959

65. Shah PM, Gramiak R, Kramer DH: Ultrasound localization of left ventricular outflow obstruction in hypertrophic obstructive cardiomyopathy. Circulation 40:3, 1969

66. Simon AL, Ross J Jr, Gault JH: Angiographic anatomy of the left ventricle and mitral valve in ideopathic hypertrophic subaortic stenosis. Circulation 36:852, 1967

67. Adelman AG, McLoughlin MJ, Marquis Y, et al: Left ventricular cine-angiographic observations in muscular subaortic stenosis. Am J Cardiol 24:689, 1969

68. Shah PM, Gramiak R, Adelman AG, et al: Role of echocardiography in diagnostic and hemodynamic assessment of hypertrophic subaortic stenosis. Circulation 44:891, 1971

69. Moreyra E, Klein JT, Shimada H, et al: Idiopathic hypertrophic subaortic stenosis diagnosed by reflected ultrasound. Am J Cardiol 23:32, 1969

70. Pridie RB, Oakley CM: Mechanism of mitral regurgitation in hypertrophic obstructive cardiomyopathy. Br Heart J 32:203, 1970

71. Ellis JG, Terneny OJ, Winters WL: Critical role of the mitral valve leaflet in hypertrophic subaortic stenosis and amelioration of the disease by mitral valve replacement. Chest 59:378, 1971

71a. Henry WL, Clark EC, Epstein SE: Asymmetric septal hypertrophy. Echocardiographic identification of the pathognomonic anatomic abnormality of IHSS. Circulation 47:225–233, 1973

72. Edler I: Atrioventricular valve motility in the living human heart recorded by ultrasound. Acta Med Scand Suppl 370:107, 1961

73. Bleifeld VW, Effert S: Ueber das ultraschallkardiogramm der trikuspidalklappe. Z Kreislaufforsch 55:154, 1966

74. Joyner CR Jr, Hey E, Berry J, et al: Reflected ultrasound in the diagnosis of tricuspid stenosis. Am J Cardiol 19:66, 1967

75. Feigenbaum H, Waldhausen JA, Hyde LP: Ultrasound diagnosis of pericardial effusion. JAMA 191:711, 1965

76. Feigenbaum H, Zaky A, Waldhausen JA: Use of ultrasound in the diagnosis of pericardial effusion. Ann Intern Med 65:443, 1966

77. Feigenbaum H, Zaky A, Grabhorn LL: Cardiac motion in patients with pericardial effusion. Circulation 34:611, 1966

78. Feigenbaum H, Zaky A, Waldhausen JA: Use of reflected ultrasound in detecting pericardial effusion. Am J Cardiol 19:84, 1967

79. Feigenbaum H: Ultrasonic cardiology. Dis Chest 55:59, 1969

80. Feigenbaum H: Echocardiographic diagnosis of pericardial effusion. Am J Cardiol 26:475, 1970

81. Feigenbaum H: Echocardiographic diagnosis of pericardial effusion by echocardiography. Ann Surg 165:826, 1967

82. Klein JJ, Raber G, Shimada H, et al: Evaluation of induced pericardial effusion by reflected ultrasound. Am J Cardiol 22:49, 1968

83. Klein JJ, Segal BL: Pericardial effusion diagnosed by reflected ultrasound. Am J Cardiol 22:57, 1968

84. Goldschlager AW, Freeman LM, Davis PJ: Pericardial effusions and echocardiography. NY J Med 7:1854, 1967

85. Rothman J, Chase NE, Kricheff II, et al: Ultrasonic diagnosis of pericardial effusion. Circulation 35, 358, 1967

86. Pridie RB, Turnbull TA: Diagnosis of pericardial effusion by ultrasound. Br Med J 3:356, 1968

87. Steinberg J, vonGal HVn, Finby N: Roentgen diagnosis of pericardial effusion. Am J Roentgenol 79:321, 1958

88. Adams DF, Blank N, Weintraub RA: Alterations in cardiac motion due to the floatation of CO_2 in the right atrium in the presence of pericardial effusion. Radiology 91:261, 1968

89. Bryk D, Kroop IG, Badow J: The effect of heart size, cardiac tamponade, and phase of the cardiac cycle on the distribution of pericardial fluid. Radiology 93:273, 1969

90. Gabor GE, Winsberg F, Bloom HS: Electrical and mechanical alteration in pericardial effusion. Chest 59:341, 1971

91. Usher B, Popp RL: Electrical alternans: Mechanism in pericardial effusion. Am Heart J 83:459, 1972

92. Goldberg BB, Ostrum BJ, Isara HJ: Ultrasonic determination of pericardial effusion. JAMA 202:927, 1967

93. Casarella WJ, Schneider BO: Pitfalls in the ultrasonic diagnosis of pericardial effusion. Am J Roentgenol 110:760, 1970

94. Soulen RL, Lapayowker MS, Gimenez JL: Echocardiography in the diagnosis of pericardial effusion. Radiology 86:1047, 1966

95. Feigenbaum H, Popp RL, Chip JN, et al: Left ventricular wall thickness measured by ultrasound. Arch Intern Med 121:391, 1968

96. Sjögren A-L, Hytonen I, Frick MH: Ultrasonic measurements of left ventricular wall thickness. Chest 58:37, 1970

97. Popp RL, Schroeder JS, Stinson EB, et al: Ultrasonic studies for the early detection of acute cardiac rejection. Transplantation 11:543, 1971

98. Troy BL, Pombo JF, Rackley CE: Measurement of left ventricular thickness and mass by endocardiography. Circulation 45:602–611, 1972

99. Troy BL, Rackley CE: Measurement of the width of the interventricular septum by echocardiography. Circulation 43 and 44 (Suppl II):52, 1971

100. Popp RL, Wolfe SB, Hirata T, et al: Estimation of right and left ventricular size by ultrasound. Am J Cardiol 24:523, 1969

101. Diamond MA, Dillon JC, Haine CL, et al: Echocardiographic features of atrial septal defect. Circulation 43:129, 1971

102. Kotler MN, Tabatznik B: Recognition of Ebstein's anomaly by ultrasound technique. Circulation 44 (Suppl II):34, 1971

103. Chester E, Joffe HS, Vecht R, et al: Ultrasound cardiography in single ventricle and the hypoplastic left and right heart symptoms. Circulation 42:123, 1970

104. Chester E, Joffe HS, Beck W, et al: Echocardiographic recognition of mitral-semilunar valve discontinuity. Circulation 43:725, 1971

105. Solinger RE, Elbl F, Minhas K: Echocardiography in normal neonates. Circulation 44 (Suppl II):228, 1971

106. Solinger RE, Elbl F, Minhas K: Echocardiography in congenital heart disease in neonates and infants. Circulation 44 (Suppl II):228, 1971

107. Ultan LB, Segal BL, Likoff W: Echocardiography in congenital heart disease. Preliminary observations. Am J Cardiol 19:74, 1967

108. Feigenbaum H, Helmen CH, Nasser WK, et al: Estimation of left ventricular diastolic volume using ultrasound. Circulation 35 and 36 (Suppl II):106, 1967

109. Feigenbaum H, Zaky A, Nasser WF: Use of ultrasound to measure left ventricular stroke volume. Circulation 35:1092, 1967

110. Feigenbaum H, Wolfe SB, Popp RL, et al: Correlation of ultrasound with angiocardiography in measuring left ventricular diastolic volume. Am J Cardiol 23:111, 1969

111. Popp RL, Harrison DC: Ultrasonic cardiac echography for determining stroke volume and valvular regurgitation. Circulation 41:493, 1970

112. Gault SH, Ross J Jr, Braunwald E: Contractile state of the left ventricle in man: Instantaneous tension-velocity-length relations in patients with and without disease of the left ventricular myocardium Circ Res 22:451, 1968

113. Lewis RP, Sandler H: Relationship between changes in left ventricular dimensions and the ejection fraction in man. Circulation 44:548, 1971

114. Murray JA, Johnston W, Reid JM: Echocardiographic determination of left ventricular performance. Proc Am Coll Physicians, 1970, p 110

115. Pombo JF, Troy BL, Russel RO: Left ventricular volumes and ejection fraction of echocardiography. Circulation 43:480, 1971

116. Pombo JF, Russell RO Jr, Rackley CE, et al: Comparison of stroke volume and cardiac output determination by ultrasound and dye dilution in acute myocardial infarction. Am J Cardiol 27:630, 1971

117. Fortuin NJ, Hood WP Jr, Sherman ME, et al: Determination of left ventricular volumes by ultrasound. Circulation 44:575, 1971

118. Gibson DG: Measurement of left ventricular volumes in man by echocardiography—comparison with biplane angiography. Br Heart J 33:614, 1971

119. Valenzuela S, Bowyer AF: Ultrasonic measurements of the ventricular response to graded upright exercise. Loma Linda School of Medicine. Proc Am Inst Ultrasound Med, 1968

120. Bowes LD, Bowyer AF: Contributions of ultrasound to the study of myocardial infarction. Loma Linda University School of Medicine. Proc Am Inst Ultrasound Med, 1968

121. Kraunz RF, Kennedy JW: Ultrasonic determination of left ventricular wall motion in normal man. Am Heart J 79:36, 1970

122. Kraunz RF, Ryan TJ: Ultrasound measurements of ventricular wall motion following administration of vasoactive drugs. Am J Cardiol 27:464, 1971

123. Fortuin NJ, Hood WP: Determination of mean velocity of circumferential fiber shortening (V_{CF}) by echocardiography. Circulation 43 and 44 (Suppl II):34, 1971

124. Paraskos JA, Grossman W, Saltz S, et al: A noninvasive technique for the determination of velocity of circumferential fiber shortening in man. Circ Res 29:610, 1971

124a. Cooper RH, O'Rourke RA, Karliner JS, et al: Comparison of ultrasound and cineangiographic measurements of the mean rate of the circumferential fiber shortening in man. Circulation 46:914–923, 1972

125. Hirata T, Wolfe SB, Popp RL, et al: Estimation of left atrial size using ultrasound. Am Heart J 78:43, 1969

126. Goldberg BB: Suprasternal ultrasonography. JAMA 215:245, 1971

127. Reid JM, Bor I: Ultrasound cardiogram of artificial mitral valves (Starr-Edwards prosthesis). Z Kreislaufforsch 58:979, 1959

128. Kingsley B, Flint GB Jr, Raber GT, et al: Another look at echocardiography. Am J Cardiol 19:108, 1967

129. Johnson ML, Paton BC, Holmes JH: Ultrasonic evaluation of prosthetic valve motion. Circulation 43 (Suppl II):3, 1971

130. Popp RL, Carmichael BM: Cardiac echography in the diagnosis of prosthetic mitral valve malfunction. Circulation 44 (Suppl II):33, 1971

131. Siggers DC, Srivongse SA, Deuchar D: Analysis of dynamics of mitral Starr-Edwards valve prosthesis using reflected ultrasound. Br Heart J 33:401, 1971

E. E. Eddleman, Jr.

4
Kinetocardiography

INTRODUCTION

With each heartbeat the precordium is set into vibration resulting from intracardiac events and positional and shape changes of the heart during the cardiac cycle. The vibrations can roughly be divided into two groups: those components which are of low- or ultralow frequency (0 to 30 Hz, i.e., cycles per second) and those which are of high frequency (approximately 30 to 2000 Hz). The low-frequency components of the first group are those produced by the movements and shape changes of the heart during ejecting and ventricular filling. The second group, or the auditory range, is caused by intracardiac events such as the opening and closing of the valves, gallop sounds, ejection clicks, and murmurs. Obviously, these frequency ranges overlap; however, they can be separated arbitrarily, as mentioned above. Phonocardiography and clinical auscultation of the heart deal with the auditory range, whereas the low-frequency movements have to be either graphically recorded or confirmed by palpation. The low-frequency movements represent a different spectrum of clinical information from that of phonocardiography.

The many different methods of recording the low-frequency precordial movements will be explained in the section on methodology, but,

This study was supported in part by the U.S. Public Health Service (HE-11310).

227

in general, they fall into two categories: absolute displacement records (kinetocardiography) and relative motion (apexcardiography). Each technique uses a different frame of reference for recording chest wall motion: the former, an external fixed point above the chest, and the latter, the chest wall itself. Both systems appear to offer similar, but somewhat different, information. This chapter deals primarily with the kinetocardiogram (absolute precordial motion).

HISTORY

The interest in precordial movements probably dates back to Marey in 1885 who first studied the movements of the precordium with the use of a capsule.[1] The system was modified by Crehore so that the vibrations of a tambour could be recorded.[2] Since that time a number of reports on isolated graphic records have appeared in the literature; however, systematic study probably began after the work of Dressler in 1933.[3] The "new" area of investigation was introduced by Johnston and Overy in 1951,[4] and since then a renewed interest has occurred, including a series of papers by Eddleman et al,[5-28] Harrison,[29-46] Luisada,[47] Schweizer,[48-50] Bertrab and Mahlich,[51-53] and the recent monographs by Rorvik,[54] Peltier,[55] and Finardi.[56] These publications offer a basis for this presentation.

KINETOCARDIOGRAPHIC METHOD

Apparatus

As stated, the kinetocardiographic method records low-frequency vibrations or movements of the precordium between direct current and approximately 30 Hz. The apparatus consists of a bellows used as a sensing device with a probe on one end.* At the end of the probe is a flat head approximately 7 mm in diameter which is placed against the chest wall for sensing the low-frequency movements. The open end of the bellows is connected by a short piece of Tygon tubing to a PM5-0.2–350 Statham strain-gauge transducer.† The entire system is mounted

---

* The bellows can be obtained from many commercial firms. The one that has been used in this laboratory has three flanges and was constructed by Kelvin & Hughes America Corporation, Annapolis, Maryland.

† The tube connected from the bellows to the strain-gauge transducer needs a three-way stopcock or some similar device so that the pressure in the system can be released to atmospheric pressure before recording.

on a rigid external frame that can easily be constructed in most machine shops.[5,25] The setup and frame are illustrated in Figure 4–1. The crucial aspect of the system is that the bellows can be placed perpendicularly against the chest wall in order to obtain pulsations from any point desired. We have now documented that there is useful clinical information not only at the point of maximum impulse but in other areas as well. It is essential that this system be mounted on an external frame in order to record absolute displacement movements of the precordium. The recording device used in our laboratory is the

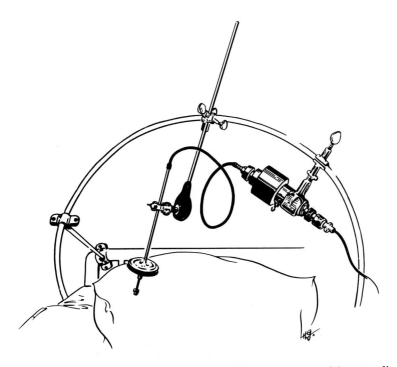

Fig. 4–1. Diagram of the kinetocardiographic apparatus used in recording low-frequency precordial movements. The bellows in the center of the photograph is connected by Tygon tubing to the PM5-0.2–350 Statham transducer mounted on the crossbar. Thus, the probe on the other end of the bellows can be placed perpendicular to any point on the chest wall to record movements at that position. Although this two-flange bellows is perfectly satisfactory, at the present time in our laboratory we are using the three-flange unit. (From Bancroft, WH Jr, Eddleman EE Jr: Methods and physical characteristics of the kinetocardiographic and apexcardiographic systems for recording low-frequency precordial motion, Am Heart J 73:756–764, 1967, with permission.)

Electronics for Medicine DR-8, but any instrument that can accept a strain-gauge transducer is sufficient. Initially, the bellows was connected to a piezoelectric transducer similar to that used for recording apexcardiograms, and this is probably satisfactory; however, the strain gauge is preferable because of the direct current response. Although the setup as shown in Figure 4–1 is a system permanently mounted to the bed, a portable apparatus has been constructed so that records can be obtained at the bedside from more critically ill patients. There is no exact design for the portable apparatus, but the external reference frame must be rigid. For this reason, there are several braces over the arm that fit across the patient's bed in order to hold the bellows system as rigidly as possible (see Fig. 4–2).

All records are obtained during normal held expiration. This is necessary because of the large movements of the chest wall during

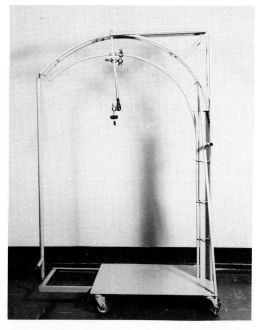

Fig. 4–2.   Portable apparatus for recording the kinetocardiogram. The detachable bar fits on the platform on the opposite side of the bed in order to stabilize the bar for mounting the bellows transducer. (From Eddleman, EE Jr, Bancroft WH Jr: Graphic recording of low-frequency precordial motion, Ala J Med Sci 8:178–183, 1971, with permission.)

breathing. Since the sensing unit goes down to direct current, the traces can be considerably distorted by respiration. This offers some problem in that the patient does have to hold his breath, but with experience the technician can easily obtain the tracing even on a dyspneic patient, since only one or two complexes are needed for analysis. The bellows is placed with slight pressure against the chest wall. The amount of pressure is not critical and does not affect the amplitude or configuration of the records as long as the contact is firm. Excessive pressure tends to dampen the system, and large outward movements may exceed the limits of the bellows; however, this artifact is easily recognized by a flat top on the curve.

The records obtained using this system are highly reproducible beat-to-beat as long as the patient is not in atrial fibrillation. In addition, they are reproducible day-to-day over a long period of time, provided the hemodynamic state does not change and provided the probe is placed at the identical point on the chest wall. This system offers an easy method which can be carried out accurately by technicians and which is reproducible beat-to-beat as well as day-by-day from many points over the chest wall.

Physical Characteristics of the System

The frequency response of the kinetocardiographic system has been described.[25] There is a resonance at approximately 75 Hz, but the system is linear up to approximately 30 Hz, with no phase shift. In addition, the system has a linear amplitude response. The length and type of the tubing make some difference, particularly in the upper frequency ranges. The tubing should be as rigid as possible, such as Tygon, and the length of the tubing between the bellows and the transducer should be kept as short as possible, preferably shorter than 20 cm.

The bellows system is somewhat rigid and offers approximately 10 pounds pressure per sq in against the chest wall; however, theoretically, this pressure should not affect the accuracy in recording displacement movements. Figure 4–3A is a record obtained by a bellows of the PMI in a normal individual, and Figure 4–3B is a record taken with a photocell which offers very little pressure against the chest wall. Note that the records are identical. Repeated recordings with a type of capacitance transducer that does not touch the chest wall are again almost identical. Thus, it is not critical to use the bellows-strain gauge as a transducer; however, in our experience it has been the easiest technique for routine use and for obtaining reproducible results. Al-

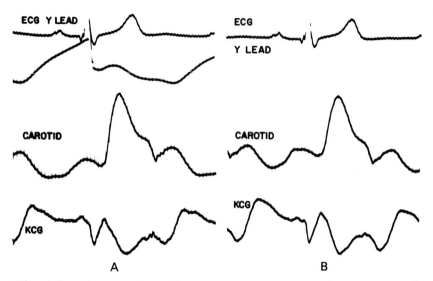

Fig. 4–3. Kinetocardiographic records obtained from the same normal subject by using the K_{45} bellows (A) as well as the K_{45} photocell (B). The photocell exhibits considerably less pressure against the chest wall than the bellows. The contour is essentially the same for each recording apparatus even though the pressure against the chest wall is different. (From Eddleman EE Jr, Harrison TR: The kinetocardiogram in patients with ischemic heart disease, Prog Cardiovasc Dis 6:189–211, 1963, with permission.)[21]

though commercial photocell pickups are available, they do have a few limitations. Often the cell is not linear over the entire sensing area. In addition, most of the transducers do not allow enough displacement of the probe to record very large movements which occur in many patients with severe heart disease. Therefore, the bellows was chosen because of its simplicity: it is easy to use and can be handled efficiently by a technician without a physician in attendance.

OTHER METHODS OF RECORDING
PRECORDIAL MOTION

There are difficulties in understanding records of precordial motion in the medical literature because of the wide variety of names, transducers, and systems that are used. There has been no standardization of the procedure, and most investigators have developed their own systems. As pointed out in the previous section, any transducer which records displacement from direct current or 0.1 Hz to 30 Hz, is linear, and is mounted from an external reference frame will produce kinetocardiograms indistinguishable from those reported in this chapter. The confusion that has arisen has resulted from three factors: (1) the use of transducers which have different frequency characteristics, (2) the use of transducers which do not sense displacement, but velocity or acceleration, and (3) the wide variety of names given to the procedure. Many publications in the literature fail to give an adequate physical description of the entire apparatus, including the recording device, which makes it very difficult for the average reader to interpret precisely what the records represent. The methods used by Schweizer[48-50] and Finardi[56] are comparable to the kinetocardiographic technique described, and the published records are identical. This cannot be said for many other systems.

In Table 4–1 an attempt has been made to characterize the properties of various systems used in recording precordial vibrations.[57-86] Note that the kinetocardiogram and the impulse cardiogram are essentially the same system with the exception that the impulse cardiogram probably has a lower frequency response. The mechanocardiogram and apexcardiogram are again essentially identical systems. On the other hand, vibrocardiography (vibrocardiogram 1 in Table 4–1) uses a linear capacitance microphone, usually with bandpass filters to alter and vary the frequency response; the very low frequency movements are not recorded. Thus, the vibrocardiographic recordings are considerably different in contour from those of the apexcardiogram or the kinetocardiogram and resemble those obtained from an accelerometer. One type of vibrocardiogram (vibrocardiogram 2 in Table 4–1) appears to be almost identical to the apexcardiogram. The precordial accelerogram recording is different from all of those described above.

There are many commercial transducers available, and only some of the common types are listed in Table 4–2. We must point out that it is not the frequency response of the transducer, but rather the characteristics of the entire system, including the recording apparatus, that generally limit the accuracy of various recording systems. For example, the Electronics for Medicine DR-8 has an upper limit of the frequency range of 2000 Hz, whereas most direct writers are considerably lower. The Siemens* mingograf direct writer can record as high as 200 Hz, whereas the Sanborn (Hewlett-Packard) direct writer, such as their electrocardiographic apparatus, is only accurate up to about 100 Hz.

* Siemens Medical of America, Atlanta, Georgia.

Table 4–1
Summary of Characteristics of Various Systems for Recording Precordial Movement

Name of System	Detailed References	Description	Type of Mount	Estimated Frequency Response	Comments
Kinetocardiogram	—	Various types of displacement transducers	From a fixed point above patient (external reference frame)	0 or 0.5–30 Hz, depends somewhat on transducer used	Recorded during held normal expiration, patient supine; records from many points over chest wall
Apexcardiogram	(See chapter 1)	Various types of displacement transducers of low frequency	On chest (relative motion)	0.5–30 Hz	Patient usually in left lateral position and apex impulse usually recorded
Mechanocardiogram	57–58	Essentially same as apexcardiogram	On chest (relative motion)	0.5–20 + Hz	Term not well accepted now

234

Impulse cardiogram	59–63	Transducer displacement—similar to KCG, but frequency range not as high	External reference frame	Approximately 0.5–10 Hz	Complex records which are difficult to analyze
Vibrocardiogram 1	64–74	Usually crystal or capacitance microphone with bandpass filters (displacement)	On chest wall (relative motion)	Varies, best estimated 5–25 or 30 Hz; higher frequency obtained by the bandpass filters	
Vibrocardiogram 2	75–76	Almost identical to apexcardiogram (displacement). Variable resistance type transducer	Chest wall (relative motion)	>1 cycles + (0–5 Hz)	
Precordial accelerogram or precordial ballistocardiogram	77–86	Usually uses an accelerometer as a transducer	Rests on chest wall	Difficult to estimate, but higher than KCG or ACG	Complex records which are difficult to interpret

235

Table 4–2
Transducer Characteristics

Transducer	Function	Frequency Response
Bellows connected to pressure strain gauge	Displacement	Linear duct current 0–30 Hz (upper limit dependent on length of connecting tubing)
Piezoelectric	Displacement	0.5–30 Hz (as used for apexcardiography). Upper limit can go above 20 KHz depending on shape of crystal
Capacitance	Displacement	20–2000 (as used for heart sound data) 1 Hz–10 KHz (Wayne Kerr distance meter)
Photocell	Displacement	dc–2000 Hz (upper limit depends on make)
Inductance	Displacement	Many types—can range from dc to 20 KHz
Inductance	Velocity	40–15 KHz
Accelerometer (All of above transducers can be made to measure acceleration by using a spring of suitable compliance and a movable mass)	Acceleration	1–30 Hz (as used in BCG); when using accelerometer for precordial movements one must be careful to correct for the angle the transducer axis makes with gravity

Note: The upper limit to the frequency response of most systems used in medicine is limited more by the recording and amplifying systems or by methods used to couple the signal source to the transducer than by the transducer itself.

If one is concentrating on low-frequency patterns, such as in the kinetocardiogram, all of these recording apparatus are sufficiently accurate. The main frequency range of the kinetocardiogram is between direct current and 30 Hz if the appropriate transducer is properly matched. In any publication on low-frequency precordial movements it is essential to include a detailed description of the transducer and the type of mounting device. For example, *the basic difference between apexcardiography and kinetocardiography is that the kinetocardiogram records absolute displacement movement of the chest wall, with a chest reference point above the patient. The apexcardiogram requires a trans-*

ducer which rests on the chest wall, and therefore records relative motion between the rim and the center portion of the chest enclosed.
It appears obvious that each system may in itself provide useful clinical information. This is well established for the apexcardiogram and kinetocardiogram, and it is quite likely that the other systems will provide useful clinical information as well. The choice of the technique should be based on the type of information desired.

NORMAL CONTOUR AND NOMENCLATURE OF THE WAVES

Figure 4–4 is a diagram of a normal kinetocardiogram; three positions are included: K_{14}, K_{24}, and K_{45}. The K_{34} trace has a contour halfway between the K_{24} and K_{45}, whereas the K_{55} record resembles a K_{45} record but is, in general, smaller in amplitude with less systolic retraction.

Nomenclature

No uniform nomenclature has yet been developed. We have attempted to present one,[26,21] which can be applied not only to normal records but also, in general, to abnormal records (Fig. 4–5). The principles used in devising a nomenclature are threefold: to keep the terminology as simple as possible; to relate the name to the mechanism responsible for the movements when reasonable; and, if the mechanism of the movement is unknown, to label it according to the positions in the cardiac cycle. If the origins of all the movements were clearly understood, a system based on mechanism would be most desirable; however, at the present time this is not possible. The designation of the point on the chest wall from which the record is obtained is simple and useful, based somewhat on the standard electrocardiographic precordial positions. Thus, the first number following K refers to a vertical line corresponding to the standard electrocardiographic precordial position, and the second number, the interspace from which it is recorded. For example, K_{14} represents the record obtained in the electrocardiographic V_1 position or in the right parasternal line in the fourth interspace, K_{24} represents the left parasternal region in the fourth interspace, K_{45} at the midclavicular line in the fifth interspace, and K_{55} in the anterior axillary line in the fifth interspace. A midepigastric record is obtained just below the zyphoid process and is designated K_{EM}.

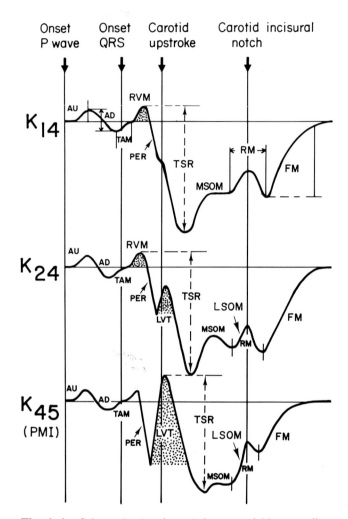

Fig. 4–4. Schematic drawing of the normal kinetocardiogram including three precordial positions, K_{14}, K_{24}, and K_{45}. The nomenclature included is based primarily on origin of movements and location within the cardiac cycle (AU, atrial upstroke; AD, atrial downstroke; TAM, terminal atrial movement; RVM, right ventricular movement (or initial outward movement); PER, preejection retraction; LVT, left ventricular thrust; TSR, total systolic retraction; MSOM, midsystolic outward movement; RM, relaxation movement; FM, filling movement; LSOM, late systolic movement).

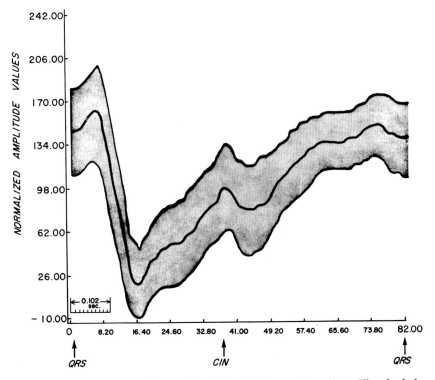

Fig. 4–5. Mean curve (K_{14} position) from 102 normal subjects. The shaded area represents 1 SD from the mean. The normalization procedure used was obtained by dividing each digital amplitude by the mean area under the curve. (From Eddleman EE Jr, Bancroft WH Jr: Quantification of the kinetocardiogram, Comput Biomed Res 1:237–250, 1967, with permission.)[26]

Normal Configuration

The normal configuration as presented in Figure 4–4 consists of three components to the atrial movements: the initial upstroke, a downstroke, and a terminal upstroke (AU, AD, TAM). This is followed by a right ventricular movement (RVM) which begins approximately 0.04 sec after the QRS complex. The movement normally is very small, is not palpable, and is of brief duration. A horizontal baseline can be drawn arbitrarily at a point on the curve 0.04 sec after the onset of the QRS complex in the electrocardiogram. This point was chosen because it usually occurs after atrial activity and before ventricular contraction. The upper limit of the duration of the baseline in normal subjects is 0.085 sec in the K_{24} position.[20] The right ventricular movement is followed by systolic retraction which begins before ejection and extends into the ejection (TSR). Over the left parasternal region, TSR is interrupted by the left ventricular thrust and is designated LVT, since this is the movement which is exaggerated in patients with left ventricular overload or hypertrophy. Systolic retraction is presumably caused by the retraction of the chest wall as the heart volume becomes smaller during ejection. The mechanics for the midsystolic outward movement (MSOM) are not clearly understood; however, it does appear to be related in some way to a pressure overload of the right ventricle. For example, this movement becomes exaggerated in patients with mitral stenosis who have high mean pulmonary artery pressures.[87] The main exception to this occurs in patients with congential heart disease, such as pulmonic stenosis, and will be discussed subsequently. There are two principal movements related to relaxation of the ventricle. The initial component is outward (late systolic outward movement (LSOM)), whereas the second movement is usually inward. The peak of the LSOM occurs close to the time of the carotid incisural notch. The relaxation movements are followed by the ventricular filling movement (FM). The onset occurs close to the time of the opening snap in patients with mitral stenosis. However, the onset cannot be taken as exactly the time when left ventricular filling begins since both left and right ventricular filling influence the movement, and the time of onset from the incisural notch varies slightly in the different precordial records. Therefore, in the kinetocardiographic traces one cannot use it as a precise time of onset of left ventricular filling.

Although the above discussion is concerned with nomenclature and description of the various major movements encountered in the kinetocardiographic records, we should point out that the evidence for the mechanism of the movements is still indirect and is based primarily on abnormalities encountered in disease states. In our laboratory we have made some attempts to correlate the various movements of the chest wall with positional and shape changes of the heart. However, to date this has been somewhat unsuccessful because of limitations in angiographic technique. With the advent of fast-filming biplane angiocardiography in the near future, additional insight should be obtained into the relationship of the cardiac movements and the shape and positional changes of the heart to the records recorded on the chest wall. This may be an important investigation since it is not clear exactly how heart movements are transmitted through the rather rigid chest wall. The chest wall has a natural frequency around 75 Hz. Thus, the low-frequency movements of the heart, from a theoretical standpoint, should be transmitted accurately to the outside. However, it is conceivable that the chest wall acting as a tight membrane might alter the signal in some fashion, a factor which needs to be elucidated.

COMPUTER PROCESSING

Since computers are now generally available in medical centers, we should present some discussion of the automatic processing of records. Automation is useful because of the large number of records that can be handled using more sophisticated types of analyses, including statistical evaluation. Kinetocardiographic records can be digitized on an A-D converter so that each amplitude throughout a series of cycles can be stored. A sampling rate of 250 times per sec is adequate to allow sufficient resolution for these low-frequency curves.

In this laboratory the records are recorded simultaneously with the electrocardiogram and the carotid pulse so that the onset of the QRS as well as the onset and end of ejection can be determined. These points in the cardiac cycle are important in order to properly identify the various waves in the kinetocardiogram. Waveform analysis of the onset of the QRS has been published by others.[88] The upstroke of the carotid pulse and the onset of ejection and the incisural notch also can be determined by several types of waveform recognition methods, one published by Kyle and Freis.[89] However, another method is used in this laboratory (Swatzell et al).* All methods so far devised have some limitations since none are entirely accurate. Thus, in our laboratory, as in others, a visual check has been built into the system so that the points in the cardiac cycle found by the computer program are displayed and can be corrected by manual intervention if necessary. Once these points are identified, the curves can then be processed in several different fashions.

Amplitude Calibration

The bellows or other types of sensing devices can be calibrated by placing the transducer on a shake table which produces a known amplitude,[25] and from this information the curve can be calibrated in either millimeters or inches. Using the previously determined factor from the shake table, each digital amplitude can then be corrected to actual amplitudes throughout the cardiac cycle. There are several other

* Swatzell RH Jr, Tucker M, Eddleman EE Jr: Computer method for determining the systolic time intervals. Comput Biomed Res 6, 1973 (in press).

methods by which the curves can be standardized in amplitude in order to compare the records from one patient to another. Each digital point can be expressed as a percentage of the total amplitude; thus, the maximum amplitude becomes 100 in all records. A third method divides each digital amplitude by the mean amplitude under the curve.[26] The last method appears to minimize the variations in thickness in the chest wall from patient to patient and completely removes any variations due to changes in the recording sensitivity. The process is performed by adding up all digital amplitudes throughout a cycle (area under curve) and dividing the area by the number of digital points throughout one cycle.

Time Normalization

One of the problems in comparing a kinetocardiographic record from one patient to another results from variations in the cardiac cycle. Thus, it is sometimes difficult to determine whether one wave is comparable to a given movement in another patient even with the same heart disease. In order for comparisons to be made, it appeared desirable that each kinetocardiographic curve should have a standard length. To do this, the heart cycle (from QRS to next QRS) is either expanded or squeezed down like an accordion, with interpolation of amplitudes between digital points, and a new curve constructed with a standard length. A heart cycle length of 0.836 sec was chosen since this represented the average cycle of a large number of normal subjects and patients. Each phase of the cardiac cycle is expanded or contracted to a fixed length. For example, the onset of the QRS to the carotid upstroke is fixed at 0.11 sec, from CU-CIN, 0.27 sec, and from CIN to the next complex, 0.44 sec, making a total of the QRS complex 0.82 sec. Thus, by amplitude and time normalization, it is possible to establish statistical limits for comparison of normal and abnormal kinetocardiograms. Figures 4–5 to 4–7 represent the mean curve from 102 normal subjects and their statistical limits. The shaded area represents 1 SD from the mean. Thus, it is possible by the use of computers to actually quantify the kinetocardiographic traces and apply statistical methods for their analysis.[26]

APPROACH TO THE INTERPRETATION

Although, as mentioned previously, the low-frequency precordial movements are related in some way to the positional, shape, and volume changes of the heart, there are several other considerations in approach-

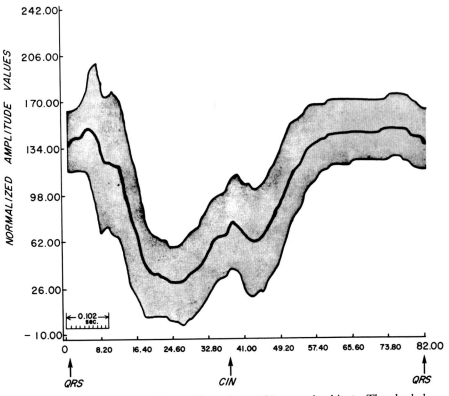

Fig. 4–6. Mean curve (K_{24} position) from 102 normal subjects. The shaded area represents 1 SD from the mean. The normalization procedure used was obtained by dividing each digital amplitude by the mean area under the curve. (From Eddleman EE Jr, Bancroft WH Jr: Quantification of the kinetocardiogram, Comput Biomed Res 1:237–250, 1967, with permission.)[26]

ing the interpretation of graphic precordial movements. These can be summarized as follows: (1) There are often small movements in the kinetocardiogram, the meaning of which is still obscure at the present time. Thus it is advisable to look at the entire record, paying particular attention to the large basic waves, as illustrated in Figure 4–4, such as the left ventricular impulse. Do not be overly concerned with every notching and small peculiar movements at the present time. The state of the interpretation has not developed to a sufficient degree to be able to attach clinical significance to the very small high-frequency components in the records. (2) As mentioned, most of the movements of the normal kinetocardiogram are inward except for the very small, initial

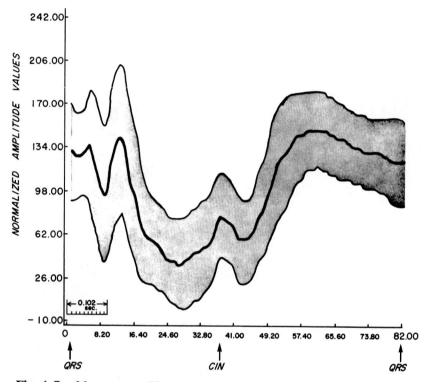

Fig. 4–7. Mean curve (K_{45} area) from 102 normal subjects. The shaded area represents 1 SD from the mean. (From Eddleman EE Jr, Bancroft WH Jr: Quantification of the kinetocardiogram, Comput Biomed Res 1:237–250, 1967, with permission.)[26]

outward atrial movement, the brief right ventricular movement and the left ventricular impulse which is normally seldom over 0.085 sec in duration as measured on a baseline as previously described. Consequently, most of the abnormal features of the kinetocardiogram are exaggerated outward movements. (3) Keep in mind that although specific disease abnormalities do affect the configuration, in general the alterations from normal are not specific enough to diagnose a given type of heart disease using the kinetocardiogram alone. (4) Functional abnormalities of the ventricle also influence the precordial movements. Consequently, the configuration is a mixture of movements related to the type of heart disease as well as to the functional state of the ventricle involved. This will be elucidated further in the chapter. For example, the atrial wave becomes larger during heart failure. (5) In addition, interpretation is dependent not only on the shape of the curve but also on the location on the precordium where the abnormalities occur. Left ventricular overload usually has a maximum impulse at the K_{45}, K_{55}, and K_{46} positions, whereas bulges caused by myocardial infarctions are more apt to be higher up over the chest wall (K_{44}, K_{34}, and rarely at K_{24}). Right ventricular abnormalities occur in the lower parasternal region of the chest, K_{14}, K_{24}, and K_{34}, although occasionally they may be present even as far as K_{45}. However, the maximum impulse is rarely in the left lateral precordial area.

Thus, in the interpretation one needs to consider the recognition of abnormal outward movements, the location of the larger movements, and the duration on the baseline. These findings must then be integrated with other manifestations of the heart disease in order to aid in achieving not only an anatomic diagnosis but functional evaluation as well. The kinetocardiogram should never be used alone in evaluating patients. The information from it must be integrated with other available clinical data. Taken in this context, the kinetocardiogram has been very useful in many clinical situations by drawing attention to abnormalities which were not previously suspected and in directing one's attention to certain disease states that may not have been considered.

LEFT VENTRICULAR ABNORMALITIES

Description of Curve

Abnormalities associated with left ventricular disease are best detected over the left lateral precordial area, usually in the K_{45}, K_{46}, and K_{55} positions. Figure 4–8 presents the location of the maximum left ventricular thrust in a group of patients with hypertension and aortic valvular disease. When there is a small left ventricular cavity and a very thick wall, the maximum impulse may be detected at K_{34} position, as in pure aortic stenosis. Figure 4–9 illustrates the abnormalities that occur in left ventricular overload. Note that the apex impulse becomes exaggerated in amplitude and prolonged in duration as severity of left ventricular overload progresses. Abnormalities occur both in pressure and flow loads of the ventricle. It has not been established whether or not the abnormal configurations as depicted in the schematic drawing (Fig. 4–9) are definitely related to an abnormal function of the left ventricle or to left ventricular hypertrophy. Nevertheless, the best way of determining the abnormality is to measure the duration of

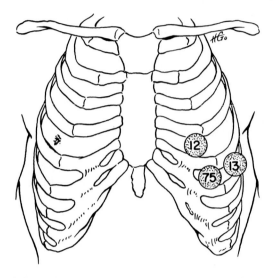

Fig. 4–8. The location of the maximum left ventricular impulse (PMI) in left ventricular overload (100 patients with left ventricular overload—hypertension and aortic valve disease). Notice that 75 percent are located in the K_{45} position, 12 percent in the K_{34} position, and 13 percent in the K_{55} position. (From Eddleman EE Jr, Harrison TR: The kinetocardiogram in patients with ischemic heart disease, Prog Cardiovasc Dis 6:189–211, 1963, with permission.)[21]

the left ventricular thrust on the arbitrary baseline, as described previously. The thrust begins before ejection and reaches a peak after the onset of ejection. In abnormal situations the duration on the baseline is 0.09 sec or greater (normal, not over 0.085 sec in 95 percent of the subjects).[20]

Functional Aspects

The configuration of the impulse is related to the type of functional abnormality as well as to the disease process. For example, in flow loads of the left ventricle such as aortic insufficiency, the amplitude is larger, but systolic retraction is more marked than usually seen in pressure loads, even though the duration is prolonged over normal in both. Pressure loads on the left ventricle produce a more sustained impulse with less total systolic retraction and in severe abnormalities the complete absence of total systolic retraction (see Fig. 4–9).

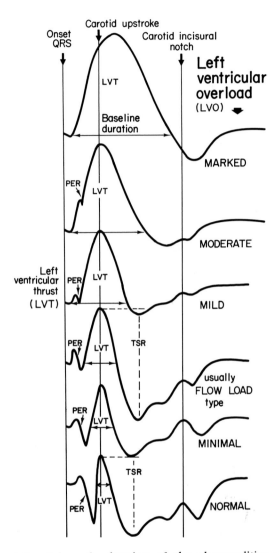

Fig. 4–9. Schematic drawing of the abnormalities encountered in the left ventricular overload. A normal curve is included at the bottom for comparison. Note that as the abnormality increases the apex impulse becomes exaggerated in amplitude, prolonged in duration along the baseline, and there is eventually an absence of the preejection retraction (PER) which occurs before the carotid upstroke.

RIGHT VENTRICULAR ABNORMALITIES

Description of Curve

The abnormalities in right ventricular disease usually occur in the lower parasternal region of the chest, K_{14}, K_{24}, and to a lesser degree in K_{34}. Figure 4–10 presents the location of the maximum outward impulse in a group of patients with mitral stenosis. A schematic drawing of the configuration is depicted in Figure 4–11. The abnormalities consist of exaggeration in amplitude and in duration of the initial right ventricular movement (greater than 0.085 sec in the parasternal region of the K_{24} record). In addition, as the abnormality progresses, total systolic retraction diminishes, and the midsystolic outward movement becomes very prominent, particularly in pressure loads.

Functional Abnormalities

The configuration of the right ventricular abnormalities depends to a large extent on the presence or absence of a pressure load on the right ventricle. For example, patients with atrial septal defect have an

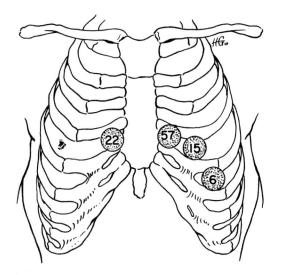

Fig. 4–10. The location of the maximum outward movement in a group of 46 patients with right ventricular overload (mitral stenosis). Note that in the majority of patients the outward movement is more prominent in the K_{24} position. (From Eddleman EE Jr, Harrison TR: The kinetocardiogram in patients with ischemic heart disease, Prog Cardiovasc Dis 6:189–211, 1963, with permission.)[21]

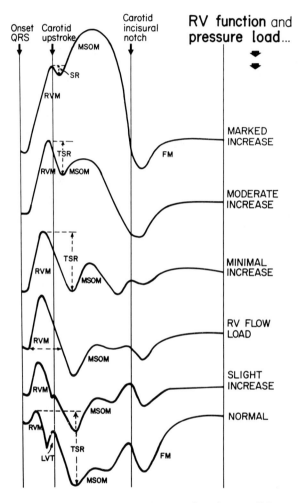

Onset Carotid
QRS upstroke

Carotid incisural notch

RV function and
pressure load...

MSOM
SR
RVM

MARKED
INCREASE

TSR
RVM MSOM
FM

MODERATE
INCREASE

TSR
RVM
MSOM

MINIMAL
INCREASE

RVM
MSOM

RV FLOW
LOAD

RVM
MSOM

SLIGHT
INCREASE

MSOM
RVM
NORMAL

TSR
LVT
FM
MSOM

Fig. 4–11. Schematic drawing of the abnormalities encountered in patients with right ventricular overload. A normal record is included for comparison. Note that as increased function in the right ventricle occurs the initial outward movement becomes larger in amplitude. The mid-systolic amplitude is markedly exaggerated in patients with right ventricular pressure load, as illustrated in this drawing.

exaggerated initial right ventricular movement (RVM) but absence of the midsystolic outward movement, with a large total systolic retraction (TSR). On the other hand, patients with pressure loads of the right ventricle, such as mitral stenosis, have not only an exaggerated right ventricular movement (RVM) but also a prominent midsystolic outward movement (MSOM), with a very small to almost absent total systolic retraction (TSR). The amplitude of the midsystolic outward movement as related to pressure load on the right ventricle will be discussed separately under the section on mitral stenosis.

Exceptions to the general description, particularly in congenital heart disease, will be discussed subsequently.

SPECIFIC ABNORMALITIES

Valvular Heart Disease

Mitral stenosis. Figure 4–12 shows a typical K_{24} record of a patient with mitral stenosis. The curve is that of a right ventricular pressure load.[8] The location on the precordium of the largest outward

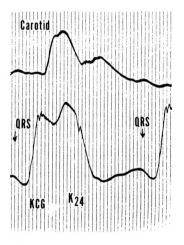

Fig. 4–12. An example of a K_{24} record from a patient with severe mitral stenosis. There is a mean pulmonary artery pressure of 68 mm Hg and mitral valve area, 0.8 cm. Notice the prominence of the initial right ventricular movement as well as the midsystolic outward movement, producing a sustained parasternal lift. This is a typical record of a patient with marked mitral stenosis.

movement usually occurs at the K_{24} area, although few occur in the K_{14}, a few in K_{35}, and fewer than 6 percent in K_{45} (see Fig. 4–10).[20] When the mean pulmonary artery pressure increases, the traces not only become exaggerated in amplitude, but there is a particular prominence to the midsystolic outward movement (MSOM). Figure 4–12 represents the curve in a patient with mean pulmonary artery pressure of 68 mm Hg; Figure 4–13 represents a patient with a mean pulmonary artery pressure of 24 mm Hg. Thus, with an increase in pulmonary artery pressure, the midsystolic outward movement (MSOM), as well as the absolute amplitude of the records, tends to become much larger. A large paradoxical heave has previously been described by Dressler as a sign of tight mitral stenosis.[90] This finding, in conjunction with other clinical data, offers a means by which functional abnormality can be assessed using noninvasive techniques.

The best evidence that the midsystolic outward movement is related to the pressure load is that this movement diminishes almost immediately after surgical correction of the valvular lesion, provided pulmonary artery pressure is reduced.[13] Figure 4–14 presents a record taken in a patient with mitral stenosis before and after mitral commissurotomy. The pulmonary artery pressure was reduced to normal

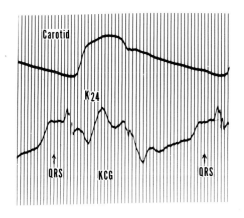

Fig. 4–13. An example of a K_{24} record from a patient with proved mitral stenosis but with only a slight elevation in mean pulmonary artery pressure. The hemodynamics are as follows: mean pulmonary artery pressure, 24 mm Hg; mean wedge pressure (or pulmonary capillary pressure), 16 mm Hg; left ventricular stroke volume, 61 cc; and calculated valve area, 2.1 cm. Note that there is only a slight exaggeration in amplitude of both the initial right ventricular and the midsystolic outward movements.

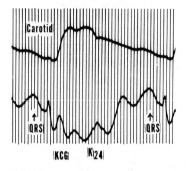

Fig. 4–14. The K_{24} record from the same patient as in Figure 4–12, following commissurotomy. The hemodynamics have returned to normal. Note that the K_{24} record now is essentially normal in contour. This illustration suggests that once the functional aspects of the mitral disease are corrected the kinetocardiogram tends to return to normal. Thus, the kinetocardiogram is highly sensitive to functional abnormalities of the ventricle.

and there was associated an immediate decrease in the midsystolic outward movement. These findings support the concept that the initial right ventricular movement is probably related to hypertrophy of the right ventricle, whereas the midsystolic outward movement reflects the pressure load.

Mitral insufficiency. Figure 4-15 is an example of the K_{34} trace of a patient with severe mitral insufficiency. The records are characterized primarily by an exaggeration of the ventricular impulse (flow-type load), and usually at the K_{34} area there is a marked exaggeration of the late systolic outward movement (LSOM), as previously reported.[9] It has become increasingly apparent that the late systolic outward movement is related to some extent to the degree of regurgitant flow. However, there are probably other factors which affect its amplitude, for example, size and compliance of the left atrium. Nevertheless, the amplitude is roughly proportional to the amount of regurgitant flow, which is illustrated in Figure 4–16 from a patient with relatively mild mitral insufficiency. This is apparent when compared to Figure 4–15. We should emphasize that patients with very minimal mitral insufficiency have an almost normal record; consequently, kinetocardiography is useful in this situation in evaluating the functional significance of systolic murmurs. For example, if a patient has a systolic murmur of long standing but still has a relatively normal pattern in

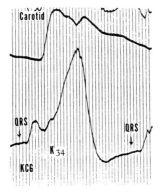

Fig. 4–15. A K_{34} record from a patient with pure mitral insufficiency with the following hemodynamics: mean pulmonary artery pressure, 26 mm Hg; left ventricular end-diastolic volume, 240 cc; left ventricular end-systolic volume, 113 cc; left ventricular stroke volume, 127 cc; forward stroke volume, only 24 cc/beat; and regurgitant flow, 103 cc/beat or 10 L/min (81 percent). Note the prominence in the late systolic outward movement in this record which is much more exaggerated than that presented in Figure 4–16 in which the regurgitant flow is considerably less.

the kinetocardiogram, then it is very unlikely that there is clinically significant regurgitation.

Since this late systolic outward movement parallels the V wave of the left atrial pressure pulse, the movement may be considered to be due to the regurgitation into the posterior chamber of the left atrium resulting in an anterior recoil or displacement of the left ventricle.

Mitral stenosis and mitral insufficiency. Mitral stenosis and mitral insufficiency are commonly associated. The kinetocardiographic pattern usually exhibits a combination of findings, as mentioned. The early systolic outward movement (RVM) peaks early in systole, it is somewhat sustained; and in addition, there is a prominent LSOM which peaks at the time of the carotid incisural notch. If there is sufficient left ventricular flow load, the patients will exhibit an abnormal exaggeration of the left ventricular impulse as well.

Aortic stenosis. The recordings from patients with aortic stenosis are not very characteristic and only demonstrate a pressure-type load on the left ventricle (see Fig. 4–17). It is important to point out that

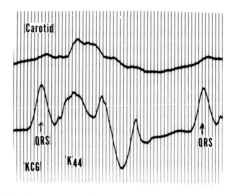

Fig. 4–16. A K_{44} record taken from a patient with mild mitral insufficiency. Hemodynamics are as follows: mean pulmonary artery pressure, 19 mm Hg; left ventricular end-diastolic volume, 208 cc; left ventricular end-systolic volume, 159 cc; total stroke volume, 49 cc/beat; forward stroke volume, 37 cc/beat; and regurgitant flow, 11 cc/beat or 0.99 L/min (23 percent). Note that the patient has a large atrial movement, somewhat prominent mid-systolic movement, and a fairly prominent late systolic outward movement reaching a peak at approximately the carotid incisural notch. This movement, although present, is not as exaggerated as in patients with severe mitral insufficiency, as illustrated in Figure 4–15.

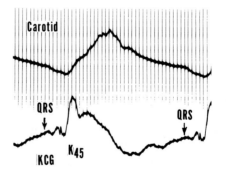

Fig. 4–17. A record taken from the K_{45} position in a patient with pure aortic stenosis. Patient had a peak gradient of 58 mm Hg and a valve area of 0.9 cm². Note that the left ventricular impulse is not markedly exaggerated in amplitude but sustained throughout systole. The typical contour of the slow rise in the carotid pulse is also noted.

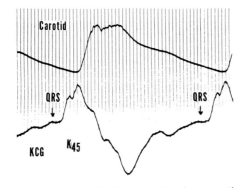

Fig. 4–18. Left ventricular impulse in a patient with severe aortic insufficiency. Note the exaggeration of the initial impulse, but there is significant systolic retraction during ejection. Hemodynamic measurements in this patient were as follows: central aortic pressure, 100/35 mm Hg; left ventricular end-diastolic volume, 667 cc; left ventricular end-systolic volume, 374 cc; left ventricular stroke volume, 293 cc; effective stroke volume, 72 cc/beat; and regurgitant flow, 221 cc/beat with 16.58 L/min (75 percent).

approximately 5 to 10 percent of patients with aortic stenosis will have a very small or absent left ventricular impulse. This finding is not understood at present. The amplitude and the duration of the left ventricular impulse are both related to the severity of the aortic valvular stenosis as measured by the aortic ventricular gradient (Eddleman et al).* In other words, the greater the amplitude and the longer the duration, the greater the chance of a high-pressure gradient across the aortic valve. However, this alone is not sufficient information to predict the gradient with any reliability. The total systolic retraction is usually reduced in patients with aortic stenosis, probably because these patients have a diminished stroke volume. The atrial waves are also exaggerated, and whether this is a reliable method of quantitation of left ventricular end-diastolic pressure is not clear at this time.

Aortic insufficiency. Figure 4–18 presents the K_{45} record from a patient with severe aortic insufficiency. Note the left ventricular flow-load type of pattern described. In aortic insufficiency the left ventricular impulse, although abnormal, is not as prolonged in duration as in aortic

* Eddleman EE Jr, Frommeyer WB Jr, Lyle DP, et al: A critical analysis of the clinical factors in estimating severity of aortic valvular disease (American Journal of Cardiology 31:687–695, 1973).

stenosis and has a configuration of a left ventricular flow load (see Fig. 4–9).[11] The impulse is exaggerated in amplitude, prolonged in duration, and followed by a rather marked systolic retraction due to the extremely large initial forward stroke volume in patients with aortic regurgitation. In patients with isolated severe and long-standing aortic insufficiency, the impulse may be completely sustained throughout systole, such as in aortic stenosis.

Combined valvular disease. Recordings from combined valvular disease (aortic stenosis, aortic insufficiency, mitral stenosis, and mitral insufficiency) become much more complex because there is evidence of both left ventricular as well as right ventricular abnormality. However, the recordings do serve a useful purpose in that the presence of a right parasternal lift as well as an abnormal left ventricular impulse is one of the more reliable means of estimating right ventricular overload as well as left ventricular overload. This is illustrated in Figure 4–19.

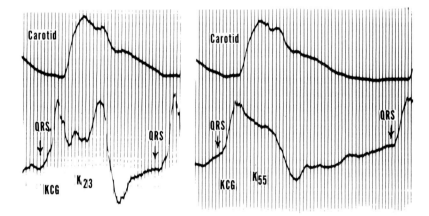

Fig. 4–19. A K_{23} and K_{55} record from a patient with mitral stenosis, mitral insufficiency, aortic stenosis, and aortic insufficiency. Patient had the following hemodynamic measurements: left ventricular end-diastolic volume, 242 cc; left ventricular end-systolic volume, 118 cc; left ventricular stroke volume, 124 cc; effective stroke volume, 54 cc/beat; regurgitant flow, 70 cc/beat or 6.16 L/min (55 percent) (regurgitant flow indicates both mitral and aortic flow); and mean gradient across the mitral valve, 13.5 mm Hg; mean gradient across the aortic valve, 26 mm Hg; and aortic peak gradient, 42 mm Hg. Note that in the K_{23} record, there is exaggeration of the right ventricular movement in addition to the late systolic outward movement indicating mitral insufficiency. The left ventricular impulse is exaggerated in amplitude, prolonged in duration, and sustained, which can be interpreted as left ventricular hypertrophy or overload.

Ischemic Heart Disease

Myocardial infarction. A previous investigation demonstrated that all the patients studied at one time or another during the course of acute myocardial infarction had an abnormal outward paradoxical movement.[14] Subsequently, approximately one-third of these diminished or either disappeared on recovery. The characteristic feature is a large sustained outward movement, as illustrated in Figure 4–20. It is most frequently located in K_{44} and K_{34}, occasionally in K_{24}, and in the mid-epigastric region (see Fig. 4–21). The paradoxical movement apparently has some relationship to the severity of the infarction since the bulges are more extensively distributed over the precordium in very large infarctions. Those patients with large and transmural infarctions even have an impulse that is almost identical to the left ventricular pressure curves (see Fig. 4-22). It is difficult to distinguish the bulges caused by myocardial infarction from severe left ventricular hypertrophy when the impulse occurs at the K_{45} or K_{55} positions. In some instances the two may coexist. The differentiation must be made from other clinical information.[21]

In addition to the paradoxical outward movements as described, patients with myocardial infarctions may also have a prominent late systolic outward movement. This usually occurs in patients who develop mitral insufficiency during the course of their disease resulting either from a rupture of the chordae tendineae or papillary muscle, or from

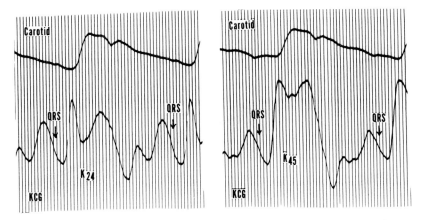

Fig. 4–20. The K_{24} and K_{45} position records from a patient with a posterior diaphragmatic myocardial infarction. Coronary angiogram revealed three-vessel coronary artery disease. There was complete occlusion of left anterior descending and left circumflex. In addition, the left diagonal branch was narrowed, along with an 80 percent narrowing of the right coronary artery. A large akinetic area was noted on the anterior left ventricular wall.

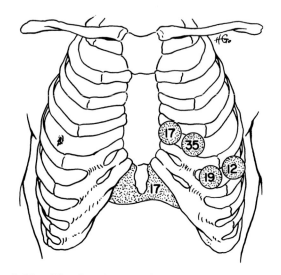

Fig. 4–21. The location of the maximum bulge in 69 patients with myocardial infarctions out of a total of 102 patients. Note that 35 percent have the maximum bulge located in the K_{34} position. (From Eddleman EE Jr, Harrison TR: The kinetocardiogram in patients with ischemic heart disease, Prog Cardiovasc Dis 6:189–211, 1963, with permission.) [21]

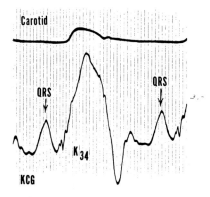

Fig. 4–22. A K_{34} record from a patient with myocardial infarction. Coronary angiograms on this patient demonstrated an almost total block of the right coronary artery with significant disease of the left coronary artery as well. Note that the paradoxical outward movement in the K_{34} record resembles that of a left ventricular pressure pulse.

dysfunction or dilatation of the mitral valve ring. Figure 4-23 illustrates a recording from a patient with ruptured chordae tendineae with mitral insufficiency, demonstrating a very prominent late systolic outward movement. The abnormality is apparently related to the degree of mitral regurgitation. However, in the very acute stage of the process some patients may not have a late systolic outward movement probably because of the small or normal size or the decreased compliance of the left atrium.

In general, the larger the infarction, the more extensive the bulges are over the precordium. It has not been documented, but it is our impression that patients with precordial bulges over the entire precordial area have a more grave prognosis than those in whom the bulges are located in one isolated area. This finding may be a useful adjunct in evaluating the subsequent course of patients with myocardial infarction.

Significant bulges and paradoxical movements may be due either to akinetic areas or to true ventricular aneurysms. At the present time there is no way to distinguish between the two. The mechanism presumably is a ballooning of the noncontractile area in the ventricular

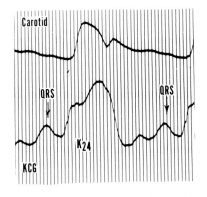

Fig. 4–23. A K_{24} record from a patient with myocardial infarction, moderate mitral insufficiency due to a ruptured chordae tendineae. Patient had the following hemodynamic measurements: left ventricular end-diastolic pressure, 189 cc; left ventricular end-systolic volume, 137 cc; mean pulmonary artery pressure, 23 mm Hg; pulmonary wedge pressure, 15 mm Hg; left ventricular stroke volume, 52 cc; ejection fraction, 0.27; and regurgitant flow, 22 cc/beat (or 42 percent). Note the prominent late systolic movement. Essentially the same configuration was present in the kinetocardiogram in the K_{34}, K_{41}, and K_{45} records.

wall as ventricular pressure increases. In addition, it is important to recognize that some paradoxical bulges may be clinically significant even though an akinetic area or an aneurysm is not demonstrated on biplane angiography. We have seen one patient with an aneurysm and an akinetic area, removed surgically, which was detected only by the presence of precordial bulges and not by biplane angiography. Thus, it is possible that the presence of these abnormal movements may offer additional information to that provided by invasive techniques such as quantitative angiocardiography.

Angina pectoris. Approximately two-thirds of patients with angina pectoris have some degree of abnormality in the kinetocardiogram. These abnormalities are difficult to describe since there is considerable variation from patient to patient. They range from large paradoxical outward movements to early systolic bulges, late systolic bulges (probably due to mitral insufficiency or to papillary muscle dysfunction), and a combination of early and late systolic bulges. About one-third of patients with angina pectoris have normal records. Clinically, the records are useful in diagnosis. An abnormal record may provide important evidence to confirm the diagnosis (Fig. 4–24 is one example).

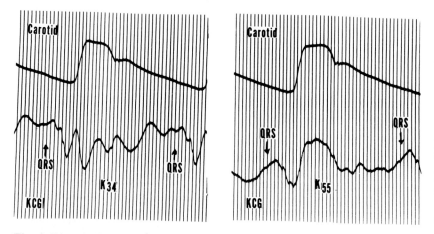

Fig. 4–24. A kinetocardiographic record showing the K_{34} and K_{55} positions from a patient with angina pectoris but no evidence of documented myocardial infarction. Coronary angiogram demonstrated coronary artery disease with complete occlusion of the right coronary artery and the left anterior descending branch. Note that the record shows a midsystolic bulge at the K_{55} area and possibly an early systolic bulge at the K_{34} area.

CONGENITAL HEART DISEASE

Atrial Septic Defect

Atrial septal defect is characterized by right ventricular flow load, as presented in Figure 4–25 which is an example of a patient with a normal pulmonary artery pressure with a large pulmonary blood flow. Notice that the abnormality is an exaggeration of the right ventricular movement followed by a marked total systolic retraction (TSR). As pulmonary artery pressure increases, total systolic retraction is diminished, and the midsystolic outward movement becomes exaggerated (Fig. 4–26). In a previous study it was possible to predict, using discriminant function analysis, whether the mean pulmonary artery pressure was greater than 25 mm Hg in patients with atrial septal defect.[23] The finding that one can discriminate between pressure and flow loads in atrial septal defect further confirms that functional abnormalities, as well as the anatomical lesion, affects the contour of the kinetocardiogram.

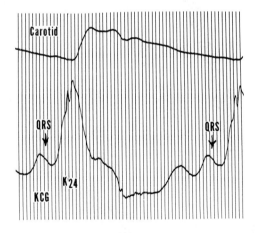

Fig. 4–25. A K_{24} record taken from a patient with atrial septal defect with a left-to-right shunt. The following hemodynamics were present on catheterization: cardiac index, 3.91 L/min/m²; pulmonary blood flow, 19.6 L/min; systemic blood flow, 7.31 L/min; mean pulmonary artery pressure, 24 mm Hg. Note the marked exaggeration of the right ventricular movement followed by a prominent systolic retraction during ejection.

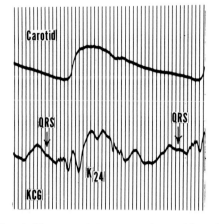

Fig. 4–26. A K_{24} record from a patient with atrial septal defect and a left-to-right shunt. The hemodynamic data are as follows: mean pulmonary artery pressure, 80 mm Hg; pulmonary resistance, 1608 dynes/sec cm^{-5}; right-to-left shunt 1.2 L/min; and cardiac index 2.51 L/min/m^2. Note the prominence of the midsystolic outward movement which is characteristic in patients with increased pulmonary artery pressure and does not retract during ejection such as that seen in Figure 4–25. In that instance the pulmonary artery pressure was within normal range with a marked left-to-right shunt.

Ventricular Septal Defect

The contour of the kinetocardiogram in ventricular septal defect is similar to that for atrial septal defect, as illustrated in Figure 4–27. Again, there is an increase in the midsystolic outward movement when the pulmonary artery pressure is elevated with a reversal of the shunt (from right to left).

Pulmonic Stenosis

The kinetocardiographic findings in pulmonic stenosis are unusual and seemingly paradoxical when compared to other congenital abnormalities. Pulmonary stenosis is characterized only by exaggeration of the initial right ventricular movement (RVM) in the parasternal region of the chest and an absence of a prominent midsystolic outward movement.* Often the contour from the pulmonic area resembles a pul-

* One would have suspected a large MSOM since the right ventricular systolic pressure is higher in these patients, based on what occurred in mitral stenosis.

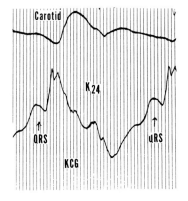

Fig. 4–27. A K_{24} record from a patient with ventricular septal defect and a left-to-right shunt. Patient demonstrated the following hemodynamic measurements: cardiac index, 5.35 L/min/m²; total pulmonary blood flow, 7.4 L/min; systemic blood flow, 5.4 L/min; mean pulmonary artery pressure, 20 mm Hg. Note the marked increase in exaggeration of right ventricular movement which is prolonged in duration and amplitude. The contour is typical of a right ventricular flow load.

monary artery pressure curve. At the apex (K_{44}, K_{45}, or K_{55} areas) there appears to be a left ventricular impulse (see Fig. 4–28).[24] Thus, the records resemble a flow-type load on the right ventricle associated with a left ventricular impulse. The explanation for the systolic retraction and the lack of the sustained impulse in the parasternal region of the chest, as one might suspect, is unknown at the present. The mechanism for what appears to be an exaggerated left ventricular impulse is assumed to be a right apex impulse rather than a left one. Nevertheless, these features along with other clinical data can be exceedingly useful. A combination of findings including a loud ejection-type murmur, heard best over the pulmonic area, right ventricular hypertrophy on electrocardiogram, what appears to be a flow-type load in the parasternal region of the chest, and a left ventricular impulse can be considered almost diagnostic of pulmonic stenosis.

Tetralogy of Fallot

The records for this group of patients vary considerably. Often there are very little abnormalities in the traces (see Fig. 4–29). It is peculiar that this congenital abnormality produces so little change in

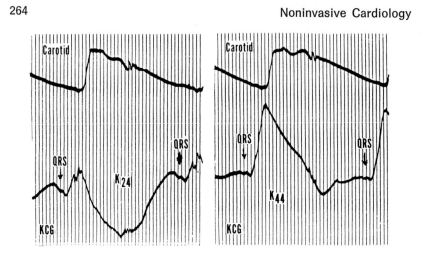

Fig. 4–28. The K_{24} and K_{44} records from a patient with mild pulmonic stenosis. Hemodynamic measurements were peak gradient, 10 mm Hg; cardiac index, 3.10 L/min/m²; and blood flow, 4.03 L/min. Note that the right ventricular movement at K_{24} is exaggerated, but the K_{44} has a moderately sustained impulse throughout ejection which resembles that of left ventricular hypertrophy.

the precordial movements, and the features as described are probably not too useful since there is such a wide variety of patterns.

Patent Ductus Arteriosus

Patent ductus is characterized by increase in flow load on both right and left ventricles. This produces an exaggeration of the right ventricular movement (RVM) followed by a marked systolic retraction and an exaggerated left ventricular thrust (see Fig. 4–30). When one considers the hemodynamics of patent ductus, this is exactly as would be expected.

Ebstein's Anomaly

This is a rare congenital abnormality; however, the features of the kinetocardiographic trace appear to be almost pathognomonic. Figure 4–31 presents the kinetocardiogram from one patient. The right precordium is characterized by two movements: a large early systolic outward movement and large mid- to late systolic outward movement, whereas the left precordium shows a marked systolic retraction almost

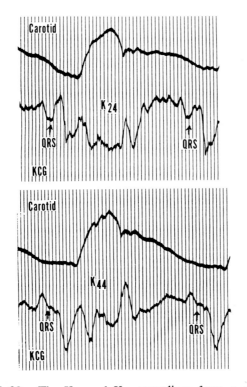

Fig. 4–29. The K_{24} and K_{44} recordings from a patient with documented evidence of tetralogy of Fallot. Patient had the following hemodynamic measurements: peak gradient across the pulmonic valve, 125 mm Hg; cardiac index, 2.56 L/min/m²; systemic blood flow, 3.99 L/min; and mean pulmonary artery pressure, 12 mm Hg. Although the patient has a number of abnormal movements in the records, there are no specific changes.

during the entire period of ejection. This produces a "rocking-type" motion of the precordium.

Eisenmenger's Syndrome

Eisenmenger's syndrome is a mixture of congential abnormalities that are difficult to characterize by kinetocardiography. Sufficient data have not been thus far accumulated to afford a consistent pattern of the recordings in patients with this syndrome.

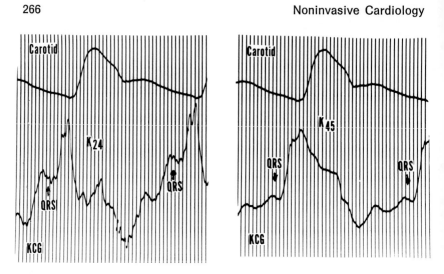

Fig. 4–30. The K_{24} and K_{45} records from a patient with patent ductus arteriosus who had a left-to-right shunt of 6.2 L/min. Additional cardiac catheterization findings were as follows: pulmonary resistance, 56 dynes/sec cm^{-5}; cardiac index, 3.00 L/min/m^2; mean pulmonary artery pressure, 20 mm Hg; and systemic blood flow, 5.10 L/min. Note the large right ventricular movement following the QRS onset in the K_{24} position and the prominence of the left ventricular thrust in the K_{45} position.

MISCELLANEOUS DISEASES

Hypertrophic Subaortic Stenosis

Hypertrophic subaortic stenosis is characterized primarily by double apex impulse (see Fig. 4–32). The second outward impulse of the left ventricular thrust does not correlate exactly in time with the late systolic outward movement noted in the carotid pulse. However, the recording of a double apical impulse along with a typical carotid pulse is considered almost pathognomonic of hypertrophic subaortic stenosis. This combination has occurred in over 90 percent of patients observed.

Myocarditis

In myocarditis there are often paradoxical outward movements present; however, these are not sufficiently characteristic of the abnormality to be clinically useful.

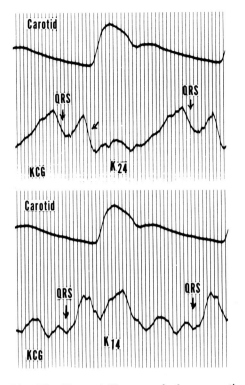

Fig. 4–31. The K_{14} and K_{24} records from a patient with Ebstein's anomaly. Note that the K_{14} position has a double systolic outward movement, whereas in the K_{24} position there is a retraction during ejection (see arrow in the K_{24} position).

Constrictive Pericarditis

It is surprising that kinetocardiographic recordings in patients with constrictive pericarditis often reveal movements that are not small or absent, but actually large (see Fig. 4–33). However, there is nothing specific in the recordings which would aid in the differential diagnosis of this disease.

SUMMARY

The kinetocardiogram, although related to movement, shape, and positional changes of the heart, appears to be related to the functional aspect of the ventricle as well. The records are clinically useful in

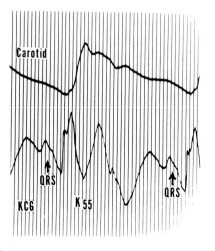

Fig. 4–32. A K_{55} record from a patient with proved hypertrophic subaortic stenosis. Note the double left ventricular impulse (two systolic outward movements). In this patient the gradient below the aortic valve ranged between 20 and 40 mm Hg.

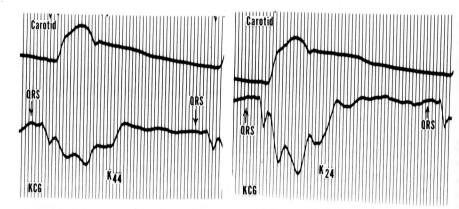

Fig. 4–33. The kinetocardiographic traces (K_{24} and K_{44} records) from a patient with constrictive pericarditis. The patient had extensive calcification of the pericardium. On cardiac catheterization the following hemodynamics were noted: cardiac index, 2.39 L/min/m²; mean pulmonary artery pressure, 20 mm Hg; mean pulmonary wedge pressure, 10 mm Hg; left ventricular pressure, 118/10 mm Hg, rising to an end-diastolic of 30 mm Hg after exercise; mean right atrial pressure, 10 mm Hg; AV oxygen difference, 7.40 vol percent; and ejection fraction, 0.38. Note that although there was extensive pericarditis and constriction in this patient, the precordial movements are still fairly prominent.

confirming the suspected cardiac diagnosis and aiding in the evaluation and quantification of functional abnormalities of the hemodynamics. In some instances the records offer a specific type of pattern.

ACKNOWLEDGMENTS

Appreciation is expressed to Mr. A. Harry Germagian and the Medical Illustration Division, Veterans Administration Hospital, Birmingham, Alabama, for the art work and illustrations used in this manuscript.

REFERENCES

1. Marey EJ: La méthode graphique dans les sciences expérimentales et principalement en physiologie et en médecine (ed 2). Paris, Masson, 1885, p 663
2. Crehore AC, Meara FS: The micrograph: An instrument which records the microscopic movements of a diaphragm by means of light interference and some records of physiological events showing the registration of sound waves including the human voice. J Exp Med 13:616–625, 1911
3. Dressler W: Die brustwandpulsationen. Wien, Austria, Verlag, 1933, p 181
4. Johnston FD, Overy DC: Vibrations of low frequency over the precordium. Circulation 3:579–588, 1951
5. Eddleman EE Jr, Willis K, Reeves TJ, et al: The kinetocardiogram I. Method of recording precordial movements. Circulation 8:269–275, 1953
6. Eddleman EE Jr, Willis K, Christianson L, et al: The kinetocardiogram II. The normal configuration and amplitude. Circulation 8:370–380, 1953
7. Eddleman EE Jr, Willis K: The kinetocardiogram III. The distribution of forces over the anterior chest. Circulation 8:569–577, 1953
8. Eddleman EE Jr, Yoe RH, Tucker WT, et al: The dynamics of ventricular contraction and relaxation in patients with mitral stenosis as studied by the kinetocardiogram and ballistocardiogram. Circulation 11:774–783, 1955
9. Tucker WT, Knowles JL, Eddleman EE Jr: Mitral insufficiency: Cardiac mechanics as studied with the kinetocardiogram and ballistocardiogram. Circulation 12:278–285, 1955
10. Eddleman EE Jr, Hefner L, Reeves TJ, et al: Movements and forces of the human heart. I. The genesis of the apical impulses. AMA Arch Intern Med 99:401–410, 1957
11. Eddleman EE Jr: Kinetocardiographic findings in aortic insufficiency. Am Heart J 53:530–541, 1957
12. Eddleman EE Jr, Reeves TJ: Kinetocardiography, in Warren JV (ed): Methods in Medical Research, vol 7. Chicago, Year Book, 1958, pp 107–118
13. Eddleman EE Jr: Kinetocardiographic changes as the result of mitral commissurotomy. Am J Med 25:733–743, 1958
14. Suh SK, Eddleman EE Jr: Kinetocardiographic findings of myocardial infarction. Circulation 19:531–542, 1959

15. Eddleman EE Jr: Ultralow frequency precordial movements—kinetocardio-grams. Am J Cardiol 4:649–651, 1959
16. Eddleman EE Jr, Thomas HD: The recognition and differentiation of right ventricular pressure and flow loads. A correlative study of kinetocardio-grams, electrocardiograms, fluoroscopy, and cardiac catheterization data in patients with mitral stenosis, septal defect, pulmonic stenosis and isolated pulmonary hypertension. Am J Cardiol 4:652–661, 1959
17. Eddleman EE Jr, Hughes ML, Thomas HD: Estimation of pulmonary artery pressure and pulmonary vascular resistance from ultra low frequency pre-cordial movements (kinetocardiograms). Am J Cardiol 4:662–668, 1959
18. Eddleman EE Jr: Cardiovascular dynamics—Technics for indirect measure-ments in Gordon BL (ed): Clinical Cardiopulmonary Physiology (ed 2). New York, Grune & Stratton, 1960, pp 158–176
19. Eddleman EE Jr, Langley JO: Paradoxical pulsation of the precordium in myocardial infarction and angina pectoris. Am Heart J 63:579–581, 1962
20. Davie JC, Langley JO, Dodson WH, et al: Clinical and kinetocardiographic studies of paradoxical precordial motion. Am Heart J 63:775–807, 1962
21. Eddleman EE Jr, Harrison TR: The kinetocardiogram in patients with ischemic heart disease. Prog Cardiovasc Dis 6:189–211, 1963
22. Eddleman EE Jr: Kinetocardiographic changes in ischemic heart disease. Circulation 32:650–655, 1965
23. Eddleman EE Jr, Holt JH, Bancroft WH Jr: Computer analysis of the kinetocardiogram from patients with atrial septal defects. Am Heart J 71:435–445, 1966
24. Holt JH Jr, Eddleman EE Jr: The precordial movements in adults with pul-monic stenosis. Circulation 35:492–500, 1967
25. Bancroft WH Jr, Eddleman EE Jr: Methods and physical characteristics of the kinetocardiographic and apexcardiographic systems for recording low-frequency precordial motion. Am Heart J 73:756–764, 1967
26. Eddleman EE Jr, Bancroft WH Jr: Quantification of the kinetocardiogram. Comput Biomed Res 1:237–250, 1967
27. Eddleman EE Jr: The effect of age on the normal kinetocardiogram. Ala J Med Sci 6:22–26, 1969
28. Eddleman EE Jr, Bancroft WH Jr: Graphic recording of low frequency pre-cordial motion. Ala J Med Sci 8:178–183, 1971
29. Harrison TR, et al: Movements of human ventricles. Trans Assoc Am Phy-sicians 66:250–256, 1953
30. Harrison TR: Palpation of the precordial impulses. Stanford Med Bull 13:385–392, 1955
31. Norman J, Harrison TR: Movements and forces of the human heart. IV. Pre-cordial movements in relation to ejection and filling of the ventricles. AMA Arch Intern Med 101:582–591, 1958
32. Harrison TR, Lowder JA, Hefner LL, et al: Movements and forces of the human heart. V. Precordial movements in relation to atrial contraction. Circulation 18:82–91, 1958
33. Harrison TR, Hughes L: Precordial systolic bulges during anginal attacks. Trans Assoc Am Physicians 71:174–185, 1958
34. Harrison TR: Precordial movements (editorial). Am J Cardiol 4:427–429, 1959

35. Harrison TR: Movements of the heart and velocity of pressure change during the first part of systole. Bull Johns Hopkins Hosp 104:290–308, 1959
36. Harrison TR: Some clinical and physiologic aspects of angina pectoris. Bull Johns Hopkins Hosp 104:275–289, 1959
37. Coghlan C, Prieto G, Harrison TR: Movements of the heart during the period between the onset of ventricular excitation and the start of left ventricular ejection. Am Heart J 62:65–82, 1961
38. Prieto G, Coghlan C, Harrison TR: Movements of the heart during the period between the onset of relaxation and the beginning of ventricular filling. Am Heart J 62:528–541, 1961
39. Skinner NS Jr, Leibeskind RS, Phillips HL, et al: Angina pectoris. Effect of exertion and of nitrites on the precordial movements. Am Heart J 61:250–258, 1961
40. Harrison TR, Coghlan C, Prieto G: Movements of the heart during ejection. Am Heart J 62:804–820, 1961
41. Harrison TR: Movements of the heart: Some clinical and physiologic considerations. Arch Intern Med 109:136–145, 1962
42. Harrison TR: The interpretation of chest pain: With especial reference to angina pectoris. World-Wide Abstracts 5:8–15, 1962
43. Harrison TR, Kelly D, Russell RO Jr, et al: The relation of age to the duration of contraction, ejection, and relaxation of the normal human heart. Am Heart J 67:189–199, 1964
44. Coleman N, Finney JO Jr, Sheffield LT, et al: Precordial movements in relation to age. Am Heart J 67:53–60, 1964
45. Harrison TR: Some present and future problems in the treatment of heart disease (T Cook Smith Lecture). J Ky Med Assoc 62:753–760, 1964
46. Harrison TR: Some unanswered questions concerning enlargement and failure of the heart (Grady Reddick Memorial Lecture). Am Heart J 69:100–115, 1965
47. Luisada AA, Magri G: Low-frequency tracings of the precordium and epigastrium in normal subjects and cardiac patients. Am Heart J 44:545–564, 1952
48. Bertrab R von, Reist P, Schweizer W: Das kinetokardiogramm beim normalen. Z Kreislaufforsch 52:553–562, 1963
49. Schweizer W, Bertrab R von, Reist P: Kinetocardiography in coronary artery disease. Br Heart J 27:263–268, 1965
50. Reist P, Schweizer W, Bertrab R von: Das kinetokardiogramm bei volum-und druckuberlastung der rechten kammer. Z Kreislaufforsch 527–536, 1965
51. Mahlich J: Ueber die Beziehung zwischen apexkardiogramm und kinetokardiogramm beim normalen. Z Kreislaufforsch 56:874–885, 1967
52. Bertrab R von, Mahlich J: Das kinetokardiogramm bei druck—und volumuberlästung des linken herzens. Z Kreislaufforsch 57:29–41, 1967
53. Bertrab R von, Mahlich J: Das kinetokardiogramm bei druck—und volumuberlästung des linken herzens. Z Kreislaufforsch 57:29–41, 1968
54. Rörvik K: Apexcardiography, Phonocardiography and Ballistocardiography— Their Diagnostic and Prognostic Significance. Oslo, Norway, Lie, 1962, p 77
55. Peltier J: Le Kinetocardiogramme: Application a l'etude des cardiopathies ischemiques. Lille Med, p 174, 1969

56. Finardi G: La Cinetocardiografia. Milano, Italy, Ambrosiana-Milano, 1968, p 187

57. Kesteloot H, Willems J, Vollenhoven E Van: On the physical principles and methodology of mechanocardiography. Acta Cardiol 24:147–160, 1969

58. Baragan J, Fernandez-Caamano F, Sozutek Y, et al: Chronic left complete bundle-branch block. Phonocardiographic and mechanocardiographic study of 30 cases. Br Heart J 30:196–202, 1968

59. Beilin L, Mounsey P: The left ventricular impulse in hypertensive heart disease. Br Heart J 24:409–421, 1962

60. Gillam PM, Deliyannis AA, Mounsey JP: The left parasternal impulse. Br Heart J 26:726–736, 1964

61. Mounsey JPD: The impulse cardiogram and the phonocardiogram. Cardiologia (Basel) 48:203–212, 1966

62. Nagle RE, Boicourt OW, Gillam PMS, Mounsey JPD: Cardiac impulse in hypertrophic obstructive cardiomyopathy. Br Heart J 28:419–425, 1966

63. Nagle RE, Tamara FA: Left parasternal impulse in pulmonary stenosis and atrial septal defect. Br Heart J 29:735–741, 1967

64. Kountz WB, Gilson AS, Smith JR: Use of the cathode ray for recording heart sounds and vibrations: Studies on normal heart. Am Heart J 20:667–676, 1940

65. Smith JR, Gilson AS, Kountz WB: Use of the cathode ray for recording heart sounds and vibrations; Studies on muscular element of the first heart sound. Am Heart J 27:17–24, 1941

66. Smith JR, Edwards JC, Kountz WB: Use of the cathode ray for recording heart sounds and vibrations; Total cardiac vibrations in one hundred normal subjects. Am Heart J 21:228–237, 1941

67. Kountz WB, Smith JR: Studies on the early recognition of myocardial disease by use of the vibrocardiogram. South Med J 35:713–719, 1942

68. Down M: Vibrocardiography—Study of vibrations in the normal heart. Australas Ann Med 5:54–61, 1956

69. Rosa LM: The "displacement": Vibrocardiogram of the precordium in the low frequency range. Am J Cardiol 4:191–199, 1959

70. Agress CM, Fields LG: New method for analyzing heart vibrations. I. Low frequency vibrations. Am J Cardiol 4:184–190, 1959

71. Agress CM, Fields LG, Wegner S, et al: The normal vibrocardiogram—physiologic variations and relation to cardiodynamic events. Am J Cardiol 8:22–31, 1961

72. Agress CM, Wegner S: The vibrocardiographic exercise test for coronary insufficiency. Am J Cardiol 9:541–546, 1962

73. Agress CM, Wegner S, Bleifer DJ, et al: The common origin of precordial vibrations. Am J Cardiol 13:226–231, 1964

74. Agress CM, Wegner S, Bleifer DJ, et al: Measurement of isometric contraction and ejection time by the vibrocardiogram. Am J Cardiol 13:340–348, 1964

75. Ueda H, Kobayashi T, Sato C, et al: Precordial low-frequency vibrocardiography. I. Method of recording. Jap Heart J 3:176–182, 1962

76. Kobayashi T, Sakamoto T, Ueda H: Precordial low-frequency vibrocardiography II. The normal configuration. Jap Heart J 3:231–239, 1962

77. Mounsey P: Precordial ballistocardiography. Br Heart J 19:259–271, 1957

78. Hollis WJ: Time relations of the precordial force-thrust and the acceleration

ballistocardiogram from a pendulum and ball bearing platform. Exp Med Surg 16:116–126, 1958

79. Hollis WJ: Preliminary observations on the relation of the precordial force-thrust to intracardiac pressure events. Exp Med Surg 16:127–137, 1958

80. Rosa LM, Constantino JP, Reich R, et al: The precordial accelerogram in normal subjects and noncardiac patients. Exp Med Surg 19:207–222, 1961

81. Rosa LM, Constantino JP, Reich R: The precordial acceleration tracing in hypertensive patients. Am J Cardiol 9:26–31, 1962

82. Rosa LM, Constantino JP, Karsak N, et al: The precordial accelerogram in ischemic heart disease—A study of middle-aged and old patients with angina pectoris; Recent and old myocardial infarction. Am J Cardiol 9:534–540, 1962

83. Rosa LM, Luisada AA: The clinical aspects of accelerography. J Maine Med Assoc 53:80–83, 1962

84. Rosa LM MacCanon DM, Inoue T: Effects of hemorrhage and shock on the precordial acceleration tracing (PACT) of the dog. Exp Med Surg 21:13–27, 1963

85. Rosa LM, Constantino JP, Harris R: Effects of physical exertion on the accelerogram in young, middle-aged and old subjects without clinical heart disease. J Am Geriat Soc 11:287–298, 1963

86. Rosa LM, MacCanon DM, Kusukawa R, et al: Analog computers in precordial pulse studies. Exp Med Surg 22:71–80, 1964

87. Eddleman EE Jr: Inspection and palpation of the precordium. In Hurst JW, Logue RB (eds): The Heart, 2nd ed, New York, McGraw-Hill, 1970, pp 192–207

88. Stallmann FW, Pipberger HV: Automatic recognition of electrocardiographic waves by digital computer. Circ Res 9:1138–1143, 1961

89. Kyle MC, Freis ED: Computer identification of systolic time intervals. Comput Biomed Res 3:637–651, 1971

90. Dressler W, Kleinfeld M, Ripstein CB: Physical sign of tight mitral stenosis. JAMA 154:49–52, 1954

Anthony N. DeMaria, Joseph A. Bonanno,
Ezra A. Amsterdam, Rashid A. Massumi,
Robert Zelis, and Dean T. Mason

5
Radarkymography

INTRODUCTION

In the analysis of cardiac border movement by noninvasive means, two general approaches have been pursued in the development of several useful techniques in patients. The first is indirect and dependent upon the effects of heart motion on extracardiac structures in apexcardiography, kinetocardiography, and ballistocardiography which are described elsewhere in this book. In the second approach, direct visualization or sensing of the heart border is carried out by various means in echocardiography, radioisotope scintillation angiography,[1-3] and in roentgenographic methods.

Concerning the radiographic techniques for evaluation of cardiovascular pulsations, fluoroscopy, the method first used, relies on subjective observer interpretation and is without measurable reference points. The objective recording of movement of the cardiac silhouette was initially afforded by the roentgenkymogram[4,5] and subsequently improved by the electrokymogram.[6,7] More recently, the addition of image intensification and closed-circuit television during fluoroscopy has allowed the development of heart motion videotracking, termed *radarkymography*.[8,9] This new method can be applied with relative ease without risk to the patient, and provides precise linear and reproducible

This work was supported in part by the National Heart and Lung Institute (HL–14780).

graphic tracings of horizontal motion from multiple external-wall sites of cardiovascular structures. Although cineangiography with radiopaque media carried out during cardiac catheterization provides the most accurate measurement of wall motion and although the magnitude of epicardial movement is substantially less than that of the endocardial surface throughout ventricular contraction, radarkymography has the advantages of being noninvasive, practical, and useful for serial studies, while still having sufficient sensitivity for reliable assessment of normal and disturbed function.

The purpose of this chapter is to consider the noninvasive techniques based on radiographic information which delineate external cardiovascular motion. Roentgenkymography and electrokymography are reviewed briefly for historical purposes and to provide background of the early investigations of heart silhouette motion. Principal emphasis is focused on the value and limitations of radarkymography in the quantification of movement of cardiovascular structures in health and disease.

ROENTGENKYMOGRAPHY

Heart motion was first recorded permanently on radiographic film by Sabat in 1911 using a single-slit screen or grid.[4] One year later, Gott and Rosenthal applied the term of *roentgenkymography* to this technique[10] which allows analysis of a preselected portion of the external cardiac border by the projection of x-rays through a narrow horizontal slit in a lead shield onto a vertically moving film. This technique was extended to examination of the entire heart approximately 25 years later when Katzman[11] and Stumpf[12] devised the multiple-slit kymograph which uses a grid consisting of a series of parallel horizontal slits in the lead shield.

With continued development by several investigators, the procedure is now carried out either with stationary film and moving parallel-slit grid (surface, plane or scanning kymography)[13] (Fig. 5–1) or by the combination of moving film and stationary horizontal grid (step or linear kymography)[14] (Fig. 5–2). In step kymography, time-motion curves are recorded in an upward direction on the film from multiple preselected points on the heart border, as the film moves vertically downward. Surface kymography, on the other hand, provides time curves in a downward direction on the film from a continuum of points throughout the entire cardiac silhouette in a single plane, with the horizontal grid moving vertically downward.

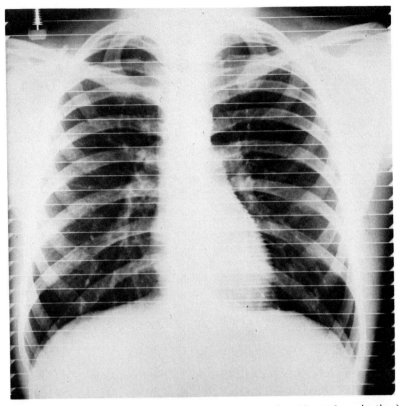

Fig. 5–1. Technique of surface roentgenkymography (frontal projection) in a normal subject (provided by Gilbert H. Alexander, M.D., Director of Diagnostic Radiology, St. Francis General Hospital, Pittsburgh, Pa.).

In practice, the grid usually consists of 20 or more 0.4-mm slits at intervals of 12 mm on the shield, most often arranged horizontally but on occasion vertically.[5] The grid or film moves 11 mm in 1.5 sec, thereby allowing parallel unexposed lines of 1-mm width which serve as a series of parallel markers on the film. The patient can be positioned in different views. The degree of radiation is high and requires 20 times the exposure for a single film compared to a standard chest roentgenogram.

A wide variety of cardiovascular diseases have been examined by roentgenkymography and an abundance of useful descriptive information has been provided.[5] The greatest value of roentgenkymography appears to be in the evaluation of cardiac calcifications and identification of pericardial abnormalities. Several problems are recognized with

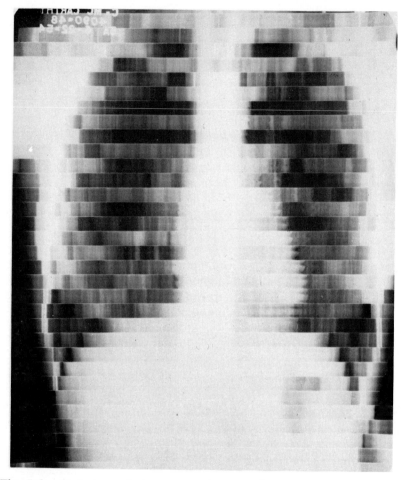

Fig. 5–2. Technique of step roentgenkymography (frontal projection) in a patient with mitral stenosis (provided by Gilbert H. Alexander, M.D., Director of Diagnostic Radiology, St. Francis General Hospital, Pittsburgh, Pa.).

this technique. Usually, it is possible to record only a few beats. The pulsations obtained on the film are small in magnitude and their time-course is indefinite. Thus, it is difficult to precisely measure the extent of movement, and careful analysis of instantaneous motion is not afforded with standard parallel-slit kymographic equipment. Moreover, the step kymogram does not examine the whole cardiac silhouette and, with the surface method, the border point recorded is not constant. The most recent advance in roentgenkymographic methodology has been application of the polykymograph[15] in development of the technique of analytic roentgenkymography which allows evaluation of graphic curves which qualitatively estimate border motion of selected portions of the cardiovascular silhouette.[16]

ELECTROKYMOGRAPHY

The need for more refined methodology in the assessment of cardiac border motion led to the development of the electrokymogram by Henny and Boone, in 1945.[6] This instrument provides continuous graphic curves throughout the cardiac cycle obtained from preselected points along the cardiac border in different views (Fig. 5–3). The apparatus consists essentially of a photomultiplier pickup unit and its

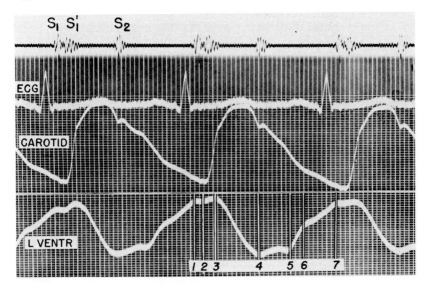

Fig. 5–3. Normal electrokymogram of lateral left ventricular (L Ventr) border (frontal projection) recorded simultaneously with phonocardiogram (top panel), electrocardiogram, and indirect carotid pulse tracing (1, onset of isovolumetric ventricular contraction; 2, completion of isovolumetric systole; 3, onset of ventricular ejection; 4, closure of aortic valve; 5, onset of rapid ventricular filling; 6, beginning of remainder of diastole following completion of rapid-filling phase and 7, completion of ventricular diastole). Thin vertical lines represent 0.02 sec and thick vertical lines 0.10 sec. (From Dack S, Paley DH, Sussman MD: A comparison of electrokymography and roentgenkymography in the study of myocardial infarction, Circulation 1: 551, 1950, with permission.)

recording galvanometer in combination with a standard fluoroscope. The component parts are arranged in the following order: x-ray tube, fluoroscopic shutter, patient under examination, the pickup unit connected laterally to the graphic recorder, and the fluoroscopic screen.[17] Directly in front of the photomultiplier tube is a narrow rectangular slit in a small lead shield which is positioned fluoroscopically over a point on the heart border, with the long axis of the opening placed in the same plane as the pulsations, and the fluoroscopic shutters coned down to the area of the shield.

The fluorescent surface of the photoelectric cell is activated by x-rays transversing the patient and passing through the slit.[6,17] The average number of x-rays reaching the phototube through the rectangular aperture varies with heart motion. Thus, during expansile lateral movement in diastole, less radiation is sensed by the fluorescent area which results in less current generated by the photomultiplier tube and the continuous line on the photographic recorder moves upward. Conversely, when the heart silhouette moves medially during the ejection phase of systole, the current developed by the photocell rises and the graphic tracing is deflected downward.

The electrokymogram has several advantages over the roentgenkymogram.[18] A continuous pulse curve is provided with ease from any area of interest on the cardiac border that can be visualized by fluoroscopy. The sensitivity of the tracing is severalfold more than that of the roentgenkymogram and is suitable for careful qualitative analysis of contour. Further, several cardiac cycles can easily be obtained consistent with the safety of the fluoroscopic procedure, and the heart

---

Fig. 5–4. Electrokymogram of the lateral wall of the left ventricle (frontal projection) in a patient with a low ventricular aneurysm and an old apical-anterolateral myocardial infarction. Border motion at the apex of the left ventricle shows paradoxical lateral motion (upward deflection on tracing between vertical lines 2 and 3) during ventricular ejection (between lines 2 and 4) which is sustained until completion of isovolumetric relaxation (line 5). Paradoxical medial movement of the ventricle apex (downward deflection on tracing) occurs during the period of rapid diastolic filling (between lines 5 and 6) of the upper left ventricle. The upper left ventricular tracing shows relatively normal border motion except for premature termination of downward deflection during ejection (1, onset of isovolumetric contraction). Also shown are the simultaneously recorded electrocardiogram, indirect carotid pulse, and aortic electrokymogram. Time lines same as in Figure 5–3. (From Dack S, Paley DH, Sussman MD: A comparison of electrokymography and roentgenkymography in the study of myocardial infarction, Circulation 1:551, 1950, with permission.)

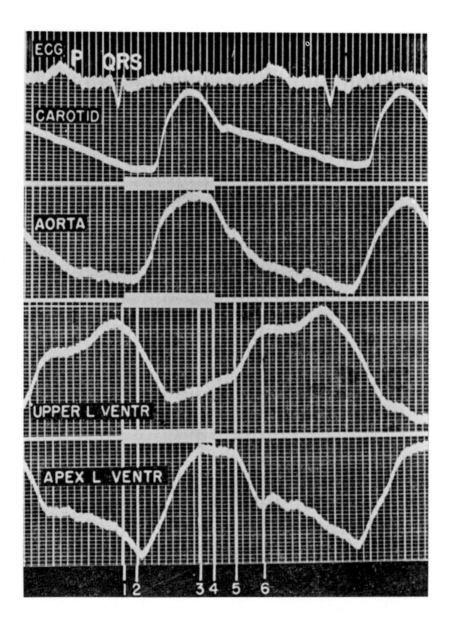

movements can be recorded simultaneously with reference tracings of other physiologic information. The electrokymogram has proved to be a valuable instrument, and a considerable amount of important information concerning directional changes of heart border motion has been obtained in various types of cardiovascular diseases.[7,19-22] Its greatest application has been in the investigation of left ventricular epicardial movement, particularly in coronary artery disease and postmyocardial infarction in which abnormal temporal patterns of segmental contraction have been clearly documented by Dack and associates (Fig. 5–4)[7,8,20] and other workers.[19,21,22] However, electrokymography has certain inherent limitations with linearity and reproducibility, and therefore the tracings are not suitable for quantification. Although still considered a useful direct qualitative technique for the evaluation of cardiovascular border motion when carried out by skilled individuals, its application has become less in the past decade, and the indirect method of apexcardiography is now the noninvasive technique generally used for objective evaluation of left ventricular pulsations.

RADARKYMOGRAPHY

The recent application of an electronic tracking system to the televised picture obtained during fluoroscopy using image intensification has provided an accuratae and practical noninvasive technique for translating cardiac pulsations into linear graphic tracings.[8,9] This new objective method of studying instantaneous movements of the cardiovascular silhouette, termed *radarkymography,* uses the Heart Motion Video Tracker, manufactured by Biotronex Laboratories, Silver Spring, Maryland (Fig. 5–5). The device electronically scans a selected portion of the cardiac image on the television monitor while the tracking circuit

---

Fig. 5–5. Heart motion videotracker system: equipment system used in recording radarkymograms. In the upper right-hand corner is an enlargement of the television (TV) monitor showing the midlateral cardiac border between the two vertical cursors of the radarkymographic videotracker. The image intensified fluoroscopic picture is recorded on videotape simultaneously with the electrocardiogram in its audio channel using the ECG modulator. Later, the cardiac image is projected on the TV monitor and the videotracker cursors are positioned manually with the radarkymograph (RKG) controls on the heart silhouette as demonstrated in the upper right-hand insert. The radarkymogram and the electrocardiogram are displayed simultaneously on the oscilloscope and their tracings recorded.

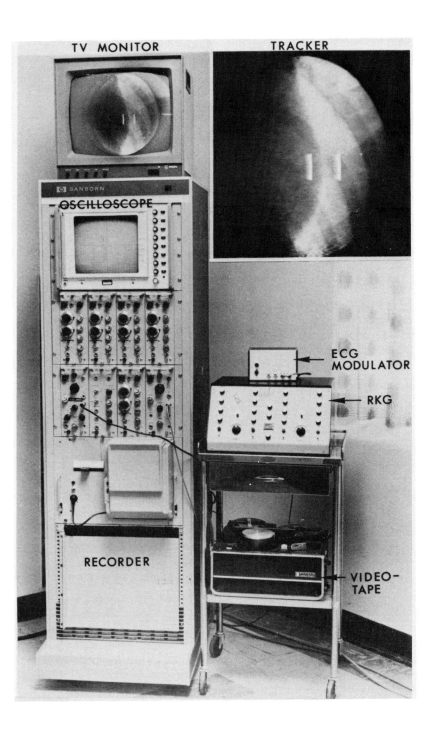

continuously produces an analog signal of border motion (Figs. 5–6 to 5–11). Since radio waves are not involved, radarkymography is somewhat of a misnomer, but rather the term signifies its track during scan characteristic of electronic loop operation.

Method

The composite system used in recording radarkymograms is illustrated in Figure 5–5. In practice, videotape recordings of the heart are obtained during image intensification fluoroscopy. In addition, the electrocardiogram serves as a reference tracing and is recorded simultaneously by means of the electrocardiographic modulator on the audio-channel of the videotape. Later, the videotape is played back on the television monitor, and a selected area of cardiac border motion is analyzed by the radarkymographic circuitry.[8,9] The resultant radarkymographic tracing is displayed, together with the taped electrocardiogram on the oscilloscope after reprocessing by the modulator, and the tracings are recorded on paper (Figs. 5–6, 5–7, 5–9, 5–11). It is also possible to directly apply the Heart Motion Video Tracker to the television screen at the time of cardiac catheterization, which allows the radarkymogram to be recorded simultaneously with several channels of pressure tracings and other physiologic variables on the oscilloscopic recorder (Fig. 5–8).

The standard television picture consists of a sequence of horizontal lines at a rate of 60 image sweeps per second. In chest fluoroscopy, the light intensity varies along each line according to the cardiac image and nearby structures, and thereby the change in tissue density at the interface between the heart border and the lungs is visible on the television monitor. This transition from dark to light is contained in the videomonitor as a voltage change, representing the edge of the cardiovascular silhouette and, in the lateral border of the left ventricle in the frontal view, the voltage spike moves medially in systole and laterally with diastole in a horizontal plane.[8,9] The desired lateral boundary of the heart is selected for electronic scan and tracking by adjusting hand-operated controls on the radarkymogram machine which position two visible cursors on the television screen (Fig. 5–5). The controls allow adjustments of cursor amplitude and width between the cursors, as well as their horizontal and vertical positioning. Also, there are gain and videoclip controls which aid in locking the electronic loop on the cardiac interface; the gain adjustment allows increased sensitivity of the loop in its sensing of the heart border and the videoclip control accentuates the border voltage spike. The picture between the vertical cursors is the specific area electronically scanned, and the vertical plane or point of predominant change in density within it is automatically tracked by the radarkymogram.

In the scanning process of the radarkymographic system, the television voltage signal of the cardiovascular border is differentiated and conditioned into a well-defined peak, the precise location of which is identified and continuously followed by the electronic tracking loop between the two cursors.[8,9] During the cardiac cycle, horizontal pulsation of the heart border produces corresponding displacement of the border voltage peak, thereby causing horizontal motion of the electronic tracking loop and cursors. This, in turn, is translated into analog voltage signals linearly proportional to organ movement which are visualized and recorded. The analog output is regulated by adjustment of the gain controls of the recorder. Inward movement of the heart border produces downward deflection of the radarkymographic tracing and outward cardiac motion is graphically recorded in an upward direction.

Manual positioning of the cursors allows sequential tracking of multiple sites of the cardiovascular silhouette and tracking of different border projections is accomplished by rotating the patient. Although horizontal tracking is most often used, the circuitry of the radarkymogram includes the capability of vertical tracking. Both single and dual channel models are available, the latter affording simultaneous tracking of two border areas. In addition to tracking of the heart and great vessel silhouette, it is possible to record the motion of small very opaque objects such as calcified cardiovascular structures and metallic clips placed on the epicardium.[23] It may also be possible to apply this technique in the study of cardiovascular inner wall motion during angiocardiography by tracking the interface between contrast medium and the myocardium or vascular surface. We should point out that radarkymography is a method different from the technique of roentgen videodensitometry in which densitometer analyses of videotape cineangiograms allows a quantitative approach to the measurement of blood flow and ventricular volume changes.[24,25]

The horizontal motion of the cardiac border can be quantitatively correlated with the vertical deflection of the radarkymographic tracing.[9,26] Thus, the tracking circuit is electronically locked on a target of contrasting interface and the graphic tracing is calibrated by relating the amplitude of its deflection to corresponding known distance of cursor movement. Cursor-loop and tracing motion are corrected for radiographic magnification by comparison with a measured metal grid fluoroscoped at midchest level and projected on the television screen.

Concerning the recording characteristics of the radarkymogram, the tracking signal obtained from the center of the television screen is completely linear with interface movement and is reduced only 5 percent at the margins of the picture.[9] In addition, the technique has been shown to be reproducible.[9,26] There is a 10 msec lag of the re- corded tracing to televised border motion.[9] The frequency response of the graphic recording is 100 percent at 10 Hz (cps) and 70 percent at 15 Hz (cps).[9] The limiting factor in regard to both response time and frequency response is the frame rate of the television camera which allows the tracking loop to sense border movement once every 17 msec.[9] With improved videomonitoring systems using faster rates of image dis- play, higher fidelity properties of radarkymography would be achieved.

Clinical Application

Radarkymography has been applied clinically in the study of border motion of the left ventricle, left atrium, and aorta.[9,26] Pulsations of the left ventricle are recorded at the high, mid- and low segments of its border in the frontal (Figs. 5–6, 5–11) and left anterior oblique (Figs. 5–9, 5–11) views and from the posterior-diaphragmatic wall in the lateral view (Fig. 5–10). The normal left ventricular radarkymo- gram consists of a triphastic pulse in each cardiac cycle (Fig. 5–6). During the phase of isovolumic contraction, small lateral outward motion of this chamber is recorded as an upward deflection (*i* wave) caused by geometric and rotational changes. The *i* wave is followed by a rapid downward deflection (*e* wave) representing medial inward movement of the left ventricle during the ejection period of systole. The subsequent expansion of the ventricle during diastolic filling is recorded as an upward deflection (*d* wave) on the radarkymogram. The normal pulsations of the aorta are opposite in direction to those of the left ventricle and comprise an upward wave during ventricular ejection and a downward motion during diastole (Figs. 5–6, 5–7, 5–9, 5–10).

In patients with aortic valvular disease, abnormal magnitude of pulse waves are observed in the left ventricular and aortic radarkymo- grams (Fig. 5–7).[9] Thus, in aortic regurgitation, there is a more rapid and greater extent of movement in both the ejection and filling waves of the left ventricular tracing (Fig. 5–7A) compared to both patients with valvular aortic stenosis (Fig. 5–7B) and to normal subjects (Fig. 5–6). Also, in the left ventricular radarkymogram of valvular aortic stenosis, the downward slope of the *e* wave during ejection is delayed relative to the normal rate of rise of the subsequent *d* wave in diastole (Fig. 5–7B) and to the normal negative slope of the *e* wave (Fig. 5–6).

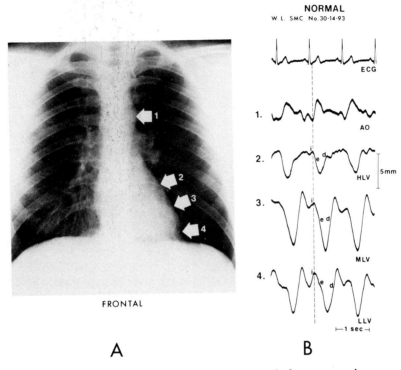

A   B

Fig. 5–6. Chest roentgenogram (A) and (B) radarkymograms in normal subject. The arrows on the roentgenogram indicate the border areas tracked and the numbered tracings indicate the corresponding radarkymograms. The vertical dashed line signifies the onset of ventricular ejection (AO, aortic arch; HLV, high left ventricle; *i*, isovolumic ventricular contraction wave; *e*, ventricular ejection wave; *d*, diastolic filling wave). The extent of border motion is indicated by the vertical calibration marker.

In the aortic radarkymogram obtained from the aortic knob, the rate of rise and amplitude of the upstroke during ejection are augmented in aortic regurgitation (Fig. 5–7A) and reduced in valvular aortic stenosis (Fig. 5–7B) compared to normal subjects (Fig. 5–6). In addition, the upstroke time of the aortic radarkymogram is prolonged in valvular aortic stenosis.[9] In contrast to valvular aortic stenosis, patients with idiopathic hypertrophic subaortic stenosis are characterized by normal upstroke times of the aortic radarkymogram.[9] In patients with coarctation of the aorta, the marked difference in upstroke excursions of aortic radarkymograms recorded proximal to the obstruction compared to those obtained at a distal site have proved useful in the identification of this condition.[9]

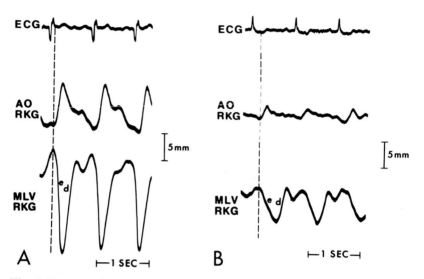

Fig. 5–7. Radarkymograms (RKG) from the aorta (Ao) and midleft ventricular (MLV) lateral border. A. Patient with aortic regurgitation. B. Patient with valvular aortic stenosis. Format and abbreviations same as in Figure 5–6.

When the left atrium is sufficiently enlarged, the left atrial radarkymogram can be recorded in the frontal view at the right heart border and in the lateral projection by tracking extrinsic-induced pulsations of the barium-filled esophagus.[9] In mitral stenosis, there is slow downward deflection of the tracing in ventricular diastole signifying impairment of left atrial emptying.[9] In contrast, the left atrial radarkymogram in mitral regurgitation is characterized by rapid negative deflection during ventricular filling and a prominent upward wave in ventricular systole.[9]

Ventricular Dyssynergy

The most important application of the radarkymogram at the present time is in the study of abnormal segmental contraction patterns of the left ventricle in patients with coronary arterial disease.[9,26] Essentially three principal types of localized disorders of the temporal sequence of ventricular systole have been observed: (1) hypokinesis, diminished extent of local inward wall movement; (2) akinesis, absence of regional wall motion; and (3) dyskinesis, paradoxical outward movement of a portion of the myocardial wall as in ventricular aneurysm. These patterns of epicardial dyssynergy detected by radarkymography are identical to the regional alterations of endocardial movement described by left ventricular cineangiography in coronary arterial disease.[27]

In a recent study using radarkymography, ventricular dyssynergy was recorded in 70 percent of patients in the period immediately following acute transmural myocardial infarction.[26] Tracings of abnormal segmental contraction were obtained over the corresponding electrocardiographic area of infarction in all patients with acute anterior and anterolateral infarctions. Since there was difficulty in recording adequately the posterior border of the left ventricle, segmental dyssynergy was not observed in this area in most patients with acute diaphragmatic infarction.[26] Prognosis was less favorable in patients with chronically persistent abnormal contraction patterns.[26] In chronic coronary arterial disease, all patients with electrocardiographic evidence of old anterior and anterolateral infarctions exhibited corresponding segmental contraction disorders by radarkymography.[26] Approximately half of patients with either old diaphragmatic infarction on electrocardiogram or left ventricular ischemia without infarction exhibited abnormal wall motion. In these patients with chronic coronary arterial disease, chest fluoroscopy failed to detect dyssynergy in half the patients in whom this abnormality was clearly demonstrated by radarkymography.[26] Further, in all patients with disturbed wall movement demonstrated by radarkymograms who underwent cardiac catheterization, left ventricular cineangiography confirmed the presence and location of abnormal segmental contraction.[26]

Figure 5–8 shows the radarkymograms in a patient with a mid- and low-wall left ventricular aneurysm, proved by selective cineangiography, and an old anterolateral myocardial infarction. The radarkymographic tracing or border motion was obtained at the time of cardiac catheterization and recorded simultaneously with the electrocardiogram and ascending intraaortic pressure pulse. The downward *e* wave movement of the high segment of the lateral left ventricle is normal except for somewhat early diminution of motion prior to aortic valve closure. In contrast, the radarkymogram of the midportion of the lateral left ventricular silhouette exhibits marked paradoxical pulsations indicating regional dyskinesis of this area (panel 2). During ejection, the onset of which is signified by the vertical dashed line, the midwall moved laterally thereby describing an abnormal upward *e* wave on the radarkymogram and, in diastole, the border moved medially as shown by the downward *d* wave.

The radarkymograms of the lateral (frontal view, A1–4) and posterolateral (left anterior oblique view, LAO, panel B5–7) borders of the left ventricle in a patient with a low left ventricular aneurysm

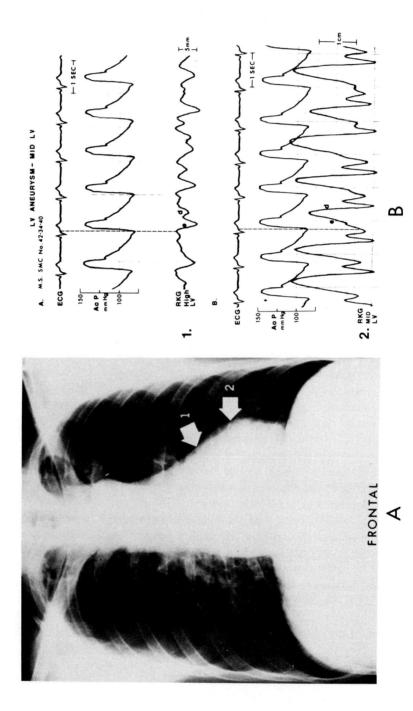

LV ANEURYSM- MID LV

A. M.S. SMC No. 42-34-40

ECG

⊢1 SEC⊣

Ao P
mm Hg
150
100

1.

RKG
High
LV

⊥5 mm⊤

B.

ECG

⊢1 SEC⊣

Ao P
mm Hg
150
100

2.

RKG
MID
LV

⊢1 cm⊣

B

FRONTAL

A

and old anterior and anterolateral myocardial infarction are shown in
Figure 5–9. The tracing of the low ventricular segment in the frontal
view exhibits localized dyskinesis with paradoxical motion of the e and
d waves (A4). In the areas adjacent to this paradoxical pulsation,
there is hypokinesis and akinesis of the midlateral ventricular wall (A3)
and the mid- and low portions of the posterolateral wall (B6 and B7).
The anterior-apical area of dyskinesis is demonstrated in the diagram
of inner wall motion obtained by left ventricular cineangiography.

Figure 5–10 shows the radarkymograms in a patient with an old
anterolateral myocardial infarction and an aneurysm of the mid and
low lateral wall of the left ventricle documented by selective cineangiography. The tracings of the mid and low posterolateral segments
(left anterior oblique view in B) and posterior diaphragmatic area
(lateral view, C5) are normal. In contrast, abnormal pulsations are
recorded on the low lateral ventricular segment as indicated by the
upward deflection of the e wave in the middle of the ejection period
(frontal view, A4). In addition, the movement of the midlateral left
ventricle appears abnormal because of the outward bulge of the e wave
in midejection and possibly also by the prominent upward e wave
deflection at the onset of ejection (A3). Since lateral displacement
may be sustained and even outward motion may take place normally
at the onset of ejection, the brief initial upward deflection of the e wave
of the high lateral left ventricle (A2) and the high posterolateral left
ventricle (B) can be considered within normal limits. The late ejection
period of each of these four segments demonstrates normal downward
motion of the e wave. Abnormal outward movements of brief duration
in different portions of the ejection phase represent regional disorders
of contractile activity and local conduction disturbances, thereby describing the pattern of ventricular asynchrony.[27] These abnormal movements reflect a disruption in the temporal sequence of contraction by
alternating zones of dyssynergy with delayed tension development and
impaired fiber shortening in different areas of the ventricle.

The radarkymograms of the left ventricle are shown in Figure
5–11 in a patient in the immediate period following acute anterior
myocardial infarction. The mid lateral wall motion exhibits dyskinesis
throughout ejection by the upward paradoxical e wave and is followed

---

Fig. 5–8. Roentgenogram (A) and (B) from a patient with a chronic left
ventricular aneurysm of the midwall and an old anterolateral myocardial
infarction. The RKG was obtained at the time of cardiac catheterization and
recorded simultaneously with the ascending intraaortic pressure pulse (AoP)
and ECG. Format and abbreviation same as in Figure 5–6.

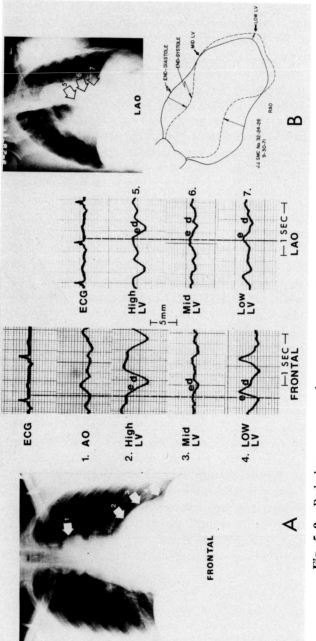

Fig. 5-9. Radarkymograms and roentgenograms from a patient with a chronic low left ventricular aneurysm and an old anterior-anterolateral myocardial infarction. A. The radarkymograms of the lateral border (frontal projection) are shown in panels 1–4. B. Radarkymogram of the posterolateral border obtained in the left anterior oblique (LAO) projection are shown in panels 5–7; and the ventricular endocardial movement in ventricular systole at the time of selective cineangiography is shown diagrammatically (RAO, right anterior oblique view). Format and abbreviations same as in Figure 5–6.

292

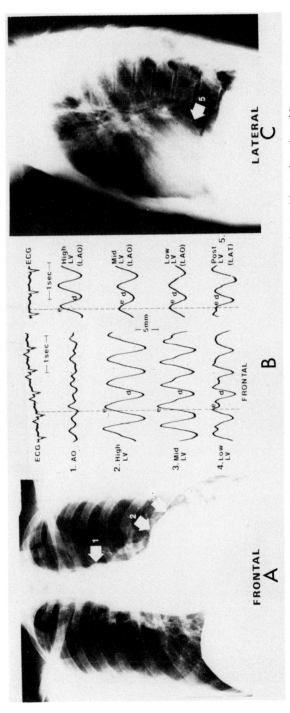

Fig. 5–10. Radarkymograms and roentgenograms from a patient with a chronic mid-low lateral left ventricular aneurysm and an old anterolateral myocardial infarction. A. The radarkymograms of the lateral border (frontal projection) are given in panels 1–4. B. Radarkymograms of the posterolateral border (LAO projection). C. Radarkymogram of the posterior surface (lateral view) is shown in panel 5. Format and abbreviations same as in Figure 5–6.

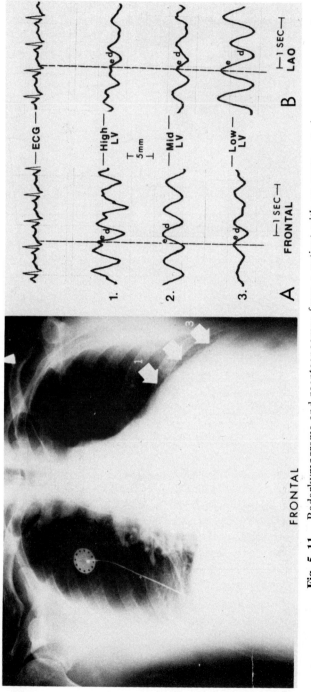

Fig. 5–11. Radarkymograms and roentgenogram from a patient with an acute anterior myocardial infarction, recorded in the immediate period following this event. A. The radarkymograms of the lateral wall (frontal projection) are demonstrated in panels 1–3. Tracing A2 demonstrates midlateral wall dyskinesis. B. Radarkymograms of the posterolateral border (LAO view). Format and abbreviations same as in Figure 5–6.

by abnormal downward diastolic deflection of the d wave (panel A2). The high and low segments of the lateral left ventricle (panels A1 and A3) and the entire posterolateral border move normally (panel B).

Ventricular Contractility

In addition to the study of border movement, radarkymography has been applied to the evaluation of left ventricular contractility. In this approach, the radarkymogram is used to noninvasively determine fiber-shortening rate of the ventricular epicardium during ejection,[28] which is similar in concept to the invasive approaches of assessing contractile state by using opaque metal epicardial markers[29] and coronary artery branch points.[30] Certain physiologic and technical difficulties would be anticipated with radarkymographic analysis of contractility. Thus, the fiber-shortening rate itself is not an independent measure of inotropic state, but rather it is influenced by ventricular loading.[31] Further, epicardial movement differs from fiber velocity within the ventricular wall and at the endocardial surface, and the segmental method of evaluation of left ventricular contractility is not feasible when contractile activity is nonuniform throughout the chamber. Further, there are some inaccuracies in the determination of fiber-shortening rate by radarkymography: since the tracking signal is not necessarily derived from the same fixed point on the epicardium, the interface is a curve rather than a straight line, and only horizontal motion is sensed. However, the study of acute interventions in experimental animals shows that the product of the negative slope and extent of displacement of the e wave of the radarkymogram correlates well with ventricular isovolumic and ejection mechanical and hemodynamic variables that are sensitive to changes in contractility.[28] Further, the value of radarkymography in the evaluation of inotropic state might be enhanced by combining these determinations of border velocity with other noninvasive measurements of cardiac function such as systolic time intervals.[32]

Limitations

Although radarkymography appears to be the best method currently available for the objective noninvasive assessment of external ventricular border motion, it is important to recognize certain limitations of this technique. Considerable experience is necessary for the successful operation of the complex and delicate control system. Further, the radarkymographic equipment is relatively expensive and requires the additional facilities of fluoroscopic image intensification and good quality closed-circuit television monitor, videotape and recorder systems. The frequency and time responses of the radarkymogram are limited somewhat by standard television cameras.[9] Radarkymography necessitates a distinct contrasting interface between the cardiovascular border and surrounding tissues, and thus it is often not possible to track satisfactorily the diaphragmatic border of the heart. Also, difficulties in tracking are encountered in conditions such as pulmonary edema, fibrosis and other lung parenchymal opacifications, pleural effusion, interfering skeletal structures, and excessive movement of the heart produced by accentuated respiration in dyspneic patients.[9,26]

Advantages

There are several advantages of radarkymography over other direct noninvasive radiographic methods in the analysis of cardiovascular pulsations. The method is objective and considerably more accurate than standard fluoroscopy. Compared to roentgenkymography and electrokymography, radarkymography is reproducible, more practical and precise, is applicable to acutely ill and immobile patients, and the patient's presence is not required after the fluoroscopic image is recorded on videotape. Further, radarkymography provides good linearity of response throughout the majority of area of the television picture,[9] allows quantification of border movement,[9,26] and provides estimation of the extent of ventricular dyssynergy.

Concerning the improved reproducibility and higher fidelity characteristics of the radarkymographic tracings compared to electrokymography, the photomultiplier tube of the latter device elicits different voltage responses dependent upon the area excited by light exposure from the fluoroscope, and the frequency response of the electrokymogram is only 70 percent at 8 Hz (cps).[33] In regard to the improved linearity of response of radarkymography, this device electronically tracks the difference in radiodensity between the heart and lung regardless of border position between the cursors, whereas duplication of cardiac border alignment in the electrokymographic aperture is imprecise. Some difficulty in interpretation is inherent in both electrokymography and radarkymography in that recorded border motion results both from rotation of the cardiac silhouette as well as displacement.[34] Although radioisotope scintillation[1-3] and echocardiography[35] afford at least a potential noninvasive approach to the evaluation of posterior ventricular and septal wall motion, movement of the inner myocardial surface, and ventricular wall thickness, radarkymography is substantially more sensitive and accurate in the analysis of external cardiac border pulsations. Although less accurate and reliable than cineangiography, radarkymography is noninvasive, the radiation dosage is small, and it is useful for serial studies.

SUMMARY

Radiographic approaches in the assessment of external cardiac border motion provide the unique combination of direct and noninvasive examination. These radiographic methods have included the development of roentgenkymography, electrokymography, and the new technique of radarkymography. Radarkymography involves electronic tracking of the fluorosopically obtained cardiovascular silhouette on a television monitor and thereby provides graphic tracings of border motion from multiple sites. The principal advantages of this method include good reproducibility, linearity of response, improved fidelity and precision, quantification of border movement, and ease of application. Its major clinical use has been in the analysis of abnormal segmental contraction of the left ventricle in coronary arterial disease. Although relatively little experience has yet been obtained with radarkymography, this method appears to be the best presently available for the noninvasive evaluation of external cardiovascular border motion.

ACKNOWLEDGMENTS

The authors gratefully acknowledge the technical contributions of John J. Stupar, Miss Kay Riggs and James G. McFarland, and the secretarial assistance of Mrs. Barbara J. Giles and Miss Kathy Quinn.

REFERENCES

1. Mason DT, Ashburn WL, Harbert JC, Cohen LS, Braunwald E: Rapid sequential visualization of the heart and great vessels in man using the wide-field anger scintillation camera: Radioisotope-angiography following the injection of technetium-99m. Circulation 39:19, 1969
2. Mullins CB, Mason DT, Ross J Jr, Ashburn WL: Determination of ventricular volume by radioisotope-angiography. Am J Cardiol 24:72, 1969
3. Zaret BL, Strauss HW, Hurley PJ, Natarajan TK, Pitt B: A noninvasive scintophotographic method for detecting regional ventricular dysfunction in man. New Engl J Med 284:1165, 1971

4. Sabat B: Ueber ein verfahren den rontgenographischen darstellung der bewegungen innerer organe (des herzens, der aorta, des zwerchfells). Livow Tygod Lekar 28:4, 1911

5. Alexander GH: The Heart and Its Action: Roentgenkymographic Studies. St. Louis, Green, 1970, pp 1–259

6. Henny GC, Boone BR: Electrokymograph for recording heart motion utilizing the roentgenoscope. Am J Roentgenol Rad Ther 54:3:217, 1945

7. Dack S, Paley DH: Electrokymography. Am J Med 12:331, 1952

8. Schuette WH, Simon AL: A new device for recording cardiac motion. Med Res Eng 7:25, 1968

9. Cohen LS, Simon AL, Whitehouse WC, Schuette WH, Braunwald E: Heart motion video-tracking (radarkymography) in diagnosis of congenital and acquired heart disease. Am J Cardiol 22:678, 1968

10. Gott T, Rosenthal J: Ueber ein verfahren zur darstellung der herzbewegung mittels rontgenstrahlen (roentgenkymographie). Munch Med Wochenschr 59:2033, 1912

11. Katzman S: The roentgen ray cardiograph. Radiology 11:134, 1928

12. Stumpf P: Die gestaltanderung des schlagenden herzens im roentgenbild. Fortschr Geb Roentgenestr 38:1055, 1928

13. Stumpf P: X-ray kymography of the heart. Br J Radiol 7:707, 1934

14. Hirsch IS, Gubner R: Application of roentgenkymography to the study of normal and abnormal cardiac physiology. Am Heart J 12:413, 1936

15. Cignolini P: Metodi e mete della chimografia cardiaca (roentgenmiografia cardiaca) Radiol Med (Torino) 19:401, 1932

16. Juliani G, Quaglia C: Atlas of Cardiovascular Kymography. Springfield, Ill., Thomas, 1965, pp 1–205

17. Henny GC, Boone BR: Electrokymograph for recording heart motion, improvised type. Am J Roentgenology and Radium Therapy 57:409, 1947

18. Dack S, Paley DH, Sussman MD: A comparison of electrokymography and roentgenkymography in the study of myocardial infarction. Circulation 1:551, 1950

19. Gillick FG, Reynolds WF: Clinical application of electrokymography. California Med 70:407, 1949

20. Sussman ML, Dack S, Paley DH: Some clinical applications of electrokymography. Radiology 53:500, 1949

21. Schwedel JB, Samet P, Mednick H: Electrokymographic studies of abnormal left ventricular pulsations. Am Heart J 40:410, 1950

22. Bartley O: Electrokymographic changes in myocardial infarction. Acta Radiologica 54:81, 1960

23. Harrison DC, Goldblatt A, Glick G, Mason DT, Braunwald E: Studies on cardiac dimensions in intact, unanesthetized man. Circ Res 13:448, 1963

24. Wood EH, Strum RE, Sanders JJ: Data processing in cardiovascular physiology with particular reference to Roentgen videodensitometry. Mayo Clin Proc 39:849, 1964

25. Smith HC, Frye RI, Donald DE, Davis GD, Pluth JR, Strum RE, Wood EH: Roentgen videodensitometric measure of coronary blood flow. Mayo Clin Proc 46:800, 1971

26. Kazamias TM, Gander MP, Ross J Jr, Braunwald E: Detection of left-ventricular-wall motion disorders in coronary artery disease by radarkymography. New Engl J Med 285, 2:63, 1971

27. Herman MV, Gorlin R: Implications of left ventricular asynergy. Am J Cardiol 23:538, 1969

28. Levitsky S, Schuette WH, Sloane RE, Mullin EM, Souther SG, Whitehouse WC, Morrow AG: Radarkymography: A noninvasive approach for evaluating myocardial contractility. Circulation 42 (Suppl III):121, 1970

29. Sonnenblick EH, Williams JF Jr, Glick G, Mason DT, Braunwald E: Studies on digitalis XV. Effects of cardiac glycosides on myocardial force-velocity relations in the non-failing human heart. Circulation 34:524, 1966

30. McDonald IG: The shape and movements of the human left ventricle during systole: A study by cineangiography and by cineradiography of epicardial markers. Am J Cardiol 26:221, 1970

31. Mason DT, Spann JF Jr, Zelis R, Amsterdam EA: Alterations of hemodynamics and myocardial mechanics in patients with congestive heart failure: Pathophysiologic mechanisms and assessment of cardiac function and ventricular contractility. Prog Cardiovasc Dis 12:507, 1970

32. Weissler AM, Harris WS, Schoenfeld CD: Bedside technics for the evaluation of ventricular function in man. Am J Cardiol 23:577, 1969

33. Zinsser HF Jr, Kay CF, Benjamin JM Jr: The electrokymograph: Studies in recording fidelity. Circulation 2:197, 1950

34. Soloff LA: Assessment of cardiac motion. New Engl J Med 285:804, 1971

35. Fortuin NJ, Hood WP Jr: Determination of mean velocity of circumferential fiber shortening by echocardiography. Circulation 44 (Suppl II):34, 1971

R. P. Lewis, R. F. Leighton,
W. F. Forester, and A. M. Weissler

6
Systolic Time Intervals

Personne n'a le tact assez fin pour sentir avec le doigt les details minu-
tieux que révèle le sphygmographe dans une seule pulsation, détails dont
chacun a certainement sa valeur et pourra servir, un jour, à préciser le
diagnostic. (Marey, 1860.)

INTRODUCTION

Soon after Ludwig adapted the kymograph for recording cardiovascular pulsations in 1847, Marey introduced the sphygmograph, an
instrument designed for graphic recording of the arterial pulse in man.[1,2]
Using this instrument, Marey reported on the numerous changes in
contour of the arterial and venous pulse which accompany cardiac
disease. His contemporary, Garrod, concentrated on the significance of
the duration of sytole.[3] He reported in 1874 on the inverse relationship
between heart rate and the duration of left ventricular ejection. Thurston, and Chapman and Lond later attempted to elucidate the relationship of the duration of systole to cycle length and to apply this
measurement to the analysis of cardiac performance in man.[4,5] As
early as 1904, Bowen used recordings of the carotid arterial pulse to

This investigation was supported in part by the National Heart and Lung
Institute (HL-05786, HL-05035, HL-05546, HE-12660 and Program Project HE-
11504) and the Central Ohio Heart Chapter of the American Heart Association
(#22-69).

measure the duration of ejection during exercise.[6] Thus, by the turn of the twentieth century, a remarkable literature suggesting use of the systolic time intervals as a measure of left ventricular performance in man had been established. When a clearer delineation of the phases of systole was enunciated in the now classical studies of Wiggers, their potential was more fully realized.[7,8] Almost half a century ago, Katz and Feil first applied modern electronic recording techniques for determining the phases of systole in the presence of left ventricular diseases.[9-11] Blumberger later reported extensive studies on the systolic intervals in a wide variety of cardiac disorders.[12]

Despite the early introduction of the method, its clinical application received little attention until recent years. In large part, this is related to the fact that the significance of the systolic time intervals as measures of left ventricular function were not critically tested in the past. It was only after the development of direct measures of left ventricular performance which could be related to the systolic time intervals in man that their significance could be appreciated in a quantitative sense. On the basis of studies in recent years, a new understanding of the use of the systolic time intervals in the analysis of the left ventricular performance in man has evolved. It is the purpose of this review to summarize these more current developments and to direct interest to clinical application of the measurement of the systolic intervals.

MEASUREMENT OF THE SYSTOLIC TIME INTERVALS

Studies in recent years have stressed measurement of three systolic time intervals (STI); total electromechanical systole (QS_2), the left ventricular ejection time (LVET), and the preejection period (PEP).[13-15] These intervals are measured from simultaneous fast-speed recordings of the electrocardiogram, the phonocardiogram, and the carotid or subclavian arterial pulsations (Fig. 6–1). A chest pneumogram is generally recorded as well. The recordings are obtained at a paper speed of 100 mm/sec. The electrocardiographic lead most clearly demonstrating the onset of ventricular depolarization has been used in the past to delineate the onset of ventricular deplorization. In more recent years an orthogonal lead system has been preferred in some laboratories. With either application, the entire electrocardiogram is first displayed so as to determine the lead which best delineates the onset of ventricular depolarization. A phonocardiographic pickup is placed over the upper precordium for recording the initial high-frequency vibrations of the second heart sound. Sounds with a fre-

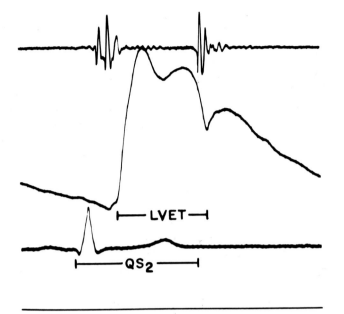

PEP = QS$_2$ – LVET

Fig. 6–1. Simultaneous tracing of electrocardiogram, phonocardiogram, and carotid arterial pulse at 100 mm/sec paper speed illustrating the measurement of QS$_2$, LVET, and the calculation of PEP (QRS$_2$, total electromechanical systole; LVET, left ventricular ejection time, and PEP, preejection period).

quency of less than 100 Hz must be attenuated by a proper filter to obtain optimum recordings of the second heart sound. The carotid or subclavian arterial pulsation is generally recorded with a funnel-shaped pickup (ID 2.3 cm) attached by polyethylene tubing (length 3 cm, ID 4 mm) to a Statham-P23Db pressure transducer. The entire system is air-filled and amplified to permit the inscription of an arterial pulse of sufficiently large amplitude to allow clear demarcation of its onset and incisura. In practice, the funnel is placed firmly over the carotid arterial pulsation just below the carotid sinus. The gauge is vented to air while pressure is applied, after which the vent is closed manually for recording of the pulse. Other transducer systems can be used for recording of the arterial pulse. The Marey capsule connected by plastic tubing to either a piezoelectric or direct-current transducer is commonly used. As pointed out recently by Kesteloot and coworkers, the transducer used in pulse recordings should have a time constant of at least 2.0 sec.[16] A flat-frequency response between 0.1 and 30 Hz is considered adequate for clinical application.

Before obtaining a permanent recording, it is advisable to scan an oscilloscopic display of the electrocardiogram, phonocardiogram, and carotid arterial pulsation to ascertain that each of the events from which the calculations are made are sharply inscribed. For best definition of the STI, the following characteristics of these recordings should be clearly delineated: (1) a clear initial depolarization force departing acutely from a flat baseline on the electrocardiogram, (2) a sharp inscription of the initial high-frequency vibrations of the aortic second sound, and (3) a clearly discernible rapid upstroke and pointed single incisural notch on the carotid arterial pulse tracing. For accurate measurement, the amplification of the carotid arterial pulse tracing should permit at least a 5-cm inscription of the upstroke of the arterial wave. The observer must be cognizant of the possibility of carotid-vertebral arterial disease in the patient to be studied. Compression of the carotid artery in such a patient may result in inadvertent depression of cerebral blood flow. In patients with established or suspected carotid-vertebral arterial disease, the carotid arterial pulsation should be avoided and the subclavian arterial pulsation substituted.

The QS_2 interval is measured from the onset of ventricular depolarization to the first high-frequency vibrations of the aortic component of the second heart sound. The LVET is measured from the beginning upstroke to the trough of the incisural notch on the carotid or subclavian arterial pulse tracing. The aortic component of the second heart sound is best defined by its relationship to the incisura of the carotid or subclavian arterial pulse. The incisura of the carotid pulse follows the high-frequency vibrations of the aortic component of the second heart sound by 10 to 45 msec (Fig. 6–1). In a recent analysis of 207 patients in this laboratory, this interval averaged 18.5 msec ± 8.2 (1 Sd). Frequently, the incisural notch falls between the aortic and pulmonic components of the second heart sound permitting easy identification of the aortic vibration. The delay in the appearance of the incisural notch relative to the second heart sound is attributed to the transmission time of the arterial pulse from the proximal aorta to the site of its detection in the carotid or subclavian artery.

The beginning upstroke of the carotid arterial pulsation is defined as the first point at which the upstroke of the carotid arterial pulsation rises above the low-frequency preejection vibrations of the arterial pulse wave. When a photographic recorder is used, diminution in the calibre of the inscription of the light beam helps define this point. It is essential to obtain an incisural notch with a sharp point for precise delineation. Failure to obtain such a point is a common source of error ($\pm$ 10 msec) and is particularly common when small carotid pulse waves are recorded. The importance of an adequate-sized carotid pulse is illustrated in Fig. 6–2. It has been our experience that in 1 to 2 percent of all patients with chronic heart disease adequate pulse tracings cannot be obtained.

The PEP is that interval from the beginning of ventricular depolarization to the beginning of left ventricular ejection. The PEP is derived by subtracting the LVET from QS_2, thereby eliminating the delay in transmission of the arterial pulse from the proximal aorta to carotid artery. An alternate derivation of PEP involves the determination of the interval from the onset of ventricular depolarization to the beginning of the upstroke of the carotid arterial pulse from which the arterial pulse transmission time (A_2-incisural interval) is subtracted. The relation of the measured STI to the cardiac cycle is illustrated in Fig. 6–3.

The determinations of QS_2, PEP, and LVET are the STI routinely

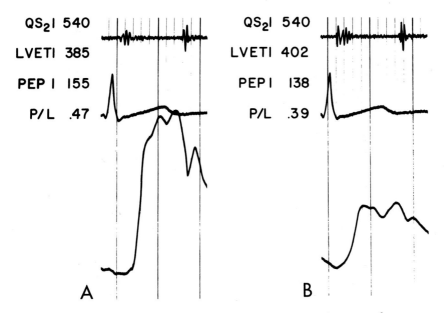

QS_2I	540		QS_2I	540
LVETI	385		LVETI	402
PEP I	155		PEP I	138
P/L	.47		P/L	.39

A   B

Fig. 6–2. The effect of a low-amplitude carotid pulse tracing upon the measured LVET in the same patient with different gain setting for the carotid tracing: A. High gain; B. Low gain. The landmarks on the low-gain trace are poorly delineated producing a 17-msec error in the measurement of the LVET. (P/L = PEP/LVET.)

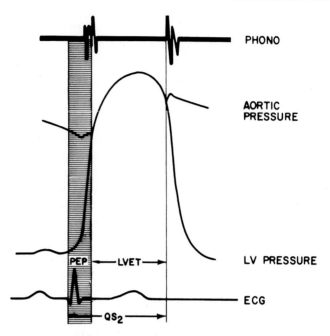

PHONO

AORTIC
PRESSURE

LV PRESSURE

ECG

PEP — LVET —

— QS$_2$ —

Fig. 6–3. Relation of the measured systolic time intervals
to the cardiac cycle. Simultaneous registration of phonocardiogram (phono), aortic pressure, left ventricular (LV)
pressure, and electrocardiogram (ECG) (S$_1$ and S$_2$, heart
sounds). (From Weissler AM et al: Bedside technics for
the evaluation of ventricular function in man. Am J Cardiol
23: 577–583, 1969, with permission.)

performed in this laboratory since their measurement relies on the
four most clearly delineated and reproducible temporal landmarks of
the cardiac cycle from externally derived recordings; namely, the onset
of ventricular depolarization, the upstroke and incisural notch of the
carotid or subclavian arterial pulse tracing, and the aortic component
of the second heart sound.

From the technical point of view, it is important to emphasize
that measurement of STI necessitates fast-speed recordings. At paper
speeds of 200, 100, 50, and 25 mm/sec, the maximal attainable limits
for measuring the STI are, respectively, 2.5, 5.0, 10, and 20 msec.
At low paper speeds (below 100 mm/sec) only large changes in STI
can be defined accurately. The recordings of STI should be obtained
along with precise time demarcations so as to facilitate the ease and
accuracy of the measurement.

Previously, the initial high-frequency vibrations of the first heart

sound were used as a landmark for subdividing the PEP into isovolumic contraction time (ICT) and electromechanical delay. However,
recent studies have shown that the first sound is inscribed at a varying
interval after the onset of left ventricular mechanical systole (approximately 45 msec).[17–19] Furthermore, the first sound is frequently not
clearly delineated in patients with heart disease. The rapid upstroke of
the apexcardiogram has been used to define ICT by external measurement.[20,21] Comparison of the QS_1 and Q-u (Q to upstroke of left
ventricular impulse on the apexcardiogram) intervals in normal subjects, subjects with heart disease and a normal QRS duration, left
ventricular conduction delays of 90 to 120 msec, and complete left
bundle branch block is given in Table 6–1. It is apparent that the
Q-u is more sensitive than the QS_1 for defining delays in left ventricular contraction. Thus, it is likely that measurement of the ICT
will permit better discrimination between the effect of the conduction
disturbance itself and left ventricular dysfunction in patients with a
prolonged QRS ($>$ 90 msec).

Previous studies have attempted to validate the LVET measurement from the carotid arterial pulsation in man by comparison with
recordings obtained simultaneously from fluid-filled catheters in the

Table 6–1
Electromechanical Delay in Chronic Heart Disease
Defined by Phonocardiogram and Apexcardiogram

Group	Type of Subject	No. of Subjects	Phonocardiogram Q-S$_1$ (msec)[a]	Apexcardiogram Q-u (msec)[b]
I	Normal	25	78 ± 2.2[c]	32 ± 1.6
II	Chronic heart disease (QRS < 90 msec)	26	77 ± 3.4	38 ± 2.4
III	Chronic heart disease (QRS 90–120)	7	77 ± 3.5	38 ± 3.4
IV	Complete left bundle branch block	6	83 ± 4.3	58 ± 5.6

[a] No significant difference between groups except Group I vs Group IV
(p < 0.05).
[b] Group I vs II, p < .05; I vs III, NS (not significant); I vs IV, p < .001.
Group II vs III, NS; II vs IV, p < .005.
Group III vs IV, p < .001.
[c] 1 SEM.

proximal aorta.[22-24] These studies have generally supported the accuracy of the measurement of LVET by the noninvasive technique. In recent studies the STI measurements derived externally have been compared to the same intervals determined from arterial and left ventricular pressure tracings obtained from a high-fidelity catheter-tip micromanometer.[25-27] In so doing, the transmission delays and lowered frequency responses inherent in fluid-filled catheters were eliminated. These studies have confirmed the accuracy of the determinations of QS_2, LVET, and PEP through a wide range of STI (Fig. 6–4 and 6–5).

Two recent studies in which the apexcardiogram was recorded simultaneously with the left ventricular pressure from a manometer-tip catheter indicate that the apexcardiogram is a valid measurement of the onset of contraction.[27,28] In another study the directly measured ICT showed a high degree of correlation with the externally derived PEP over a wide variety of hemodynamic interventions.[26] This is probably true because of the constancy of the interval between the onset of the Q wave and onset of left ventricular contraction in the absence of intraventricular conduction disturbances.

Similar studies of the aortic component of the second heart sound have been conducted. Although the precise timing of closure of the

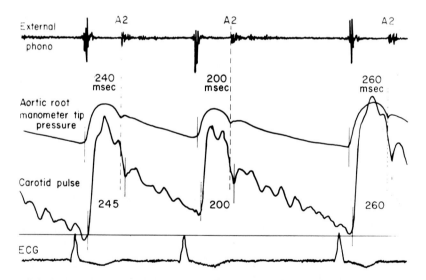

Fig. 6–4. Simultaneous recordings of external phono, ECG, external carotid, and aortic root pressure from a high-fidelity manometer tip catheter in a patient with atrial fibrillation. The delay in the carotid is apparent. The LVET from the two arterial pulses is nearly identical. The initial high-frequency vibrations of A_2 correspond exactly with the aortic incisural notch.

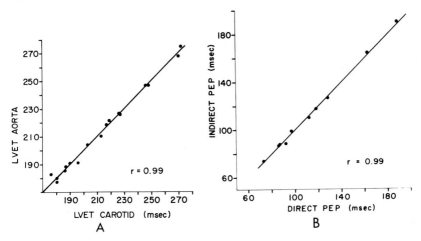

Fig. 6–5. Correlation between simultaneous systolic time intervals (STI) obtained from a high-fidelity manometer-tip catheter in the aorta or left ventricle and external measurements. A. The LVET from the aorta and carotid is compared in 17 patients. B. The PEP obtained directly from the left ventricular pressure pulse is compared to the PEP obtained indirectly from external tracings in 10 patients.

aortic valve is still not clear, it is known that the incisural notch and initial vibrations of A_2 occur simultaneously approximately 10 msec after the left ventricular aortic pressure crossover. This is true in all disease states except aortic valve disease (see later section). In an animal study, the incisural notch and A^2 were shown to occur precisely at the peak deceleration of forward aortic flow under a wide variey of hemodynamic conditions.[29] The conclusion was that the aortic closure sound provided a faithful measure of the termination of left ventricular ejection. Finally, in a study of five patients in atrial fibrillation, a beat-to-beat analysis over a wide variety of RR intervals showed that the left ventricular aortic pressure crossover occurred at the same position relative to peak pressure on the left ventricular pressure pulse.[30]

   In applying STI measurements, it is of utmost importance to define a normal range of variation relative to heart rate. In the range of heart rate from 40 to 110 beats per min, the durations of QS_2, LVET, and PEP are related linearly to heart rate.[13,14,31] Willems and Kesteloot have tested various mathematical expressions of the relationship between LVET and heart rate in man.[32] When normal subjects are considered, variability about the linear equation describing the relationship between heart rate and LVET at rest and during exercise is virtually the same as that for hyperbolic, exponential, or polynomial equations.

When extremes of heart rate are considered through the inclusion of observations in patients with heart block and supraventricular tachycardia, the relationship between heart rate and LVET is only slightly better expressed in exponential, hyperbolic, or polynomial equations than in linear equations. Hence, for practical purposes, the linear equation would appear to provide the best expression of the relationship of LVET to heart rate.

Linear regression equations relating STI and heart rate have been derived in this laboratory from observations on normal individuals.[13] The regression equations derived from data obtained between the hours of 8:00 to 10:00 AM in 211 normal supine basal subjects ranging in age from 19 to 65 are shown in Table 6–2. The QS$_2$ and LVET are slightly longer (ave + 11 msec) in women. In children, no significant difference in STI between the sexes has been found. However, for any heart rate all the STI are shorter in children than adults.[33,34] The intervals increase with age from infancy to puberty; this increase is independent of changes in heart rate during maturation.

In applying the STI clinically, deviations from the normal regression equations are expressed in two ways: (1) calculating the predicted normal interval for the observed heart rate from the appropriate regression equation and subtracting the measured interval from this value or (2) calculating the corresponding STI-index; QS$_2$I, ETI, and PEPI (Table 6–2). The STI-indices (in milliseconds) are obtained by transposition of terms of the regression equation and calculated as the sum of the measured interval and the product of the observed heart rate and the appropriate normal regression slope. In fact, the indices are

Table 6–2
Regression Data: Systolic Time Intervals
in Normal Subjects

Systolic Interval	Sex	Regression Equation STI-Index	Standard Deviation
Total electromechanical systole (QS$_2$)	Male	QS$_2$ = −2.1 HR + 546	14
	Female	QS$_2$ = −2.0 HR + 549	14
Preejection period	Male	PEP = −0.4 HR + 131	10
	Female	PEP = −0.4 HR + 133	11
LV ejection time	Male	LVET = −1.7 HR + 413	10
	Female	LVET = −1.6 HR + 418	10

Abbreviations: QS$_2$, total electromechanical systole; PEP, preejection period; LVET, left ventricular ejection time; HR, heart rate; STI, systolic time interval.

the corresponding Y intercepts of the regression equations, i.e., the measured interval extrapolated to zero heart rate, assuming a normal regression slope. Thus, for men, the QS_2I is the measured $QS_2 + 2.1$ times observed heart rate; the ETI is the measured LVET $+ 1.7$ times observed heart rate; and the PEPI is the measured PEP $+ 0.4$ times heart rate. When compared to the normal index, the calculated value yields a quantitative measure of the deviation in the STI corrected for heart rate. The calculation of the STI-indices offers a convenient expression for studying serial changes and facilitates comparisons among patients. *Throughout this presentation, designations of alteration in PEP, LVET, and QS_2 denote changes which are corrected for heart rate.*

During the assumption of the upright posture in normal individuals, there is a prolongation of the PEP and abbreviation in LVET, associated with a slight abbreviation of QS_2.[35,36] At a 90° passive head-up tilt, the mean lengthening of PEP is 35 msec, whereas LVET shortens by 40 msec.

There is a diurnal decrease in LVET and QS_2, unaccompanied by significant change in PEP, in normal subjects.[37] This effect appears to reach its maximum between 4:00 and 8:00 PM and averages 8 and 10 msec for LVET and QS_2, respectively. The interpretation of the STI among patients with cardiac disease must take this slight but definite diurnal variation into account.

In order to properly interpret variations in the STI when serial studies are performed, it is necessary to know the extent of day-to-day variability of the STI in individual subjects. Thirty-three normal subjects were studied daily for 4 to 10 days. The mean values and standard deviations for each subject were calculated and from these results the mean standard deviation of each STI for the entire group was determined. These were ± 6.2 msec for the QS_2, ± 5.2 msec for the LVET, and ± 4.3 msec for the PEP. These small standard deviations indicate the remarkable consistancy of the STI in normal subjects.

It is not always practical to perform routine STI between the hours of 8:00 and 10:00 AM. Furthermore, many patients undergoing STI measurements may be apprehensive since they know they are having a "heart test." This could result in adrenergic stimulation which was minimal or absent in the 211 normal volunteers from which the original regression equations were obtained. For practical purposes, we have found that the magnitude of the changes induced by psychogenic stimulation, diurnal variation, and short rest period are small (Figs. 6–6 and 6–7). Consequently, in our laboratory routine STI are performed from 8:00 to 3:00 PM with a 5-min rest period before the actual measurement. However, for investigative studies these variables should be rigorously controlled.

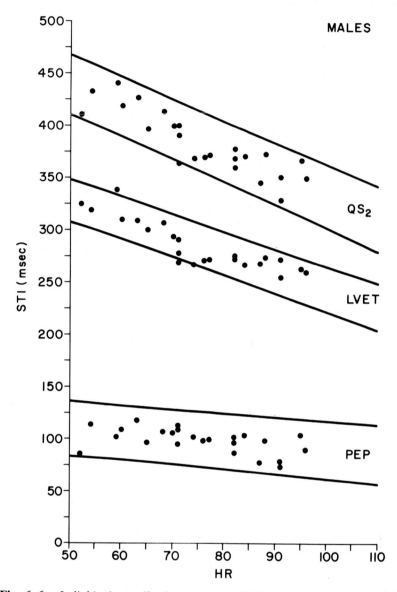

Fig. 6–6. Individual systolic time intervals (STI) obtained from 26 male patients who subsequently proved to have no heart disease. Ninety-five percent confidence intervals for QS$_2$, LVET, and PEP obtained from regression data for 121 normal volunteers are superimposed.[13] The patients were studied as part of a cardiac evaluation. The STI were measured between 8:00 AM and 3:00 PM after a 5- to 15-min rest period. The values obtained under these circumstances were not statistically different from those of normal volunteers.

312

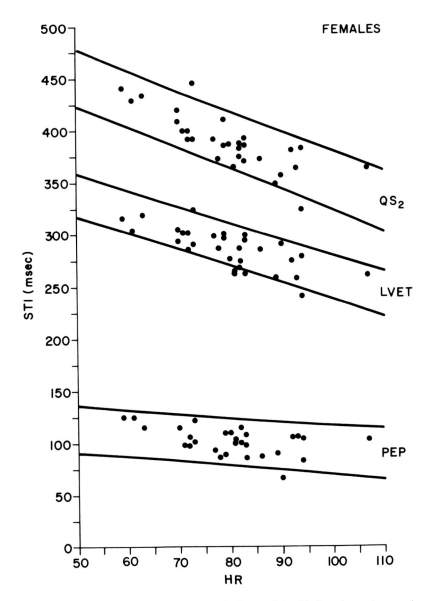

Fig. 6–7. Similar data to Figure 6–6 obtained in 31 female patients who proved to have no heart disease. The STI of the patients were not statistically different than those obtained from 90 normal female volunteers.

In the adult population, a slight increase in the PEP occurs with advancing age.[38] With the exception of a minimal prolongation in the late decades of life,[39] the duration of LVET corrected for heart rate varies remarkably little with age. The slight prolongation of PEP and LVET with advancing age is accompanied by significant prolongation of QS_2 in older subjects.[40]

PHYSIOLOGICAL BASIS FOR SYSTOLIC
TIME INTERVAL MEASUREMENTS

That changes in the duration of the phases of systole parallel other hemodynamic alterations was first clearly described by Frank.[41] He noted in the frog heart that with increased left ventricular filling, there was an abbreviation in the isovolumic phase, a prolongation of ejection and delayed aortic valve closure, all of which were accompanied by an increased stroke volume. Frank noted, in addition, that with increasing afterload there was prolongation of isovolumic contraction and abbreviation in left ventricular ejection whereas total systole diminished or remained unchanged. The increase in afterload was accompanied by a diminution in ventricular stroke volume. These early experiments, suggesting a close relationship between the duration of the phases of systole and changes in preload and afterload, were elaborated in the studies of Wiggers and Katz in the dog heart and by Peserico in the frog heart.[7,8,11,42]

Studies in more recent years have been designed to separate more completely the independent contributions of heart rate, stroke volume, and aortic pressure to the duration of the STI. Braunwald et al confirmed the close quantitative relationship between left ventricular stroke volume and duration of ejection in the isolated dog heart preparation.[43] When heart rate and stroke volume were maintained constant, increasing aortic pressure was noted not to affect the duration of ejection except at extremes of mean aortic pressure (175 to 200 mm Hg), when a lengthening of the LVET was noted. In an exquisitely controlled study on the isolated dog heart by Wallace and coworkers, the effects of changes in stroke volume, arterial pressure, and heart rate on the duration of ICT, LVET, and mechanical systole, measured from the left ventricular and aortic pressure pulses, were again examined.[44] When heart rate and aortic pressure were maintained constant, changes in left ventricular stroke volume induced by alterations in left ventricular filling were accompanied by concordant changes in LVET and inverse changes in ICT, whereas the duration of mechanical systole remained constant or changed only slightly. When heart rate and stroke volume were maintained constant, increases in aortic pressure were accompanied by an increase in ICT, and the LVET decreased. The duration of mechanical systole under these circumstances remained unchanged or decreased. These changes in the duration of the systolic phases with increasing mean aortic pressure were not influenced by beta blockade with dichlorisoproterenol. When heart rate was increased while mean aortic pressure and stroke volume were maintained constant, there was a concordant diminution in the ICT, LVET, and the duration of mechanical systole. The effects of increases in mean aortic pressure and heart rate on the STI were uninfluenced by beta blockade. When mean aortic pressure, stroke volume, and heart rate were maintained constant, sympathetic cardiostimulation and cardiac glycosides tended to produce an abbreviation in all STI. The above studies on the effects of acute hemodynamic interventions on the isolated dog heart established an important physiologic background on which to base further investigations in man.

Early studies by Lombard and Cope confirmed the inverse relationship between heart rate and LVET in man.[45] These investigators noted that for any level of heart rate the assumption of the upright posture was accompanied by an abbreviation in the LVET, an effect which was attributed to a lowering in stroke volume. Studies by Weissler and associates demonstrated the close relationship among LVET, heart rate, and stroke volume in normal human subjects.[22] In a graphic series of investigations, Greenfield and Harley investigated the relationship between beat-to-beat alterations in stroke volume, measured by a catheter flowmeter in the proximal aorta, and changes in the PEP and LVET in patients with atrial fibrillation and atrioventricular dissociation.[46,47] In these studies, wherein stroke volume varied spontaneously at a time when alterations in intrinsic contractility and afterload were minimal, the inverse relationship between stroke volume and PEP and the direct relationship between stroke volume and LVET were conclusively demonstrated. On the basis of these and other studies attempting to isolate the independent contributions of changes in heart rate, stroke volume, pre- and afterload, and altered inotropic states in man, the following relationships in normal intact subjects have been confirmed: (1) Increases in heart rate, occurring spontaneously or induced by pharmacologic agents or atrial pacing, are accompanied by abbreviations in the QS_2 and LVET.* Abbreviation of the PEP accompanies an increase in heart rate induced by adrenergic cardiostimulation but not that due to vagal blockade or atrial pacing.[49-51] (2) Increases in

* Refs. 13, 14, 48–50.

stroke volume caused by enhanced ventricular filling are accompanied by a lengthening of the LVET and abbreviation of the PEP, while in general, the QS_2 is unaltered.[22,46,47] (3) Transient increases in afterload induce prolongation of both LVET and PEP, whereas transient decreases in afterload lengthen the LVET and abbreviate the PEP.[48,51–53] (4) Pharmacologic interventions that have a positive inotropic effect associated with little change in afterload are accompanied by abbreviations in QS_2, LVET, and PEP.*

The effects of acute alterations in afterload on the LVET and QS_2 in man are not entirely consistent with previous experimental studies in the isolated heart. Whereas the LVET and the duration of systole tend to diminish with increased afterload in the intact and isolated dog heart, increases in arterial pressure induced by intravenous administration of methoxamine are accompanied by lengthening of the PEP, LVET, and QS_2 in the intact man. These changes in STI with pharmacologically induced increases in arterial pressure in man have been demonstrated by Shaver and associates to occur at a time when heart rate is held constant.[52] It is possible that the lengthening of the STI during such pharmacologic vasoconstrictor activity may, in part, be explained by baroreceptor stimulation with increased vagal and decreased cardiosympathetic activity. In limited observation, however, these responses in LVET and QS_2 to increased afterload were not appreciably altered by atropine or beta blockade. The PEP lengthening during methoxamine infusion was blocked by atropine.[52] Present evidence, therefore, supports the thesis that increased afterload itself prolongs all systolic phases in man. In general, the data of Shaver and associates indicate a 1-msec increase in LVET for each millimeter of mercury increase in mean sysolic pressure induced by methoxamine. However, a chronic increase in blood pressure has a much less striking effect on the STI, the major effect being on the PEP.[13,39,57,58]

In recent years much attention has been focused on the PEP as a potential measure of intrinsic myocardial contractile performance. Consideration of several hemodynamic factors are pertinent to the use of the PEP in interpreting left ventricular dynamics. The major determinants of the duration of the PEP are the left ventricular end-diastolic pressure (LVEDP), the aortic diastolic pressure and the rate of left ventricular pressure development (LV dp/dt) from onset of mechanical systole to the opening of the aortic valve. In acute experiments, these factors have been demonstrated to contribute to the PEP.[59,60] In controlled studies, heart rate itself appears not to influence the PEP except

* Refs. 37, 48, 51, 54–56.

when it is accompanied by changes in the above factors. In considering the role of LVEDP itself, one must recognize that sudden increases in LVEDP are accompanied by increasing ventricular end-diastolic fiber stretch, a change which of itself induces increases in the rate of left ventricular pressure development (Starling effect). In considering the rate at which left ventricular pressure is developed (LV dp/dt) during the preejection period, one must recognize that both the total force developed by the left ventricular wall and the volume of the ventricle are important determinants. Thus, for a given total force generated by the left ventricle during the isovolumic phase of systole, the dp/dt will vary inversely with the initial volume of the chamber.

The above considerations are pertinent to the interpretation of PEP changes in chronic disorders of left ventricular performance. In states of sustained left ventricular decompensation, a prolonged PEP is often associated with an elevated LVEDP and volume whereas aortic diastolic pressure remains essentially unchanged or slightly increased. The pressure developed by the left ventricle during the isovolumic phase of systole (end-diastolic to aortic diastolic pressure) is hence generally less than normal except when diastolic hypertension is a major factor in the disease process. The prolonged PEP in these circumstances is therefore accounted for by a decrease in the rate of left ventricular pressure developed throughout the PEP. Although this decrease in LV dp/dt during the PEP is essentially related to an ineffective rate of force generated by the left ventricle during isovolumic systole, one cannot readily ascertain whether this is caused by a decrease in intrinsic contractile performance of the myocardium or to other factors such as inadequate hypertrophy, excessive LV end-diastolic volume, or myocardial dyssynergy. Thus, a prolongation of PEP in chronic heart failure is a reflection of an overall change in left ventricular chamber performance which cannot and should not be attributed to any of these factors, i.e., diminished intrinsic contractile performance, without due consideration to other variables such as ventricular volume, mass, and synergy. Like the stroke volume or ejection fraction the PEP is, in fact, a measure of overall left ventricular performance during isovolumic systole and does not necessarily reflect the intrinsic contractile properties of the left ventricle.

Many of the above studies in man have focused on the effects of acute interventions on the duration of the phases of systole. Of pertinence to the clinical application of the STI are the effects of the sustained hemodynamic alterations associated with left ventricular disease. Earlier studies on changes in STI among patients with cardiac disease demonstrated the presence of a prolonged PEP and an abbreviated

LVET relative to heart rate.* These studies suggested that the changes in STI may reflect the fall in stroke volume in chronic heart failure. In recent years application of quantitative techniques for hemodynamic evaluation of cardiac performance in man has permitted more critical evaluation of these relationships. Among patients with heart disease caused by coronary arteriosclerosis, hypertension, and primary myocardial disease in whom all medications had been withheld, the pattern of change in the STI noted above, namely, a prolongation of PEP and abbreviation of LVET while QS_2 remained normal, was confirmed.[13,14] Among individuals with a reduced cardiac output, the magnitude of the deviations in PEP and LVET correlated closely and significantly with the stroke volume and cardiac output. Among those patients with functionally mild disease (NYHA classes I to II), in whom cardiac output and stroke volume were diminished only slightly, the deviations in PEP and LVET were relatively small, whereas among patients with functionally severe disease (classes III to IV) the deviations from normal in PEP and LVET were marked (Fig. 6–8). Of additional interest was the observation that among those patients in whom cardiac output and stroke volume ranged within normal limits, significant deviations in PEP and LVET were nonetheless frequent. Thus, although the changes in STI might accompany alterations in stroke volume and cardiac output, they probably were not causally related to these hemodynamic events. Rather, it appeared that the changes in STI were the direct result of the overall changes in left ventricular performance. These observations provided evidence that the STI reflect not only transient hemodynamic changes but accompany sustained alterations in left ventricular performance as well.

In studies on the significance of systolic time intervals as a measure of left ventricular performance, investigators have frequently used the correlation technique wherein changes in STI are related to other measures of left ventricular performance such as the end-diastolic pressure and volume, the ejection fraction, the stroke volume, and the cardiac output. In considering this approach, one must be cognizant that in left ventricular disease, various cardiac performance characteristics are altered in parallel. The correlation technique merely quantitates the closeness of these associated changes. A high degree of correlation does not establish a cause and effect relationship between the measured variables; rather it indicates the proximity of the magnitude of change in the variables tested. Thus, one should not erroneously attribute a change in any systolic interval to another physiologic variable solely on the basis of a close correlation. Further, it is hazardous

* Refs. 12, 22, 61, 62.

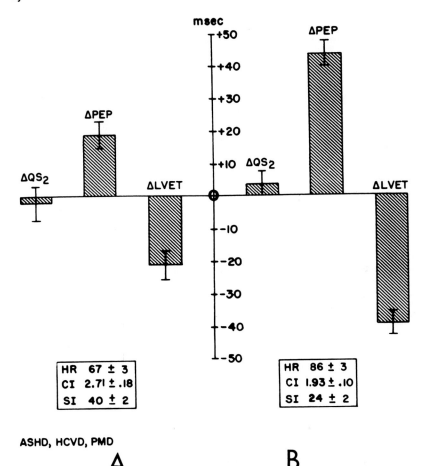

Fig. 6–8. Systolic time intervals in heart disease. A. Mean deviations from normal in QS₂, PEP, and LVET in 11 patients with functional classes I to II. B. Mean deviations from normal in QS₂, PEP, and LVET in 23 patients with functional classes III to IV heart disease: arteriosclerotic heart disease, hypertensive cardiovascular disease, and primary myocardial disease (CI, cardiac index; HR, heart rate; SI, stroke index). (Adapted from Weissler AM et al: Bedside technics for the evaluation of ventricular function in man, Am J Cardiol 23: 577–583, 1969, with permission.)

to quantitate any independent physiologic variable from the change in a systolic interval even when the correlation is high. Since the measured physiologic variables reflect different fundamental aspects of the left ventricular contractile apparatus, it should not be surprising that the STI change when other variables do not and vice versa. The various factors which influence the STI are summarized in Table 6–3.

Table 6–3
Factors Affecting the Systolic Time Intervals

Systolic Interval	Increase	Decrease
Preejection period	↓ LV *dp/dt* LV conduction defect Acute ↑ in arterial pressure ↓ venous return Negative inotropic agents	Aortic valve disease Low LV isovolumic systolic pressure Acute ↓ in arterial pressure ↑ venous return Positive inotropic agents
LV ejection time	Acute ↑ in arterial pressure ↑ venous return Aortic valve disease	LV dysfunction ↓ venous return Positive inotropic agents Negative inotropic agents
Total electromechanical systole	LV conduction defect Aortic valve disease Acute ↑ in arterial pressure	Positive inotropic agents
Preejection period/ LV ejection time	Negative inotropic agents ↓ venous return LV conduct defect LV dysfunction	Positive inotropic agents ↑ venous return Aortic valve disease

CLINICAL APPLICATION OF SYSTOLIC TIME INTERVALS

Of greatest importance to the clinical application of STI measurements is the fact that they afford quantitation of left ventricular performance which can be derived without penetration of the body's surface. This permits repeated observations with little or no disturbance to the patient. As noted previously, left ventricular dysfunction characteristically produces lengthening of the PEP and diminution in the LVET with little change in the QS_2. As we will discuss in this section, the presence of valvular disease, drugs, or certain other conditions may

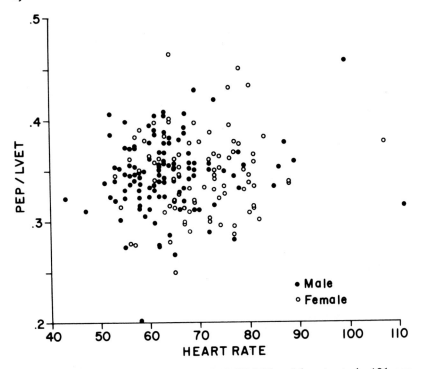

Fig. 6–9. The relationship between PEP/LVET and heart rate in 121 normal male and 90 normal female volunteers. No statistically significant relationship of PEP/LVET to heart rate is demonstrable.

alter these relationships and must be considered when STI are interpreted.

Evaluation of Left Ventricular Performance in Chronic Nonvalvular Heart Disease

Recently the ratio of the PEP to the LVET has become popular as a single expression of ventricular performance from STI,[14,15] Others have used the inverse of this ratio or related the LVET to subintervals of the PEP.* Either the ratio PEP/LVET or its variants has the advantage of encompassing deviations in both basic intervals, the PEP and LVET, and may reflect abnormality when neither measure is clearly beyond normal. Furthermore, the ratio is uninfluenced by heart rate within the range of 40 to 110 beats per min (Fig. 6–9).

* Refs. 12, 61, 62, 64–67.

Finally, because digitalis shortens both the PEP and LVET, the ratio is more useful in identifying abnormal left ventricular performance than either PEP or LVET alone in patients receiving digitalis (see section on digitalis).[68]

Diminished left ventricular performance results in an increase in the PEP/LVET.[14] When this ratio is correlated with cardiac index and stroke index, a significant and close relationship is found among patients with arteriosclerotic, hypertensive, and primary myocardial disease (Fig. 6–10).[14] There is a better correlation of PEP/LVET with stroke index than with cardiac index. Further studies have identified patients, mostly functional class II in whom the cardiac index or stroke index is normal, but in whom the PEP/LVET is clearly abnormal (Fig. 6–11).[63] This suggests that the PEP/LVET is a more sensitive index of left ventricular dysfunction than is the cardiac index or stroke index. Many patients with left ventricular dysfunction maintain a normal cardiac index simply by compensatory tachycardia. In others, it may relate to increased left ventricular end-diastolic volume which allows ejection of a normal-sized stroke volume with a less than normal extent of fiber shortening.[63]

Since the PEP/LVET has appeared to be a more sensitive indicator of ventricular performance than the cardiac output, several recent studies have correlated this ratio with more fundamental direct expressions of ventricular function. Garrard and associates correlated the PEP/LVET with the left ventricular ejection fraction determined by quantitative angiography, left ventricular end-diastolic pressure, and left ventricular end-diastolic volume (Table 6–4).[69] Of these parameters of left ventricular performance, the ejection fraction was most closely correlated with the PEP/LVET ($r = 0.90$, $p < 0.01$). This relationship was obtained in patients with valvular and nonvalvular heart disease with a wide variation in functional impairment (Fig. 6–12). Thus, in a variety of chronic heart diseases the PEP/LVET closely reflects the ejection fraction. In a similar study, Thomas and coworkers found an overall correlation of -0.70 between the PEP/LVET and ejection fraction.[70] Other authors have described a similar relationship between changes in the PEP and the ejection fraction, but it is apparent that deviations in the PEP correlate less well than the PEP/LVET with direct measures of left ventricular performance (Table 6–4).[71,72]

At present there are few studies correlating changes in STI with various isovolumic contractility indices. Ahmed and coworkers have reported significant correlations between the PEP/LVET and the ejection fraction, contractile element velocity at peak isometric stress, and

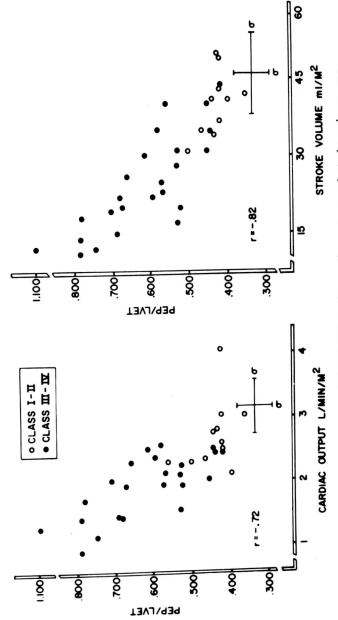

Fig. 6–10. The relation of PEP/LVET to the cardiac output and stroke volume, corrected for body surface area, among 34 patients with heart disease. Bars represent 1 SD from the mean normal value for the PEP/LVET and the flow measurements. (From Weissler AM et al: Bedside technics for the evaluation of ventricular function in man, Am J Cardiol 23:577–583, 1969, with permission.)

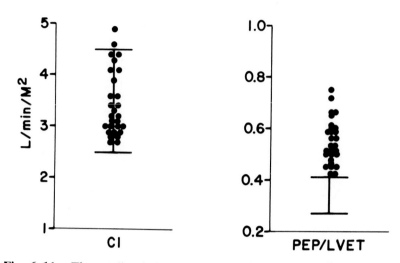

Fig. 6–11. The cardiac index (CI) and PEP/LVET in 28 class II patients with normal cardiac index and abnormal PEP/LVET. The 2 SD-range for both variables is indicated.

Table 6–4
Correlation Matrix for 68 Patients with
Various Cardiac Disorders[a,b]

Systolic Interval	End-Diastole Volume	Ejection Fraction	Left Ventricular End-Diastolic Pressure
Δ Preejection period	0.63	−0.77	0.44
Δ Left Ventricular ejection time	−0.34	0.60	0.35
Preejection period/ left ventricular ejection time	0.68	−0.90	0.57

Source: Adapted from Garrard et al: The relationship of alterations in systolic time intervals to ejection fraction in patients with cardiac disease, Circulation 42:455–462, 1970, with permission.
[a] All figures represent correlation coefficients (r values).
[b] All figures are significant to p < 0.01.

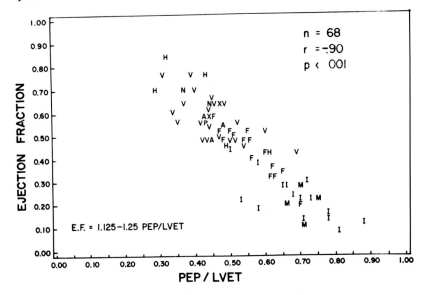

Fig. 6–12. The relationship of PEP/LVET to ejection fraction. The linearity of the relationship is expressed by the regression equation EF = 1.125 − 1.25 PEP/LVET (SD from regression = 0.08) (V, mitral valve disease; F, mitral valve disease with atrial fibrillation; I, ischemic heart disease; M, primary myocardial disease; H, idiopathic hypertrophic subaortic stenosis; X, aortic insufficiency; P, acute pericarditis). (From Garrard CL Jr et al: The relationship of alterations in systolic time intervals to ejection fraction in patients with cardiac disease, Circulation 42:455–462, 1970, with permission.)

the Frank-Levison contractility index in patients with left ventricular myocardial disease.[73] In subjects with valvular heart disease, intracardiac hunts, and cor pulmonale, no close correlations between PEP/LVET and these indices were found. A close correlation between the change in the QS_2 and maximum left ventricular $dp/dt/P$ following digitalis has been shown.[74]

The importance of preload in the interpretation of abnormal STI in chronic congestive heart failure has recently been reported.[75] In a large series of patients followed serially during diuresis, over 50 percent exhibited a deterioration in the PEP/LVET as therapy proceeded. This was attributed to diminished filling pressure for a noncompliant left ventricle. Thus, proper interpretation of the STI in patients with chronic heart failure requires that excessive diuresis be considered as a potential contributory factor to the abnormal PEP/LVET.

We must stress that the presence of left ventricular disease does not imply that STI will be abnormal. Patients with clinically recognizable primary myocardial disease nearly always have abnormal STI. However, in patients with old myocardial infarction the STI may be normal following recovery. Similarly, many patients with chronic hypertension have normal STI. Such patients usually have minimal symptoms and presumably have developed adequate compensatory hypertrophy. Thus, STI are highly useful in assessing the adequacy of left ventricular compensation in the presence of established heart disease.

Coronary Artery Disease

Chronic coronary artery disease. The STI reflect left ventricular performance in chronic coronary artery disease and therefore do not necessarily relate closely to the symptom of angina pectoris nor to pathology of the coronary arteries. Although we have noted reversible abnormality of the PEP/LVET during acute coronary insufficiency, the changes, if any, in the STI during a typical anginal attack have not been described. Between anginal episodes, the PEP/LVET is normal if left ventricular performance is normal. Perry noted a correlation of −0.76 between PEP/LVET and the ejection fraction in 15 patients.[76] McConahay noted a correlation of −0.58 in 32 patients which improved to −0.67 when the postexercise value of PEP/LVET was used.[77] In a larger series of 80 patients with a wider range of ejection fractions (8 to 81 percent) we have found a correlation of −0.85 (Fig. 6–13).

Büyükoztürk noted that the QS_2 was abbreviated in patients with chronic coronary artery disease.[79] This was most pronounced in those with poor collateral vessels visualized on the coronary arteriogram. We have noted the same phenomenon. The QS_2 was significantly shortened in 78 patients with chronic stable angina and 21 with old myocardial infarction (on no drugs) compared to a control group with chest pain and normal coronary arteries. This phenomenon, which was attributed to a hyperadrenergic state in patients with chronic coronary artery disease, has been shown to exist during acute myocardial infarction.[102]

Exercise Testing

Exercise studies with STI have as yet revealed no clear cut pattern of change.* In part this is because the measurements have been made in both the supine and erect positions, and because variable exercise

* Refs. 32, 57, 66, 67, 80–87.

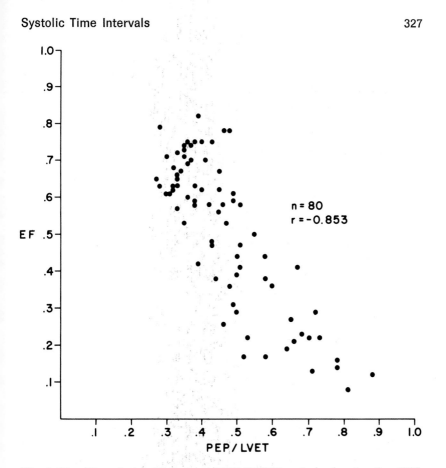

Fig. 6–13. The relationship between PEP/LVET and ejection fraction (EF) in 80 patients with documented chronic coronary artery disease. The majority of patients were receiving digitalis. The EF was calculated from a single-plane RAO cine by the area-length method.[166]

loads have been used, some of which have measured the STI during exercise, whereas others have used variable time periods following exertion. Furthermore, normal regression equations to correct for heart rate following exertion are not yet available.

Several investigators, each using a different exercise protocol have noted that the LVET is relatively prolonged during or after exercise in patients with angina compared to normal controls.[83,84,86] This phenomenon is not affected by beta adrenergic blockade.[87] In a recent series, prolongation of the LVET after maximal exercise (corrected by postexercise regression equations obtained from normal subjects) identified an additional 27 percent of patients with significant coronary artery disease in whom no significant ischemic changes occurred on the electrocardiogram.[78] The physiologic explanation of this phenomenon is unclear but inability of the ischemic ventricle to respond to inotropic stimulation has been suggested.[85,87]

Myocardial Revascularization

Reports indicate that the PEP/LVET improved after saphenous vein graft surgery in a group of patients with significant left ventricular dysfunction preoperatively.[88] One study suggested that serial STI were useful in determining if graft closure occurred. Another study showed that the STI pre- and postoperatively correlated well with direct measures of ejection fraction and dp/dt.[89] Patients with normal left ventricular performance before surgery were unchanged after surgery unless a postoperative myocardial infarction occurred.

Acute Myocardial Infarction

Acute myocardial infarction represents a special situation compared to chronic heart disease and the recent literature has become confused regarding the usefulness of the STI in this disorder.[58,90–103] In most patients there is a striking increase in catecholamine output which profoundly influences the STI.[104–111] Furthermore, there may be a striking reduction in left ventricular isovolumic pressure (aortic diastolic pressure minus left ventricular end-diastolic pressure) owing to reduced left ventricular diastolic distensibility or systemic hypotension, or both.

Virtually all investigators have noted a marked shortening of the STI in the early stages of myocardial infarction. Recently, reports have shown that the reduced QS_2 correlates closely with the increase in catecholamine excretion in these patients (Fig. 6–14).[102] The typical pattern of prolonged PEP, short LVET, and normal QS_2 characteristic of left ventricular dysfunction noted in chronic heart disease is therefore modified in acute myocardial infarction. Indeed, a normal PEP is abnormally long in this situation and may be associated with a diminished left ventricular dp/dt.[112]

In spite of these considerations the PEP/LVET ratio appears to be a useful measure of left ventricular performance in acute myocardial infarction. A high degree of correlation with the cardiac index and stroke index has been reported.[90,100] Others have shown that patients with more severe myocardial infarction assessed clinically have more severe shortening of the LVET and prolongation of the PEP.[93,96,99,100]

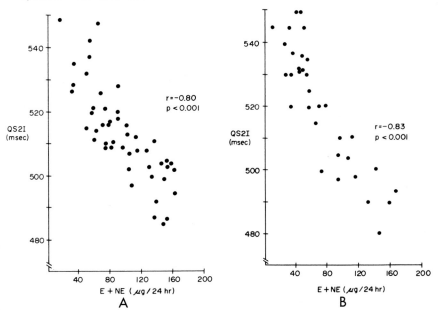

Fig. 6–14. The relationship between QS$_2$I and 24-hour urinary excretion of epinephrine (E) and norepinephrine (NE). A. In 24 patients with documented acute myocardial infarction (AMI). B. In 27 patients admitted to the Coronary Care Unit in whom no AMI was documented. The upper limit of normal for E + NE is 70 μg/24 hr. A similar close relationship between increased excretion of catecholamines and shortening of the QS$_2$I exists for both groups. Most patients in the AMI group were studied both at admission and at discharge. (From Lewis RP et al: Shortening of electromechanical systole as a manifestation of excessive adrenergic stimulation in acute myocardial infarction, Circulation 46:856–863, 1972, with permission.)

The fact remains that many patients with acute myocardial infarction have a normal PEP/LVET, even though all STI are short. This perhaps reflects the fact that in many patients normal cardiac performance is maintained in spite of the acute insult to the myocardium.[103] This is particularly true for nonhypertensive patients experiencing their first infarction in the majority of whom no clinical heart failure occurs.[78]

Several investigators have stressed the value of serial STI measurements. Failure of abnormal STI to return toward normal is a bad prognostic sign.[93,96,100] Persistence of an abnormal PEP/LVET at 3 weeks usually indicates that postinfarction heart failure will be a problem.[78]

The STI have not proved to be a highly sensitive predictor of mortality although most of those who do not survive have severe derangement of the STI.[93,96,113] This is to be expected since left ventricular failure is not the sole cause of mortality in acute myocardial infarction.

When cardiogenic shock supervenes, the STI may be less useful. As noted above, these patients have high levels of catecholamine secretion (or exogenous administration) and a narrowed range of left ventricular developed pressure. These factors tend to shorten the PEP. The proposed index of $(\Delta P/\Delta T)/LV$ filling pressure obtained from measuring the STI and left ventricular filling pressure directly or indirectly may be more useful in this setting.[113] However, serial measurement of the LVET may also be useful.[93,96,100]

Since abnormalities of the PEP/LVET are usually associated with other clinical signs of left ventricular dysfunction (S3 gallop, circulatory congestion), these patients are clearly candidates for digitalis therapy (Fig. 15). However, Rahimitoola has recently showed that some patients

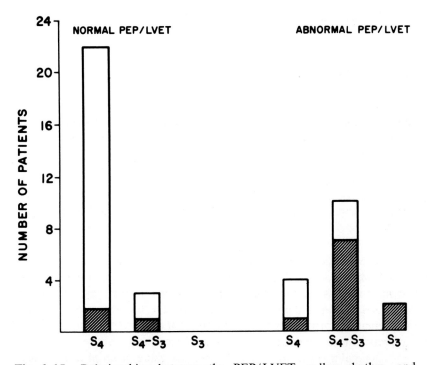

Fig. 6–15. Relationships between the PEP/LVET, gallop rhythm, and clinical evidence of circulatory congestions (CHF) in 41 patients with documented acute myocardial infarction. All patients studied had gallops. Those with a normal PEP/LVET had infrequent S_3 gallops and a low incidence of CHF whereas those with an abnormal PEP/LVET usually had both a S_3 gallop and CHF (cross-hatch areas represent patients with clinical congestive heart failure).

with a normal PEP/LVET 3 to 5 weeks after infarction may have persistence of an increased LVEDP.[114] This is reflected by the high incidence of gallop rhythm in these patients.[115] The elevated LVEDP can be significantly reduced by ouabain without other obvious hemodynamic changes. Thus digitalis may be of benefit even for some patients with a normal PEP/LVET following a myocardial infarction. Whether such patients require permanent digitalis therapy is as yet not known.

Hypertensive Cardiovascular Disease

In chronic hypertensive disease with compensated left ventricular performance, the PEP and LVET are usually normal.[13] As left ventricular failure supervenes, there is prolongation of the PEP and abbreviation of LVET.[13] When the arterial diastolic pressure is extremely elevated, the lengthening of PEP is slightly to moderately greater than that expected from diminished left ventricular performance alone.[13] In patients with severe hypertension, the QS_2 has been found to be prolonged.[116] However, in younger individuals with evidence of hyperkinetic circulation the QS_2 may be short, possibly reflecting excessive catecholamine stimulation or hyperresponsiveness.[78]

Valvular Heart Disease

Measurements of STI appear most useful in the evaluation of patients with myocardial disease. Several studies have suggested their usefulness in patients with valvular heart disease, as well. Indeed, a promising area of investigation is the assessment by STI measurement of the effects of open-heart surgery on left ventricular performance in valvular disease.

Aortic stenosis. Previous studies have indicated that severe aortic stenosis is often accompanied by a prolongation in LVET.[117-122] The mechanism of the prolonged LVET is not clear since the stroke volume is either normal or decreased. It may in part reflect the relatively low points of onset of ejection and closure of the aortic valve on the left ventricular pressure pulse. A delay in the inscription of the incisural notch and A_2 has also been demonstrated. Such a delay is prominent in the right-sided circulation both in normal subjects and in disease states.[123,124] Normally the left-sided delay is less than 10 msec.[123] Figure 6–16 illustrates a patient with significant isolated aortic stenosis studied with two high-fidelity manometer-tip catheters. The incisura shows a 50-msec delay from the aortic left ventricular crossover. The physiologic basis of the delay is not clear, but such factors as an altered

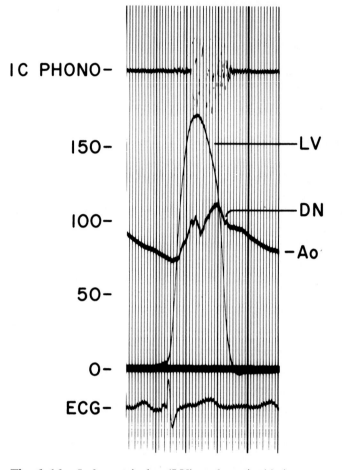

Fig. 6–16. Left ventricular (LV) and aortic (Ao) pressures and intracardiac (IC) phonocardiogram obtained from two high-fidelity manometer-tip catheters in a patient with significant aortic stenosis. The time lines are 20 msec apart (DN, incisural). There is a 50-msec delay between the LV pressure and the inscription of the notch.

flow pattern during ejection and the presence of poststenotic dilatation leading to increased capacitance of the aorta may be responsible.[19,123] Recently, Parisi and associates have shown that a high degree of correlation exists between the cardiac index and LVET in aortic stenosis in spite of the prolongation of the LVET ($r = -0.90$, $p < 0.01$).[120]

The PEP is usually shortened in aortic stenosis. This is probably related to a combination of the rapid rate of rise in left ventricular pressure during isovolumic systole and a relatively small isovolumic pressure gradient. Parisi and coworkers have shown that the PEP correlates closely with left ventricular dp/dt (r $= -0.97$, p < 0.01).[120] The short PEP and prolonged LVET result in a PEP/LVET lower than normal.

If the LVET is significantly prolonged, the QS_2 may be prolonged. This produces the well-known phenomenon of paradoxical splitting of the second heart sound. Left ventricular decompensation in aortic stenosis produces the expected shortening of the LVET and lengthening of the PEP.[121,122] Thus a prolonged LVET may be shortened to the normal range and a short PEP may be lengthened to the normal range. Treatment of left ventricular decompensation may restore the prolonged LVET and short PEP.[78]

Patients with aortic stenosis present certain technical difficulties in measuring STI. In those with calcific aortic stenosis a clearly discernible aortic second sound is frequently impossible to obtain, so that the QS_2 and PEP cannot be measured. The carotid or subclavian arterial pulse may show a poorly delineated incisural notch so that LVET cannot be obtained.

Perhaps the most useful application of STI in patients with suspected aortic stenosis is in the detection of hemodynamically significant aortic valve disease.[121,122] In a patient with a systolic ejection murmur, a long QS_2 and LVET and short PEP strongly suggest significant left ventricular outflow obstruction. In a patient with a murmur of aortic stenosis and evidence of left ventricular decompensation by clinical examination, a marked shortening of the LVET argues against severe valvular aortic stenosis as the primary cause of the left ventricular failure.

Idiopathic hypertrophic subaortic stenosis. Recent studies have suggested that the duration of the LVET may be useful in predicting the presence or absence of significant outflow obstruction in this disorder. Outflow obstruction prolongs the LVET as in valvular aortic stenosis.[125–128] Maneuvers which increase the outflow gradient, such as catecholamines, may paradoxically lengthen the LVET in these subjects (Fig. 6–17). More studies with simultaneous STI and direct measurements of outflow obstruction are required to determine the ultimate usefulness of this observation. In some subjects with no resting outflow obstruction, the QS_2 is abnormally short suggesting a hyperadrenergic state.[78]

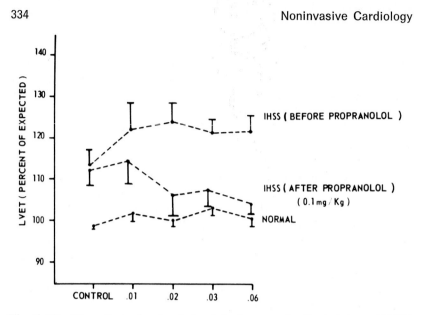

Fig. 6–17. The effect of epinephrine infusion rate (μg/kg/min) on LVET corrected for heart rate in normal subjects and patients with idiopathic hypertrophic subaortic stenosis (IHSS). Before propranolol, epinephrine produces a lengthening of the corrected LVET. This response is abolished following propranolol. Indeed a progressive normalization of the corrected LVET occurs after propranolol probably owing to the salutory effect of isolated alpha adrenergic stimulation. (From Salzman SH et al: Epinephrine infusion in man. Standardization, normal response, and abnormal response in idiopathic hypertrophic subaortic stenosis, Circulation 43:137–144, 1971, with permission.)

Aortic regurgitation. Earlier studies have documented that patients with a significant aortic regurgitation have a prolongation of LVET.[22,118–120] This has been attributed to the large left ventricular stroke volume. However, a prominent incisural delay has also been noted and may contribute to the prolongation of the LVET.[78] Characteristically, the PEP is strikingly reduced and this is probably related to the low systemic diastolic blood pressure. The PEP/LVET is also reduced below normal. Many patients with free aortic regurgitation do not have a demonstrable incisura in the central arterial pulse tracing, and the LVET cannot be measured. As in aortic stenosis, left ventricular decompensation tends to "normalize" the PEP, LVET, and PEP/LVET.

Mitral stenosis. The recent study by Garrard and coworkers demonstrated that the relationship between the PEP/LVET and ejection fraction is retained in patients with mitral stenosis.[69] However, if patients with mitral stenosis are compared to patients with left ventricular disease (ischemic heart disease and primary myocardial disease) and similar levels of cardiac output, those with mitral stenosis have less severe abnormalities in STI and ejection fraction (Table 6–5). Mitral stenosis appears unique in that a low cardiac index may be accompanied by a normal ejection fraction and normal STI. When the PEP/LVET ratio is significantly increased in patients with mitral stenosis, the ejection fraction is usually reduced.[69,78,129] That some patients with mitral stenosis and low cardiac output have relatively normal left ventricular function defined both by STI and left ventricular ejection fraction, whereas others do not, suggests that chronically impaired left ventricular filling per se is not the main factor responsible for deviations in STI when present in this disease. These data suggest that the patient with mitral stenosis and abnormal ventricular function may be identified by STI. Studies with pre- and postoperative assessment of left ventricular function following mitral valve surgery are required to confirm this hypothesis.

Mitral regurgitation. The STI in mitral regurgitation are less well understood than in other valve lesions. This may in part reflect the various etiologies for this lesion. Mitral regurgitation is frequently accompanied by considerable intrinsic left ventricular disease. It is of interest that in spite of the large left ventricular stroke volume, a prolonged LVET is distinctly uncommon.[69,78,118] Indeed, the STI are often normal. This might be because ejection of blood into the left

Table 6–5

PEP/LVET and Cardiac Output in Patients with
Mitral Stenosis and Left Ventricular Disease

Disease	No. of Patients[a]	Preejection Period/LV Ejection Time	Cardiac Index (L/min/m²)
Isolated mitral stenosis	35	0.43 ± 0.14^c $p < 0.001$	2.8 ± 0.67
Left ventricular disease[b]	50	0.60 ± 0.13	2.6 ± 0.82

    [a] All patients in sinus rhythm.
    [b] Left ventricular disease refers to patients with ischemic heart disease or primary myocardial disease.
    [c] 1 SD.

atrium may occur prior to opening of the aortic valve. In our experience, the presence of abnormal STI (prolonged PEP, shortened LVET, increased PEP/LVET) is strongly suggestive of abnormal left ventricular function in the patient with mitral regurgitation.

An interesting phenomenon occurs after mitral valve replacement.[78] Those patients with a normal PEP/LVET preoperatively usually develop a marked increase of the ratio after surgery, whereas there is lesser change in those whose initial PEP/LVET was abnormal. Indeed the change in the PEP/LVET after surgery correlates with the preoperative ejection fraction (r = 0.80, p < 0.001). The explanation for this phenomenon is not yet known. It is possible that elimination of the mitral regurgitation unmasks significant left ventricular dysfunction. However, it is also possible that the abnormal PEP/LVET is a reflection of an underloaded ventricle. Since left ventricular dilatation does not immediately regress after surgery, an inordinately high cardiac output would occur in the postoperative period if the ventricle continued to empty with a normal ejection fraction as it had before surgery. Thus, it is likely that circulatory adjustments occur which limit left ventricular performance in the early postoperative period. Serial studies in these patients demonstrated that as the heart size decreased, the PEP/LVET tends to return to normal. In patients with dominant left ventricular disease, the PEP/LVET is relatively unaltered by surgery. This same phenomenon is also noted in aortic regurgitation.

Pericardial Disease

Systolic time intervals offer several diagnostic aids in patients with pericardial disease. In the presence of pericardial tamponade, marked respiratory variations in LVET (up to 50 to 60 msec) can be demonstrated.[130] Such variations in LVET presumably represent the variations in stroke volume which are responsible for pulsus paradoxicus.[131] Since the changes in LVET may occur in the absence of detectable respiratory change in arterial pressure, measurement of STI may offer a more quantitative and precise method of establishing the presence of cardiac tamponade than does the detection of pulsus paradoxicus with a sphygmomanometer. However, it should be noted that in subjects with chronic heart or lung disease but without pericardial effusion, respiratory variations of LVET above the normal 5 to 10 msec can be seen.[132,133] In a study of 110 such patients the mean variation of LVET with respiration was 18 msec ± 7 (1 SD) and was independent of heart rate.[78]

A second application of STI in pericardial disease is in the detection of left ventricular dysfunction. In a patient with clinical evidence of acute pericarditis, this may suggest the presence of underlying myocarditis.

In patients with chronic constrictive pericarditis, we have documented a normal LVET despite a markedly elevated venous pressure and signs of congestion. Such patients usually have a normal cardiac index. In the presence of severe circulatory congestion, the finding of a normal LVET should lead one to suspect pericardial constriction as a possible cause of the congested state.

Conduction Defects

Right bundle branch block in the absence of left ventricular dysfunction does not alter left ventricular STI. Left ventricular conduction defects do prolong the PEP but may not alter the LVET. A recent study indicated that patients with so-called bilateral bundle branch block pattern (left axis deviation and right bundle branch block) had similar prolongation of the PEP to those with complete left bundle branch block.[134] Patients with either left axis deviation or right bundle branch block alone had normal values. However, another study showed slight prolongation of the PEP with isolated left axis deviation.[135]

The mechanism of the PEP prolongation in left ventricular conduction defects remains unclear. Some studies have indicated that the major prolongation is in the electromechanical delay (Q to onset of left ventricular contraction), whereas other studies have suggested that prolonged ICT is the major abnormality.* In part, the problem may be related to the various ways in which subintervals of the PEP have been studied, using either the apexcardiogram or the first heart sound to determine the onset of isovolumic contraction. As noted earlier, the apexcardiogram appears to offer the more reliable approach to delineating the electromechanical delay. It is probable that both a delay in the electromechanical interval and prolongation of ICT account for the prolongation of the PEP in most patients with left ventricular conduction defects. However, we as well as others have encountered patients with classic complete left bundle branch block in whom the electromechanical delay as defined from the apexcardiogram is normal. Thus, the measurement of the PEP alone is not sufficient to characterize left ventricular performance in significant left ventricular conduction defects.

Data from studies of five patients by atrial pacing, synchronous pacing, and right ventricular pacing all at the same heart rate are listed in Table 6–6. The latter two forms of pacing induce a form of com-

* Refs. 134, 136–147.

Table 6–6
Effect of Three Techniques of Artificial Cardiac Pacing on the STI in Six Subjects

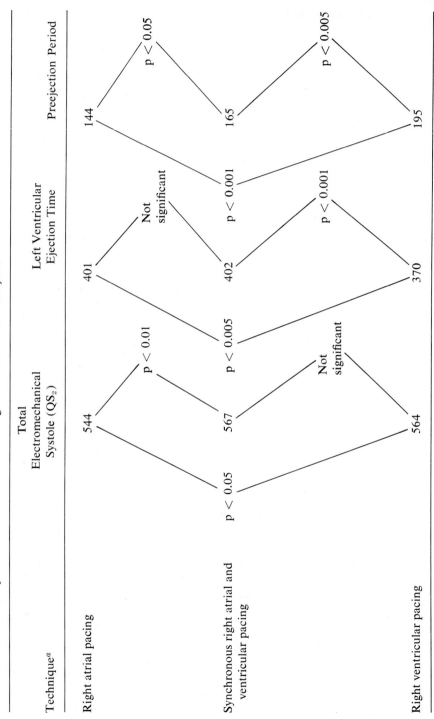

Technique[a]	Total Electromechanical Systole (QS_2)	Left Ventricular Ejection Time	Preejection Period
Right atrial pacing	544	401	144
Synchronous right atrial and ventricular pacing	567	402	165
Right ventricular pacing	564	370	195

Right atrial pacing vs. Synchronous right atrial and ventricular pacing:
QS_2 $p < 0.01$; Left Ventricular Ejection Time Not significant; Preejection Period $p < 0.05$

Synchronous right atrial and ventricular pacing vs. Right ventricular pacing:
QS_2 Not significant; Left Ventricular Ejection Time $p < 0.001$; Preejection Period $p < 0.005$

Right atrial pacing vs. Right ventricular pacing:
QS_2 $p < 0.05$; Left Ventricular Ejection Time $p < 0.005$; Preejection Period $p < 0.001$

plete left bundle branch block since the pacing catheter lies in the right ventricle. It is easy to see that when atrial pacing and synchronous pacing are compared, the LVET does not shorten, whereas the PEP prolongs during synchronous pacing. Synchronous pacing retains the benefit of atrial systole. However, when the effect of atrial systole is acutely removed, as with ventricular pacing, the LVET shortens and the PEP prolongs further. In this instance, the additional prolongation of the PEP (and decrease in the LVET) is most likely related to an acute reduction in preload related to the loss of the increment in ventricular filling owing to atrial systole. Thus in conduction defects, particularly when these are transients, both hemodynamic and electrophysiologic factors may influence the STI; a fact which should always be considered in interpretation of the STI in this type of situation.

Arrhythmias

Atrial fibrillation. Previous studies have demonstrated that the LVET is directly related to the duration of the antecedent R-R interval in patients with atrial fibrillation.[46,148] The relationship is curvilinear with less than expected lengthening of the LVET at longer R-R intervals. It may be linearized if cycle length is expressed as 60/R-R of the previous beat.[148] This is because of the nonlinear relationship between the R-R interval and the heart rate calculated from the R-R interval (60/R-R).

The PEP is also related to the previous R-R. However, the PEP lengthens rather than shortens with shorter R-R intervals.[30] This is in marked contrast to sinus rhythm wherein the PEP shortens slightly with increasing heart rate. The lengthening of the PEP (like the shortening of the LVET) is more striking with R-R intervals of less than 0.8 sec. This relationship may be somewhat linearized by expressing cycle length as 60/R-R of the previous beat.[30]

The "paradoxical" increase in the PEP at faster heart rates is probably related to two factors: the greater isovolumic pressure which must be developed and a diminished preload. We have studied five patients with atrial fibrillation with high-fidelity manometer-tip catheters in the left ventricle. Multiple beats of varying R-R intervals were analyzed. There was a high degree of linear correlation (> 0.8) between the PEP and developed pressure (aortic diastolic pressure minus left ventricular end-diastolic pressure) and PEP and maximum LV $(dp/dt)/P$.

Flessas et al studied 13 patients by beat-to-beat analysis of STI, left ventricular volumes, and velocity of fiber shortening.[149] PEP varied inversely with the ejection fraction (r = −0.94), velocity of fiber shortening (r = 0.67), and end-diastolic volume (r = −0.94). Thus shorter R-R intervals were associated with smaller end-diastolic volume, diminished contractile effort, and a long PEP. The LVET was directly related to stroke volume (r = 0.94). The PEP/LVET was inversely related to the ejection fraction (r = −0.94).

Since the PEP lengthens and the LVET shortens, the PEP/LVET increases with diminishing cycle length in atrial fibrillation.[30] The rate of increase in PEP/LVET is minimal at RR intervals > 0.8 (HR below 75), but increases markedly above the heart rate (0.0054/beat, p < 0.001) (Fig. 6–18).

When subjects were studied before and after restoration of sinus rhythm, investigators found that the PEP/LVET obtained by averag-

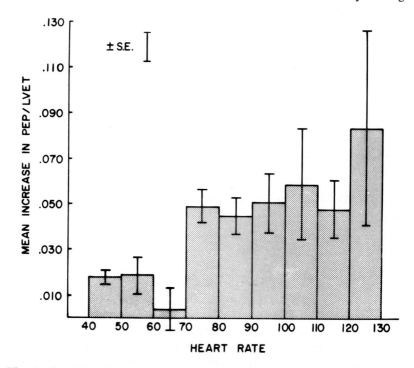

Fig. 6–18. Mean increase in the average PEP/LVET per beat for decades of heart rate from 40 to 130 in 19 subjects with atrial fibrillation. The heart rates for each beat were obtained from the preceding R-R interval (60/R-R) and a wide range of heart rates was present in each subject. For beats with a calculated heart rate above 70 there is a nearly constant increase in the PEP/LVET of 0.05 per decade (see text).

ing only beats below heart rate 75 was identical to that in sinus rhythm (0.35 versus 0.37).[30] This is in contrast to a PEP/LVET of 0.46 ($p < 0.05$) obtained when all beats in atrial fibrillation were averaged. Thus, STI calculated by averaging all beats can underestimate potential left ventricular performance and this error can largely be eliminated by measuring only those beats below heart rate 75.

In patients with mitral stenosis and atrial fibrillation, there is diastolic dependence of the LVET throughout the range of heart rate so the LVET remains linearly related to heart rate even at slower rates. In other types of cardiac disease, the LVET tends to increase less as the heart rate slows below 75. Following cardioversion, the LVET is increased for a given heart rate except when mitral stenosis is present.[150,151] This observation probably reflects the beneficial effect of atrial systole which is mitigated in mitral stenosis and as such may be a useful tool to assess the benefit of sinus rhythm.

Other arrhythmias. Few studies of tachyarrhythmias other than atrial fibrillation have been performed.[32] Major drawbacks are that adequate preload cannot be assumed, and there is question concerning the type of regression equation for correction for heart rate at rapid rates. The value of STI in tachyarrhythmias thus remains to be explored.

Premature ventricular contractions characteristically result in a prolonged PEP and shortened LVET. Of interest, it is usually demonstrable that the postextrasystolic beat shows a shorter PEP and longer LVET than normal beats. This is probably because of enhanced diastolic filling and possibly postextrasystolic potentiation, as well. The adverse effect of ventricular tachycardia on the PEP and LVET is illustrated in Figure 6–19.

When atrioventricular dissociation is induced by ventricular pacing, beats with a physiologically timed atrial systole exhibit a longer LVET than those which lack the atrial booster pump effect. This has been reported in both valvular and nonvalvular disease.[152–154] The longer LVET is caused by a larger stroke volume.

Atrial pacing. When atrial pacing is used to increase heart rate, the PEP does not shorten.[155] The failure of the PEP to shorten with atrial pacing has been attributed to a larger pressure differential between left ventricular end-diastolic pressure and aortic diastolic pressure, which counteracts a slight increase in the rate of rise of pressure development.[49]

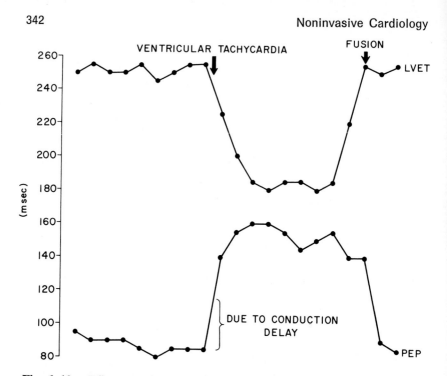

Fig. 6–19. Effect of "slow" ventricular tachycardia (VT) (heart rate 92) compared to sinus rhythm (heart rate 90) in a patient with acute myocardial infarction. The LVET and PEP are not corrected for heart rate. The onset of the VT is indicated by an arrow. It terminated with a fusion beat (Fusion). The increase in the PEP which could be attributed solely to the increased QRS duration of 35 msec during VT is indicated within the bracket. There is an obvious deterioration of the LVET and PEP during VT which cannot be attributed to the conduction abberation alone.

Miscellaneous

Pulsus alternans. During pulsus alternans, the QS_2 remains relatively constant, whereas the PEP lengthens and the LVET shortens during the weakened beat.[156,157]

Amyl nitrite inhalation. Following amyl nitrite inhalation in normal subjects, the LVET lengthens and the PEP shortens. In patients with ischemic heart disease, the LVET and PEP do not change.[53] The differences could not be related to heart rate or diastolic pressure level, and this suggested that a lack of increase in stroke volume was responsible in patients with ischemic heart disease.

Thyroid disease. Amidi and coworkers studied the ICT, LVET, and PEP in normal, hyperthyroid, and hypothyroid subjects.[158] A pattern of short ICT and LVET was present in hyperthyroid subjects and prolongation of these intervals was present in hypothyroid subjects. The mechanisms of the prolongation of LVET in hypothyroidism despite a low stroke volume remains unexplained. The short STI in hyperthyroidism were not affected by catecholamine depletion with reserpine.

EFFECTS OF DRUGS ON SYSTOLIC TIME INTERVALS

Drugs Which Affect the Autonomic Nervous System

The responses of the heart to drugs which affect the autonomic nervous system are uniquely revealed by observing changes in systolic time intervals. Slightly over a half century ago Wiggers observed shortening of STI when catecholamines were infused into animals.[8] Subsequently, Raab and coworkers elicited similar alterations in STI in humans following intravenous infusion of sympathomimetic agents.[50]

When the effects of specific sympathomimetic drugs on STI have been examined, certain differences have been noted. The shortening of PEP induced by isoproterenol infusion in doses up to 2.5 μg/min is related linearly to the dose of the drug.[51] Infusion of epinephrine results in a shortening of PEP similar to that induced by isoproterenol. A greater dose of epinephrine, however, is required to produce the same shortening of PEP. Thus, an infusion of epinephrine at 5.0 μg/min results in a 30 msec abbreviation of PEP which is of the same magnitude as that induced by isoproterenol at 2.5 μg/min.[48]

By contrast isoproterenol and epinephrine have differing effects on LVET. In most normal individuals isoproterenol induces a shortening of LVET which is greater than that expected for the increased heart rate.[51] Epinephrine infusion, however, causes no shortening of LVET when it is corrected for heart rate.[48]

When heart rate is held constant by atrial pacing in patients with heart disease, there is no change in the duration of LVET in response to an infusion of isoproterenol in the dose range of 0.5 to 2.0 μg/min, in spite of the enhanced stroke volume. There is shortening of PEP in response to isoproterenol infusion when heart rate is held constant with pacing. The shortening of PEP in response to isoproterenol during atrial pacing is virtually identical to that observed when heart rate is allowed to increase.[159] Thus both in normal subjects and in patients with heart disease shortening of PEP appears to provide a more sensitive and consistent reflection of the positive inotropic effects of the catecholamines than does shortening of LVET. The variation in response of LVET to these maneuvers may well be related to the greater dependence of LVET on the alterations in heart rate, stroke volume, and afterload which accompany the positive inotropic effects of catecholamines on the left ventricle, as originally pointed out by Raab and coworkers.[50]

It should be noted that the shortening of PEP and LVET which accompanies pharmacologic adrenergic stimulation of the heart probably results from a change in either the slope of the regression equation relating heart rate to the STI or to a change in magnitude of the STI independent of a slope change, or both. Since quantitative data on the contribution of each of these factors have not been published to date, the validity of correcting the durations of STI for changes in heart rate induced by catecholamine infusion is not yet established.

An abbreviation of STI has also been noted in individuals without heart disease but with increased endogenous sympathetic activity, including subjects under emotional tension, psychotic patients, patients who fear they are experiencing an acute myocardial infarction, and patients with pheochromocytoma.[50,51,102] The response of the PEP to a beta-sympathetic blocking agent has been used to confirm that such individuals have excessive endogenous sympathetic activity. Excessive PEP lengthening has been found in such individuals in response to a 10-mg dose of propranolol administered intravenously, in contrast to a slight (average 10 msec) lengthening of PEP induced in normal subjects by propranolol.[51,160]

Beta-blocking drugs other than propranolol vary in their effect on the duration of PEP, depending on the specific agent used. Some drugs have no effect and others actually result in slight shortening when PEP is corrected for heart rate.[160] The reasons for the slight but consistent lengthening of PEP induced by propranolol in contrast to the effect of other beta-blocking agents on PEP have not been elucidated. Such lengthening may be related to the nonspecific myocardial depression induced by propranolol, which may not be caused by other beta-blocking agents; or it may be that the other agents have a less potent beta-blocking effect on the myocardium. Propranolol causes a slight shortening of LVET when this interval is corrected for the slowing in heart rate induced by the drug.[48]

The beta-blocking effects of propranolol on the myocardium are best shown in normal subjects by infusing challenge doses of isoproterenol before and after administration of propranolol. The results of

such studies have shown that the effects of these two agents on PEP
are competitive throughout a wide dosage range for each agent (Fig.
6–20).[51]

The duration of the beta-blocking effects of propranolol has been
tested by observing the responses of PEP and heart rate to repeated
dosage levels of isoproterenol infused into normal subjects. After virtually complete beta blockade, a clear difference has been found in the
rates of dissipation of chronotropic and inotropic blocking effects. Thus

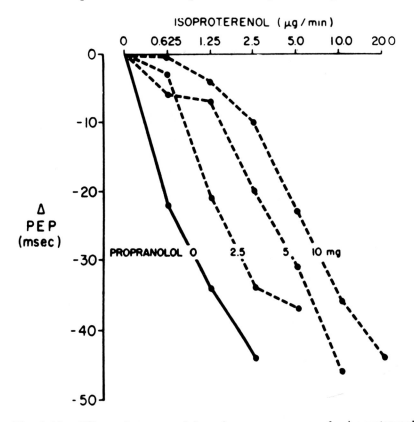

Fig. 6–20. Effects of propranolol on dose-response curve for isoproterenol
in a normal subject. Each curve was obtained on a separate day. The first
curve (solid line) was obtained after a placebo, the second after 2.5 mg
of intravenous propranolol, and the next two after 5 and 10 mg or intravenous propranolol, respectively. Increasing doses of propranolol shift the
isoproterenol dose-response curve in parallel fashion to the right. (From
Harris WS et al: Effects of adrenergic receptor activation and blockade on
the systolic preejection period, heart rate, and arterial pressure in man,
J Clin Invest 46:1704–1714, 1967, with permission.)

at 24 hr after the intravenous administration of either 5 or 10 mg of propranolol, the heart rate response to an isoproterenol infusion is still depressed, whereas the PEP response is not.[161]

In contrast to the inhibition of the shortening effect of isoproterenol on PEP observed in beta-blocked subjects, the infusion of catecholamines which have both alpha- and beta-stimulating properties such as epinephrine or norepinephrine results in an actual lengthening of PEP after propranolol administration (Fig. 6–21).[48,51] This response

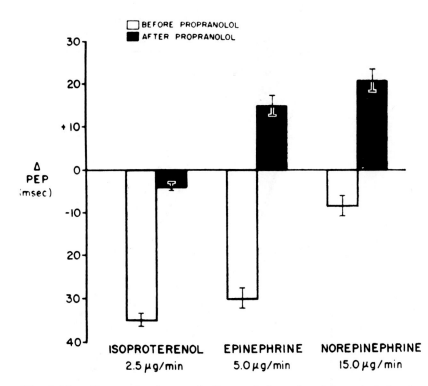

Fig. 6–21. Changes in the preejection period produced by catecholamine infusions. Isoproterenol was given intravenously to 25 normal subjects, epinephrine to 10 and norepinephrine to 15. Each subject received the same agent before and after 10 mg of intravenous propranolol. The bars represent mean changes from control (±SE) resulting from catecholamine infusion. The changes before propranolol are measured from control values before propranolol; those after propranolol from control values after propranolol. All changes from control shown are significant. (From Harris WS et al: Effects of adrenergic receptor activation and blockade on the systolic preejection period, heart rate, and arterial pressure in man, J Clin Invest 46:1704–1714, 1967, with permission.)

is apparently caused by the uncovering of alpha-receptor stimulation in the presence of beta blockade and is accompanied by a slowing of heart rate. The latter response is presumably vagal in origin.

Catecholamines which stimulate only alpha receptors and agents which exhibit nonadrenergic vasoconstricting properties result in lengthening of both PEP and LVET.[51] Atropine blocks the PEP prolongation induced both by the alpha-stimulating effects of methoxamine and norepinephrine after propranolol as well as the vasoconstrictor effects of angiotension.[52,162] Studies show this blocking effect of atropine to be dose related.[163] Thus the prolongation of PEP accompanying alpha-adrenergic stimulation is dependent, at least in part, on simultaneously induced vagal impulses to the heart. In patients with autonomic insufficiency who lack vagal efferents to the heart, PEP prolongation cannot be induced by the administration of norepinephrine after propranolol.[163]

Atropine alone results in slight shortening or in no change in the duration of PEP.[50,51] Thus the effects of atropine are similar to those of atrial pacing in that the duration of PEP remains relatively unchanged despite an increase in heart rate.[49,51]

The infusion of methoxamine into normal individuals induces a lengthening of LVET even when reflex bradycardia is prevented by maintaining a constant heart rate with atrial pacing. Since cardiac output and stroke volume remain unchanged in this situation, the methoxamine effect on LVET is apparently predominantly caused by an increase in afterload.[52]

The effects on the duration of PEP of catecholamines which have both alpha- and beta-stimulating properties are variable depending on the relative predominance of the respective receptor stimulation and of the concordant vagal response. Thus norepinephrine infused in a dose of 7.5 $\mu g/min$ results in lengthening of PEP, whereas at higher doses of 15 and 22.5 $\mu g/min$, there is abbreviation of PEP (Fig. 6–22). When propranolol is administered to block the beta-stimulating effects of norepinephrine, PEP is lengthened by infusion of norepinephrine at each dose level.[51] When the vagal effects of norepinephrine are blocked with atropine, a shortening of PEP occurs. This shortening occurs even with low doses of norepinephrine and despite an even greater pressor response.[162] The infusion of epinephrine which normally causes an abbreviation of PEP, a reflection of its dominant beta-receptor effect, induces lengthening of PEP following beta-adrenergic receptor blockade.

The effect of levodopa on the duration of PEP has recently been examined since this drug has been shown to have cardiovascular side-effects, apparently caused by dopamine which is released following decarboxylation of the amino acid. In a small group of patients, a dose-

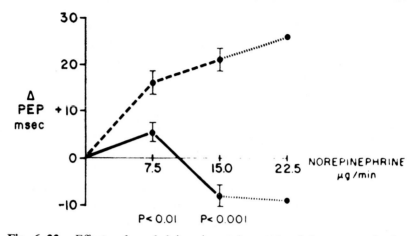

Fig. 6–22. Effects of graded insusions of norepinephrine on preejection period in 12 normal subjects. Norepinephrine was given to each subject before (solid line) and after (dashed line) intravenous propranolol (10 mg). Three of these subjects received an additional dose of 22.5 μg/min (finely broken line). (From Harris WS et al: Effects of adrenergic receptor activation and blockade on the systolic preejection period, heart rate, and arterial pressure in man. J Clin Invest 46:1704–1714, 1967, with permission.)

dependent shortening of PEP was noted following intravenous administration of levodopa.[164] This response was blocked by the oral administration of propranolol. After 3 months of continuous levodopa therapy, PEP shortening occurred either not at all or to only a slight degree, suggesting the development of tolerance.

The response of STI to an alpha-blocking agent, phentolamine, has been studied in normal subjects. Although the infusion of this drug was associated with no changes in QS_2 interval, heart rate or arterial pressure, a significant shortening of PEP and the calculated ICT occurred with lengthening of LVET. Because of the shortening of PEP, investigators postulated that phentolamine has a positive inotropic effect despite the lengthening of LVET. This pattern of change in STI is similar to that seen with epinephrine infusion.[165]

Digitalis

Early observations of Wiggers and Stimson indicated that the positive inotropic effects of digitalis on the left ventricle of the dog were accompanied by abbreviation in the phases of systole.[167] Investigations of the response in the STI to the cardiac glycosides in man were prompted by the implications of this observation. These studies on the effects of the digitalis glycosides on the STI have been reviewed in a recent symposium.[168] It was first necessary to take into account the well-known effects of heart rate on these intervals. Initial studies on the effects of digitalis were therefore designed to ascertain whether digitalis alters the relationships between heart rate and the STI.[37] Studies on 17 normal subjects demonstrated that Cedilanid-D induced an abbreviation in all of the STI without altering the slope of the regression equations relating to heart rate. It is notable that the alterations in STI following administration of the digitalis glycosides to normal subjects occurs in the absence of a change in cardiac output, whereas mean arterial pressure and peripheral resistance rise slightly.[55] An important question pertinent to the interpretation of the STI responses concerns the independent effect of the increase in peripheral resistance which accompanies the glycoside response. Studies in recent years on the effects of pharmacologically induced increases in peripheral resistance in man demonstrate an actual lengthening in STI.[48,51,52] Hence, the abbreviation in systole following digitalis cannot be explained on the basis of its peripheral vascular effects. Indeed, the shortening of STI following digitalis occurs despite the potentially antagonistic effect of an increase in peripheral resistance in normal subjects.

The abbreviation in STI following the administration of Cedilanid-D follows a time course reminiscent of that for the clinical response to this agent.[168,169] The responses in QS_2 and LVET corrected for heart rate and diurnal abbreviation in the STI are shown in Figure 6–23. The response is characterized by a prompt abbreviation which is well developed within the first 20 min following administration of the drug and is followed by a slight additional effect which progresses to a maximum at 2 hr. When the response in STI is followed during the subsequent 5-day period, a progressive dissipation in the Cedilanid-D effect is apparent so that predrug levels are approached on the fourth to fifth day following drug administration (Fig. 6–24). When the dissipation of the response to Cedilanid-D among normal subjects is plotted on a logarithmic coordinate against time, it proves to be exponential. From this logarithmic representation of the data, the physiologic half-life of Cedilanid-D has been calculated to be 30 to 42 hr.

These observations on the response to Cedilanid-D prompted additional studies to test whether the magnitude of the response in STI bears a quantitative relationship to the positive inotropic effect of digitalis. In this regard, research has shown that the responses in QS_2 and LVET, during the initial 2 hr after intravenous administration of Cedilanid-D, are dose dependent (Fig. 6–25).[168,169] Further, the di-

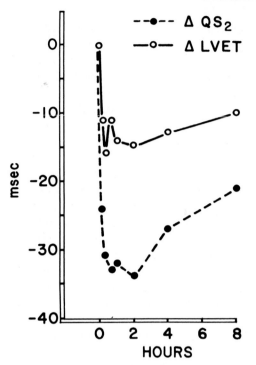

Fig. 6–23. The mean responses in QS₂ (ΔQS₂) and LVET (ΔLVET) following Cedilanid-D (1.6 mg IV) in 18 normal subjects during the first 8 hr following drug administration. (From Weissler AM et al: Comparative responses to the digitalis glycosides in man, in Marks BM, Weissler AM (Eds.): Basic and Clinical Pharmacology of Digitalis. Fort Lauderdale, Florida, Thomas, 1972, pp 260–280, with permission.)

minution in QS_2 parallels the increase in left ventricular contractile response as measured by the ratio of the maximum left ventricular $(dp/dt)/P$ (Fig. 6–26). On the basis of these observations, it would appear that the responses in STI to the digitalis glycosides offer an accurate expression of their positive inotropic effects.

Additional studies of the STI responses to the digitalis glycosides have been directed toward comparisons of the responses to various commonly used glycoside preparations.[168–170] In Figure 6–27 the onset of the shortening of the QS_2 (corrected for molecular weight of the glycoside) is shown for five commonly used glycosides. Since the curves are exponential, the time constant (the point at which 63 percent of the total effect is achieved) can be calculated for each curve and

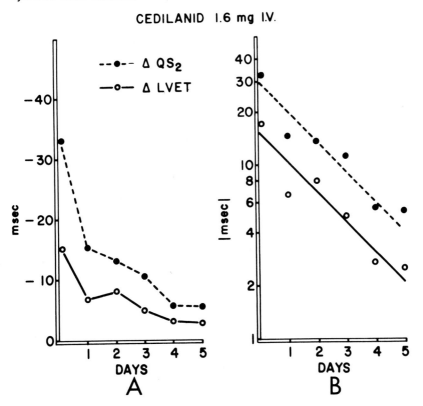

Fig. 6–24. Dissipation of the mean responses in QS_2 (ΔQS_2) and LVET ($\Delta LVET$) following Cedilanid-D (1.6 mg IV) in eight normal subjects plotted on linear (A) and semilogarithmic (B) coordinates. (From Weissler AM et al: Comparative responses to the digitalis glycosides in man, in Marks BM, Weissler AM (Eds.): Basic and Clinical Pharmacology of Digitalis. Fort Lauderdale, Florida, Thomas, 1972, pp 260–280, with permission.)

provides a quantitative measure of the rapidity of onset of inotropic effect (Table 6–7). The time constant for acetyl strophanthidin could not be calculated but is obviously very short, and the drug effect is completely dissipated in 1 hr.

When the dissipation of the responses of each of the glycosides are expressed on semilogarithmic coordinates, a quantitative comparison of the rates of disappearance of their physiologic responses can be made. The results are listed in Table 6–7.

The exponential pattern of the dissipation of the response to the various glycosides is similar to that for the decay of serum levels fol-

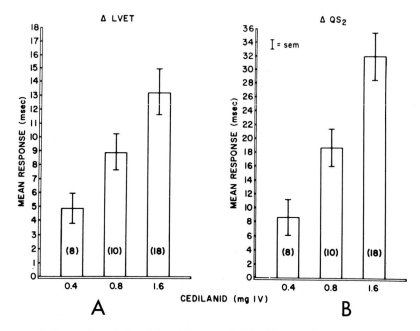

Fig. 6–25. The relationship of dose of Cedilanid-D to the mean responses. A. Response to Cedilanid-D in left ventricular ejection time (ΔLVET). B. Response in total electromechanical systole (ΔQS₂) to Cedilanid-D. The responses represent the mean decrease in each systolic time interval during the first 2 hr after drug administration. The numbers in parentheses refer to the number of subjects studied. (From Weissler AM et al: Comparative responses to the digitalis glycosides in man, in Marks BM, Weissler AM (Eds.): Basic and Clinical Pharmacology of Digitalis. Fort Lauderdale, Florida, Thomas, 1972, pp 260–280, with permission.)

Table 6–7
Left Ventricular Response to Digitalis Glycosides

Digitalis Glycoside	Time Constant (min)	Physiologic Half-Life (hr)
Ouabain	5.8 ± 0.6	23
Cedilanid-D	7.2 ± 3.3	36–42
Digoxin	23 ± 2.3	33–42
Digitoxin	56 ± 10.0	>100

Data derived from studies on systolic time interval responses.

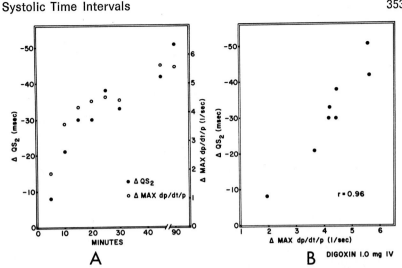

Fig. 6–26. A. Relation between the change in QS_2 (ΔQS_2) and maximum $(dp/dt)/P$ of the left ventricle (Δ max $dp/dt/P$) for 90 min following intravenous administration of 1.0 mg digoxin in one subject. The dp/dt was recorded with a high-fidelity manometer-tipped catheter. B. The high degree of correlation between the two variabes is shown. (From Weissler AM et al: Comparative responses to the digitalis glycodies in man, in Marks BM, Weissler AM (Eds.): Basic and Clinical Pharmacology of Digitalis. Fort Lauderdale, Florida, Thomas, 1972, pp 260–280, with permission.)

lowing the administration of radioactive-labeled glycosides. Recently, Wilson and coworkers have demonstrated an inverse relationship between the plasma level of digitoxin and the LVET during the early hours after a single "digitalizing dose."[171] Shapiro and coworkers have demonstrated a similar inverse relationship between blood levels and the effects of digitoxin and digoxin on the STI during the period immediately following intravenous administration.[172] This inverse relationship between the initial cardiac effects and blood levels is explained by the delayed equilibration between serum and tissue levels of the glycoside following a single intravenous dose. After the maximum response to digitoxin is reached, presumably at a time when tissue and blood levels equilibrate, the subsequent dissipation in glycoside serum levels and STI occurs in parallel. In studies on the effects of digoxin, the calculated half-lives for the excretion of this glycoside using radioactive-labeled digoxin and dissipation of the response in QS_2 were virtually identical.[172,173] In similar studies by Bush and coworkers using radioactive-labeled digitoxin, a close temporal association between the

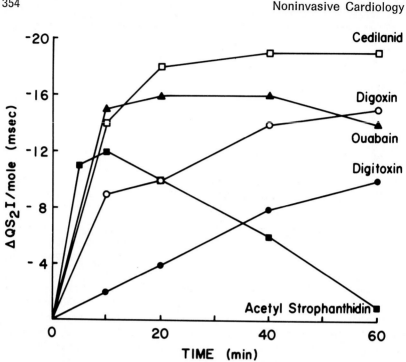

Fig. 6–27. The onset of inotropic effect (ΔQS_2I) following an intravenous digitalizing dose of 5 digitalis glycosides. The ΔQS_2 is corrected for the molecular weight of the glycoside (see text).

dissipation in the responses in QS_2 and the disappearance of the glycoside from the serum was confirmed.[174] It appears therefore that once equilibrium between plasma and tissue levels of the glycosides is achieved, the subsequent excretion of the glycoside is paralleled by a diminution in the cardiac response as measured by the STI. Since the responses in STI reflect the contractile response of the drug, it may be inferred that the serum levels reflect the concentration of the glycoside at active sites in the myocardium. To date, the latter hypothesis has not been tested directly.

The response of the QS_2 following the digitalis glycosides has been used for a comparison of the magnitude and temporal course of the effects of digoxin and digitoxin by the oral and intravenous routes (Fig. 6–28 and 6–29).[78] These studies have shown a clear delay and decrease in the cardiac response to digoxin when the drug is administered by the oral route. In contrast, the ultimate response to digitoxin is virtually identical by the oral and intravenous routes although the intravenous preparation exhibits a more rapid onset of activity. A recent

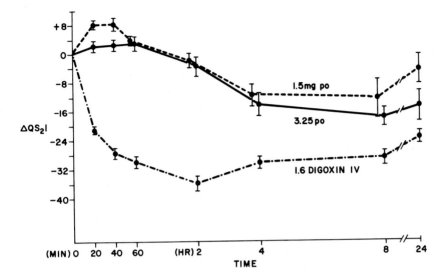

Fig. 6–28. The change in QS_2 ($\Delta QS_2 I$) following two oral (po) doses and one intravenous (IV) dose of digoxin. The IV dose produces a more rapid onset of activity and the ΔQSI is significantly greater than either oral dose through 24 hr. These is no significant difference between the two oral doses except at 24 hr.

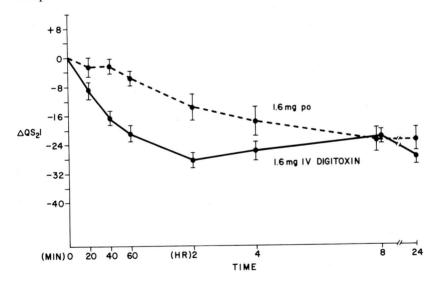

Fig. 6–29. The change in QS_2 ($\Delta QS_2 I$) following oral (po) and intravenous (IV) doses of 1.6 mg of digitoxin. The IV dose has a significantly more rapid onset of activity, but by 4 hr the total effect of the doses by the two routes is statistically indistinguishable.

report indicate that digoxin elixir is more rapidly absorbed than digoxin tablets.[175]

Of pertinence to the clinical application of STI measurements for the study of digitalis effect is the response among patients with congestive heart failure. Recent studies of Cedilanid-D in patients with clinically conspicuous congestive heart failure have confirmed that the abbreviations in QS_2 and PEP are comparable among patients with congestive heart failure and normal subjects.[68] The responses in QS_2 proved to be the most specific reflection of the cardiac effect of the glycosides when compared to other STI and various hemodynamic measures. The response in LVET among patients with heart failure is more variable than that in normal subjects. Among those individuals with greatest increase in cardiac output and stroke volume following Cedilanid-D, there is less abbreviation in LVET; i.e., the stroke volume response influences that of LVET. When cardiac output and stroke volume are increased greatly following Cedilanid-D, the LVET may actually lengthen, despite an abbreviation in QS_2. Preliminary observations indicate that among patients with heart failure, the dissipation of the response in STI is not as uniform as that among normal subjects; excretion appears to be normal in some patients and prolonged in others.[78]

The effect of the digitalis glycosides on the STI is of pertinence to the interpretation of changes in the intervals in patients with heart failure who are receiving the drug. The mean responses in QS_2, LVET, and PEP following full digitalization with Cedilanid-D (1.6 mg IV) are, respectively, 30, 15, and 15 msec. The PEP/LVET is relatively less affected by the glycosides than either PEP or LVET alone. Since the effects of heart failure on the STI are rarely completely reversed by the glycosides, it is usual to observe the pattern of a prolonged PEP, abbreviated LVET, and increased PEP/LVET in patients with heart failure who are on maintenance doses of the drug. In Figure 6–30 the response of the PEP/LVET in patients with heart failure is compared to normal subjects receiving the drug.

The abbreviation in QS_2 induced by the glycosides often is helpful in revealing the presence of a glycoside effect on the left ventricle. It has been our experience that excessive abbreviation in QS_2 (often of 50 msec or greater) accompanies other evidence of digitalis intoxication. It is notable that the PEP/LVET usually reflects the presence of residual left ventricular dysfunction, even when the clinical effects of digitalis intoxication are evident.

Recently, Levy and associates studied the effect of oral digoxin elixir in normal infants and infants with congestive heart failure.[176]

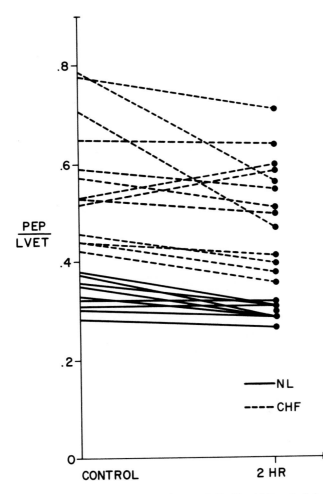

Fig. 6–30. The effect of 1.6 mg of Cedilanid-D administered intravenously upon the PEP/LVET in normal subjects and patients with chronic congestive heart failure (CHF). The mean decrease in the PEP/LVET of 0.05 is significant (p < 0.01) for normals. In patients with CHF the change in PEP/LVET was frequently greater, and the mean change was not statistically significantly different from normal. The PEP/LVET did not return to normal levels following Cedilanid-D in those patients with initial levels of 0.5 or greater.

In contrast to adults, the major shortening occurred in the PEP. The study also showed that a significant positive inotropic effect could be achieved by a much smaller dose than is commonly used.

Other studies on the effects of the digitalis glycosides have demonstrated an antagonism of the shortening in the LVET induced by Cedilanid-D by the intravenous infusion of Na_2EDTA.[177] The reversal of the abbreviation in systole following the glycoside parallels the lowering in serum calcium induced by the chelating agent.

The responses in STI have been used in a comparative study of the effects of digitoxin and pentaformylgitoxin.[178] On the basis of the responses in LVET, corrected for heart rate, pentaformylgitoxin demonstrated a less potent response than digitoxin, although the temporal course is virtually the same for the two drugs. In general, a single oral dose of 2.1 mg pentaformylgitoxin induced an abbreviation in LVET equivalent to that of 1.4 mg digitoxin.

SUMMARY

The systolic time intervals offer a conveniently derived and repeatable noninvasive measure of left ventricular performance in man. Among normal persons the systolic time intervals are so regulated as to remain within narrow limits relative to heart rate. Recent knowledge of their hemodynamic determinants and the responses to cardioactive agents has elucidated the interpretation of changes occurring in acute and chronic cardiovascular disease. Although much investigation is needed for a more comprehensive understanding of their clinical application, the studies summarized in this review support continued use of these measures in the evaluation and testing of left ventricular performance in man.

REFERENCES

1. Marey EJ: De l'emploi du sphygmographe dans le diagnostic des affections valvulaires du coeur et des aneuismes des arteres; extrait d'une note de M. Marey. C R Acad Sci (D) Paris 51:813–817, 1860
2. Ludwig C: The influence of respiratory movements on blood flow in the aorta. Arch Anat Physiol Wiss Med 242, 1847
3. Garrod AH: On some points connected with the circulation of the blood, arrived at from a study of the sphygmograph-trace. Proc Roy Soc London 23:140–151, 1874–1875

4. Thurston E: The length of the systole of the heart, as estimated from sphyg-mographic tracings. J Anat Physiol 10:494–501, 1876

5. Chapman PM, Lond MD: Abstract of the Goulstonian Lectures on the Physics of the Circulation. Br Med J 1:511–515, 1894

6. Bowen WP: Changes in heart rate, blood pressure and duration of systole resulting from bicycling. Am J Physiol 11:59–77, 1904

7. Wiggers CJ: Studies on the consecutive phases of the cardiac cycle. I. The duration of the consecutive phases of the cardiac cycle and the criteria for their precise determination. Am J Physiol 56:415–438, 1921

8. Wiggers CJ: Studies on the consecutive phases of the cardiac cycle. II. The laws governing the relative durations of ventricular systole and diastole. Am J Physiol 56:439–459, 1921

9. Katz LN, Feil HS: Clinical observations on the dynamics of ventricular systole. I. Auricular fibrillation. Arch Intern Med 32:672–692, 1923

10. Feil HS, Katz LN: Clinical observation on the dynamics of ventricular systole. II. Hypertension. Arch Intern Med 33:321–329, 1924

11. Katz LN: Observations on the dynamics of ventricular contraction in the heart-lung preparation. Am J Physiol 80:470–484, 1927

12. Blumberger K: VI. Die untersuchung der dynamik des herzens beim men-schen. Ergeb Inn Med Kinderheiks 62:424–531, 1942

13. Weissler AM, Harris WS, Schoenfeld CD: Systolic time intervals in heart failure in man. Circulation 37:149–159, 1968

14. Weissler AM, Harris WS, Schoenfeld CD: Bedside technics for the evaluation of ventricular function in man. Am J Cardiol 23:577–583, 1969

15. Weissler AM, Garrard CL Jr: Systolic time intervals in cardiac disease. Mod Conc Cardiovasc Dis 40:1–8, 1970

16. Kesteloot H, Willems J, Van Vollenhoven E: On the physical principles and methodology of mechanocardiography. Acta Cardiol 24:147–160, 1969

17. DiBartolo G, Nunez-Day D, Muiesan G, et al: Hemodynamic correlation of the first heart sound. Am J Physiol 201:888–892, 1961

18. Sarnoff SJ, Gilmore JP, Mitchell JH: Influence of atrial contraction and relaxation on closure of mitral valve. Observations on effects of autonomic nerve activity. Circ Res 11:26–35, 1962

19. Luisada A, MacCanon DM: The phases of the cardiac cycle. Am Heart J 83:705–711, 1972

20. Oreshkov V: Indirect measurement of isovolumetric contraction time on the basis of polygraphic tracing (apexcardiogram, carotid tracing, and phono-cardiogram). Cardiologia 47:315–322, 1965

21. Kumar S, Spodick DH: Study of the mechanical events of the left ventricle by atraumatic techniques: Comparison of methods of measurement and their significance. Am Heart J 80:401–413, 1970

22. Weissler AM, Peeler RG, Roehll WH Jr: Relationships between left ven-tricular ejection time, stroke volume and heart rate in normal individuals and patients with cardiovascular disease. Am Heart J 62:367–378, 1961

23. Robinson B: The carotid pulse. II. Relation of external recordings to carotid aortic and brachial pulses. Br Heart J 25:61–68, 1963

24. Benchimol A: A study of the period of isovolumic relaxation in normal sub-jects and in patients with heart disease. Am J Cardiol 19:196–206, 1967

25. Metzger CC, Chough CB, Kroetz FW, et al: True isovolumic contraction

time: Its correlation with two external indexes of ventricular performance. Am J Cardiol 25:434–442, 1970

26. Martin CE, Shaver JA, Thompson ME, et al: Direct correlation of external systolic time intervals with internal indices of ventricular function in man. Circulation 44:419–431, 1971

27. Bush CA, Lewis RP, Leighton RF, et al: Verification of systolic time intervals and the true isovolumic contraction time for the apexcardiogram by micromanometer catheterization of the left ventricle and aorta. Circulation (Abstr) 42 (Suppl III):121, 1970

28. Kesteloot H, Willems J: Relationship between the right apexcardiogram and the right ventricular dynamics. Acta Cardiol 22:64–89, 1967

29. Brough RD, Talley RC: Temporal relation of the second heart sound to aortic flow in various conditions. Am J Cardiol 30:237–241, 1972

30. Sherman JA, Lewis RP: Systolic time intervals in atrial fibrillation. Circulation (Abstr) 45 and 46 (Suppl II):220, 1972

31. Weissler AM, Harris LC, White GD: Left ventricular ejection time index in man. J Appl Physiol 18:919–923, 1963

32. Willems J, Kesteloot H: The left ventricular ejection time. Its relation to heart rate, mechanical systole and some anthropometric data. Acta Cardiol 22:401–425, 1967

33. Harris LC, Weissler AM, Manske AO, et al: Duration of the phases of mechanical systole in infants and children. Am J Cardiol 14:448–455, 1964

34. Golde D, Burstin L: Systolic phases of the cardiac cycle in children. Circulation 42:1029–1036, 1970

35. Stafford RW, Harris WS, Weissler AM: Left ventricular systolic time intervals as indices of postural circulatory stress in man. Circulation 41:485–492, 1970

36. Fontana ME, Wooley CF, Lewis RP: Postural angiographic studies in man (submitted for publication)

37. Weissler AM, Kamen AR, Bornstein RS, et al: Effect of deslanoside on the duration of the phases of ventricular systole in man. Am J Cardiol 15:153–161, 1965

38. Harrison TR, Dixon K, Russell RO Jr, et al: Relation of age to the duration of contraction, ejection and relaxation of the normal human heart. Am Heart J 67:189–199, 1964

39. Willems JL, Roelandt J, De Geest H, et al: Left ventricular ejection time in elderly subjects. Circulation 42:37–42, 1970

40. Slodki SJ, Hussain AT, Luisada AA: The Q-II interval: III. Study of the second heart sound in old age. J Am Geriatr Soc 17:673–679, 1969

41. Frank O (trans Chapman CB, Wasserman E): On the dynamics of cardiac muscle. Am Heart J 58:282–317, 1959

42. Peserico E: The influence of mechanical factors of the circulation upon the heart volume. J Physiol 65:146–156, 1928

43. Braunwald E, Sarnoff SJ, Stainsby WN: Determinants of duration and mean rate of ventricular ejection. Circ Res 6:319–325, 1958

44. Wallace AG, Mitchell JH, Skinner NS, et al: Duration of the phases of left ventricular systole. Circ Res 12:611–619, 1963

45. Lombard WP, Cope OM: The duration of the systole of the left ventricle of man. Am J Physiol 77:263–295, 1926

46. Greenfield JC Jr, Harley A, Thompson HK, et al: Pressure-flow studies in man during atrial fibrillation. J Clin Invest 47:2411–2421, 1968

47. Harley A, Starmer CF, Greenfield JC Jr; Pressure-flow studies in man: Evaluation of the duration of the phases of systole. J Clin Invest 48: 895–905, 1969

48. Harris WS, Schoenfeld CD, Brooks RH, et al: Effect of beta adrenergic blockade on the hemodynamic responses to epinephrine in man. Am J Cardiol 17:484–492, 1966

49. Leighton RF, Zaron SJ, Robinson JL, et al: Effects of atrial pacing on left ventricular performance in patients with heart disease. Circulation 40: 615–622, 1969

50. Raab W, Paula e Silva P de, Starcheska YK: Adrenergic and cholinergic influences on the dynamic cycle of the normal human heart. Cardiologia 33:350–364, 1958

51. Harris WS, Schoenfeld CD, Weissler AM: Effects of adrenergic receptor activation and blockade on the systolic pre-ejection period, heart rate and arterial pressure in man. J Clin Invest 46:1704–1714, 1967

52. Shaver JA, Kroetz FW, Leonard JJ, et al: The effect of steady-state increases in systemic arterial pressure on the duration of left ventricular ejection time. J Clin Invest 47:217–230, 1968

53. Sawayama T, Ochiai M, Marumoto S, et al: Influence of amyl nitrite inhalation on the systolic time intervals in normal subjects and in patients with ischemic heart disease. Circulation 40:327–335, 1969

54. Leighton RF, Polumbo RA, Zaron SJ, et al: Determinants of the shortening of left ventricular pre-ejection period induced by isoproterenol. Clin Res (Abstr) 17:513, 1969

55. Weissler AM, Gamel WG, Grode HE, et al: Effect of digitalis on ventricular ejection in normal human subjects. Circulation 29:721–729, 1964

56. Shiner PT, Harris WS, Weissler AM: Effects of acute changes in serum calcium levels on the systolic time intervals in man. Am J Cardiol 24: 42–48, 1969

57. Jones WF, Foster GL: Determinants of duration of left ventricular ejection in normal young men. J Appl Physiol 19:279–283, 1964

58. Hodges M, Halpern BL, Friesinger GC, et al: Left ventricular pre-ejection period and ejection time in patients with acute myocardial infarction. Circulation 45:933–942, 1972

59. Reeves TJ, Hefner LL, Jones WB, et al: The hemodynamic determinants of the rate of change in pressure in the left ventricle during isometric contraction. Am Heart J 60:745, 1960

60. Talley RC, Meyer JF, McNay JL: Evaluation of the pre-ejection period as an estimate of myocardial contractility in dogs. Am J Cardiol 27:384, 1971

61. Jezek V: Clinical value of the polygraphic tracing in the study of the sequence of events during cardiac contraction. Cardiologia 43:298–316, 1963

62. Margolis C: Significance of ejection period/tension period as a factor in the assessment of cardiac function and as a possible diagnostic tool for the uncovering of silent coronary heart disease: Study of 111 cases. Dis Chest 46:706–713, 1964

63. Lewis RP, Marcus DR, Garrard CL, et al: Abnormal systolic time intervals

with normal cardiac output in chronic myocardial disease. Circulation (Abstr) 42 (Suppl III):65, 1970

64. Hishimoto Y, Matsuura T, Kitizama T, et al: Clinical considerations on the duration of left ventricular systole. Jap Circ J 32: 1417–1426, 1968

65. Agress CM, Wegner S: Determination of stroke volume from left ventricular isovolumic contraction and ejection time. Jap Heart J 9:339–348, 1968

66. Aranow NS: Isovolumic contraction and left ventricular ejection time. Am J Cardiol 26:283–290, 1970

67. Aranow WS, Bowyer AF, Kaplan MA: External isovolumic contraction time and left ventricular ejection time/external isovolumic contraction time ratios at rest and after exercise in coronary artery disease. Circulation 43:59–65, 1971

68. Weissler AM, Schoenfeld CD: Effect of digitalis on systolic time intervals in heart failure. Am J Med Sci 259:4–20, 1970

69. Garrard CL Jr, Weissler AM, Dodge HT: The relationship of alterations in systolic time intervals to ejection fraction in patients with cardiac disease. Circulation 42:455–462, 1970

70. Thomas D, Basta L, Kioschos M: Factors influencing the validity of systolic time intervals in estimating left ventricular ejection fraction. Circulation (Abstr) 45 and 46 (Suppl II):230, 1972

71. Sutton R, Hood WP Jr, Craige E: Correlation of pre-ejection period with left ventricular ejection fraction. Clin Res (Abstr) 13:28, 1970

72. Kroetz FW, Kioschos JM, Mozena D, et al: Correlation of left ventricular pre-ejection period with left ventricular ejection fraction in patients with heart disease. Proceedings of the Central Society for Clin Res (Abstr) 42:70, 1969

73. Ahmed SS, Levinson GE, Schwartz CJ, et al: Systolic time intervals as measures of the contractile state of the myocardium in man. Circulation 46:559–571, 1972

74. Bush CA, Lewis RP, Leighton RF: The effect of rapid digitalization on left ventricular function in man. Submitted for publication

75. Boudoulas H, Lewis RP, Weissler AM: Use of systolic time intervals as a measure of left ventricular performance during therapy of congestive heart failure. Circulation (Abstr) 43 and 44:144, 1971

76. Perry JM Jr, Garrard CL: Systolic time intervals-relation to severity of coronary artery disease and left ventricular dysfunction. Circulation (Abstr) 41 and 42 (Suppl III):121, 1970

77. McConahay DR, Martin MM, Cheitlin MD: Resting and exercise systolic time intervals. Correlations with ventricular performance in patients with coronary artery disease. Circulation 45:529–601, 1972

78. Lewis RP, Weissler AM: Unpublished observations

79. Büyüköztürk K, Kimbiris D, Segal BL: Systolic time intervals. Relation to severity of coronary artery disease, intercoronary collateralization and left ventricular dyskinesia. Am J Cardiol 28:183–190, 1971

80. Agress CM, Wegner S, Nabakura S, et al: Comparison of the ejection time-heart rate relationships in normal and ischemic subjects. Jap Heart J 6:497–510, 1965

81. Frank MN, Kinlaw WB: Indirect measurement of isovolumetric contraction time and tension period in normal subjects. Am J Cardiol 10:800–806, 1962

82. Cummings GR, Edwards AH: Indirect measurement of left ventricular function during exercise. Can Med Assoc J 89:219–221, 1963

83. Miller JB, Miels W, Salzman SH: Systolic time intervals during muscular exercise in normals and patients with angina pectoris. Circulation (Abstr) 42 (Suppl III):65, 1970

84. Pouget JM, Harris WS, Mayron BR, et al: Abnormal responses of the systolic time intervals to exercise in patients with angina pectoris. Circulation 43:289–298, 1971

85. Pigott VM, Spodick DH, Rectra EH, et al: Cardiocirculatory responses to exercise: Physiologic study by noninvasive techniques. Am Heart J 82: 632–641, 1971

86. Whitsett TL, Naughton J: The effect of exercise on systolic time intervals in sedentary and active individuals and rehabilitated patients with heart disease. Am J Cardiol 27:352–358, 1971

87. Lopez-Arostegui F, Bhaduri V, Harris WS, et al: Effect of beta adrenergic receptor blockade on responses of systolic time intervals to exercise: Diagnostic differences between normal and angina patients. Circulation (Abstr) 43 and 44:196, 1971

88. Johnson A, O'Rourke RA: Effect of myocardial revascularization on systolic time intervals in patients with left ventricular dysfunction. Circulation (Abstr) 43 and 44:103, 1971

89. Boudoulas H, Lewis RP, Karayannacos PE, et al: Effect of saphenous vein graft surgery upon left ventricular function. Am J Cardiol (Abstr) 31:123, 1973

90. Schoenfeld CD, Robinson JL, Weissler AM, et al: The left ventricular systolic time intervals in acute myocardial infarction. Clin Res (Abstr) 15: 411, 1967

91. Toutouzas P, Gupta D, Samson R, et al: Q-second sound interval in acute myocardial infarction. Br Med J 31:462–467, 1969

92. Inoue K, Young GM, Grierson AL, et al: Isometric contraction period of the left ventricle in acute myocardial infarction. Circulation 42:79–90, 1970

93. Diamont B, Killip T: Indirect assessment of left ventricular performance in acute myocardial infarction. Circulation 42:579–592, 1970

94. Samson R: Changes in systolic time intervals in acute myocardial infarction. Br Heart J 32:839–846, 1970

95. Bennett ED, Smithen CS, Sowton GE: Systolic time intervals in acute myocardial infarction. Am J Cardiol (Abstr) 26:625, 1970

96. Heikkila J, Luomanmake K, Pyorala K: Serial observations on left ventricular dysfunction in acute myocardial infarction. II Systolic time intervals in power failure. Circulation 44:343–354, 1971

97. Jain SR, Lindahl J: Apex cardiogram and systolic time intervals in acute myocardial infarction. Br Heart J 33:578–584, 1971

98. Dowling JT, Sloman G, Urquhart C: Systolic time interval fluctuations produced by acute myocardial infarction. Br Heart J 33:765–772, 1971

99. Hamosh P, Cohn JN, Engelman K, et al: Systolic time intervals and left ventricular function in acute myocardial infarction. Circulation 45:375–381, 1972

100. Fabian J, Epstein N, Coulshed N, et al: Duration of phases of left ven-

tricular systole using indirect methods. II Acute myocardial infarction. Br Heart J 34:882–889, 1972

101. Austin TW, Ahuja SP, Boughner DR: Atraumatic study of left ventricular events following acute myocardial infarction. Am J Cardiol 29:745–748, 1972

102. Lewis RP, Boudoulas H, Forester WF, et al: Shortening of electromechanical systole as a manifestation of excessive adrenergic stimulation in acute myocardial infarction. Circulation 46:856–863, 1972

103. Rama BW, Myers NH, Wallace AG, et al: Hemodynamic findings in 123 patients with acute myocardial infarction on admission. Circulation 42:567–577, 1970

104. Valori C, Thomas M, Shielingford J: Free noradrenaline and adrenaline excretion in relation to clinical syndromes following myocardial infarction. Am J Cardiol 20:605–617, 1967

105. Klein RF, Troyer WG, Thompson HK, et al: Catecholamine excretion in myocardial infarction. Arch Intern Med 122:476–482, 1968

106. Januszewicz A, Sznajderman M, Wocial D, et al: Urinary excretion of free norepinephrine and free epinephrine in patients with acute myocardial infarction in relation to its clinical course. Am Heart J 76:345–352, 1968

107. Hayashi KD, Moss AJ, Yu PN: Urinary catecholamine excretion in myocardial infarction. Circulation 40:473–481, 1969

108. Griffeths J, Leung F: The sequential estimation of plasma catecholamines and whole blood histamine in myocardial infarction. Am Heart J 82:171–179, 1971

109. Januszewicz W, Sznajderman M, Ceswecka-Sznajderman M, et al: Plasma free fatty acid and catecholamine levels in patients with acute myocardial infarction. Br Heart J 33:716–718, 1971

110. Siggers DC, Salter C, Fluck DC: Serial plasma adrenaline and noradrenaline levels in myocardial infarction using a new double isotope technique. Br Heart J 33:878–883, 1971

111. Lukomsky PE, Aganov RG: Blood plasma catecholamines and their urinary excretion in patients with acute myocardial infarction. Am Heart J 83:182–188, 1972

112. Diamond G, Forrester JS, Chatterjee K, et al: Mean electromechanical $\Delta P/\Delta T$. On indirect index of the peak rate of rise of left ventricular pressure. Am J Cardiol 30:338–342, 1972

113. Agress CM, Wegner S, Forrester JS, et al: An indirect method for evaluation of left ventricular function in acute myocardial infarction. Circulation 46:291–297, 1972

114. Rahimitoola SH, Di Gilio MM, Sinno MZ, et al: Effect of ouabain on impaired left ventricular function during convalescence after acute myocardial infarction. Circulation 44:866–876, 1972

115. Hill JC, O'Rourke RA, Lewis RP, et al: The diagnostic value of the atrial gallop in acute myocardial infarction. Am Heart J 78:194–201, 1969

116. Shah PM, Slodki SJ: The Q-II interval. A study of the second heart sound in normal adults and in systemic hypertension. Circulation 29:551–561, 1964

117. Benchimol A, Dimond EG, Shen Y: Ejection time in aortic stenosis and mitral stenosis. Am J Cardiol 5:728–273, 1960

118. Moskowitz RL, Wechsler BM: Left ventricular ejection time in aortic and mitral valve disease. Am J Cardiol 15:809:814, 1965
119. Benchimol A, Matsuo S: Ejection time before and after aortic valve replacement. Am J Cardiol 27:244–248, 1971
120. Parisi AF, Salzman SH, Schecter E: Systolic time intervals in severe aortic valve disease. Changes with surgery and hemodynamic correlations. Circulation 44:539–547, 1971
121. Sherman JA, Lewis RP, Fontana ME, et al: Use of left ventricular ejection time in assessing the severity of aortic stenosis. Circulation (Abstr) 43 and 44:225, 1971
122. Bonner AJ, Tavel MD: Systolic time intervals in congestive heart failure due to aortic stenosis. Circulation (Abstr) 45 and 46 (Suppl II):133, 1972
123. Shaver JA: Personal communication
124. Curtis EI, Matthews RE, Shaver JE: Mechanism of normal splitting of the second heart sound. Circulation (Abstr) 45 and 46 (Suppl II):64, 1972
125. Cohn K, Hancock EW: Effect of amyl nitrite and isoproterenol on the ejection time in hypertrophic subaortic stenosis. Clin Res (Abstr) 14:123, 1966
126. Wigle ED, Auger P, Marquis Y: Muscular subaortic stenosis. The direct relation between the intraventricular pressure difference and the left ventricular ejection time. Circulation 36:36–44, 1967
127. Salzman SH, Wolfson S, Jackson B, et al: Epinephrine infusion in man. Standardization, normal response, and abnormal response in idiopathic hypertrophic subaortic stenosis. Circulation 43:137–144, 1971
128. Turner HS, Philips VK, Leighton RF: Idiopathic subvalvular aortic stenosis: A case report in a pilot. Aerosp Med 43:200–203, 1972
129. Aranow WS, Kaplan MA, Ellestad M: Prediction of left ventricular contractility in mitral valve disease by EICT and LVET/EICT measurements. Clin Res (Abstr) 17:226, 1969
130. Carter WH, McIntosh HD, Orgain ES: Respiratory variation of left ventricular ejection time in patients with pericardial effusion. Am J Cardiol 29:427–431, 1972
131. Shabetai R, Fowler NO, Guntheroth WG: The hemodynamics of cardiac tamponade and constructive pericarditis. Am J Cardiol 26:480–489, 1970
132. Pigott VM, Spodick DH: Effects of normal breathing and expiratory apnea on duration of the phases of cardiac systole. Am Heart J 82:786–793, 1971
133. Lange RL, Botticelli JT, Tsagaris TJ, et al: Diagnostic signs in compressive cardiac disorders. Constrictive pericarditis, pericardial effusion and tamponade. Circulation 33:763–377, 1966
134. Baragan J, Tsrnandez F, Coblence B, et al: Left ventricular dynamics in complete right bundle branch block with left axis deviation of QRS. Circulation 42:797–804, 1970
135. Broder G, Polansky BJ: Prolongation of pre-ejection period in left anterior hemiblock. Circulation (Abstr) 43 and 44 (Suppl II):145, 1971
136. Coblentz B, Harvey RM, Ferrer MI, et al: The relationship between electrical and mechanical events in the cardiac cycle of man. Br Heart J 11:1–22, 1949
137. Leatham A: Splitting of the first and second heart sounds. Lancet 2:607–614, 1954

138. Braunwald E, Morrow AG: Sequence of ventricular contraction in human bundle branch block. Am J Med 23:205–211, 1957

139. Bourassa MG, Birteau GM, Allenstein BJ: Hemodynamic studies during intermittent left bundle branch block. Am J Cardiol 10:792–799, 1962

140. Leighton RF, Ryan JM, Goodwin RS, et al: Incomplete left bundle branch block. The view from transseptal intraventricular leads. Circulation 36: 261–274, 1967

141. Oravetz J, Wissner S, Argano B, et al: Dynamic analysis of heart sounds in right and left bundle branch blocks. Circulation 36: 275–283, 1967

142. Baragon J, Fernandez-Caamano F, Sozutek Y, et al: Chronic complete bundle branch block: Phonocardiographic and mechanocardiographic study of 30 cases. Br Heart J 30:196–202, 1968

143. Silie M: Etude phonomecanocardiographique des blocs de branche: A propos de 106 observations (Thesis) Lyon, Imprimerie Bosc Fereres, 1969

144. Santos DE, DeLapaz A, Pietras RJ, et al: The apexcardiogram in left bundle branch block. Br Heart J 31:693–699, 1969

145. Adolph RJ, Fowler NO, Tanaka K: Prolongation of isovolumic contraction time in left bundle branch block. Am Heart J 78:585–591, 1969

146. Haft JL, Herman MW, Gorlin R: Left bundle branch block. Etiologic, hemodynamic and ventriculographic considerations. Circulation 43:279–287, 1971

147. D'Cunha GF, Friedberg HD, Jaume F: The first sound in intermittent left bundle branch block. Am J Cardiol 27:447–449, 1971

148. Schoenfeld CD, Cohen S, Taguchi JT, et al: Relationship between cycle length and left ventricular ejection time in atrial fibrillation. Clin Res (Abstr) 11:26, 1963

149. Flessas AP, Pomposiello JC, Connelly GP, et al: Determinants of systolic time intervals in the human heart. Circulation (Abstr) 43 and 44 (Suppl II):165, 1971

150. Krohn BG, Magidson O: Left ventricular ejection time following cardioversion. Am J Cardiol 18:729–737, 1966

151. Tavel ME, Baugh DO, Feigenbaum H, et al: Left ventricular ejection time in atrial fibrillation. Circulation 46:744–752, 1972

152. Kroetz FW, Leonard JJ, Shaver JA, et al: The effect of atrial contraction on left ventricular performance in valvular aortic stenosis. Circulation 35: 852–867, 1967

153. Heidenreich FP, Thompson ME, Shaver JA, et al: Left atrial transport in mitral stenosis. Circulation 40:545–554, 1969

154. Thompson ME, Metzger CC, Shaver JA, et al: Assessment of left atrial function immediately following cardioversion. Circulation (Abstr) 42 (Suppl III):59, 1970

155. Leighton RF, Weissler AM, Weinstein PB, et al: Right and left ventricular systolic intervals. Effects of heart rate, respiration, and atrial pacing. Am J Cardiol 27:66–72, 1971

156. Harris LC, Nghien Qx, Schreiber MH, et al: Severe pulsus alternans associated with primary myocardial disease in children. Observations on clinical features, hemodynamic findings, mechanism, and prognosis. Circulation 34:948–961, 1966

157. Spodick DH, St Pierre JR: Pulsus alternans: Physiologic study by noninvasive techniques. Am Heart J 80:766–777, 1970

158. Amidi M, Leon DF, de Groot NJ, et al: Effect of the thyroid state on myocardial contractility and ventricular ejection rate in man. Circulation 38: 229–239, 1968

159. Leighton RF, Polumbo RA, Zaron SJ, et al: The use of systolic time intervals in predicting hemodynamic effects of isoproterenol. Clin Res (Abstr) 18:317, 1970

160. Hunt D, Sloman G, Clark RM, et al: Effects of beta-adrenergic blockade on the systolic time intervals. Am J Med Sci 259:97–113, 1970

161. Rich JM, Robinson JL, Weissler AM: Differential blocking effect of propranolol on the chronotropic and inotropic actions of isoproterenol. Submitted for publication

162. Harris WS, Weissler AM, Brooks RH, et al: The effect of vagal influences on the pre-ejection period in man. J Clin Invest (Abstr) 46:1067, 1967

163. Harris WS, Weissler AM, Brooks RH: Vagal influence on left ventricular contraction in man: A cause for prolongation of the pre-ejection period. Clin Res (Abstr) 14:426, 1966

164. Whitsett TL, Goldberg LI: Effects of levodopa on systolic pre-ejection period, blood pressure, and heart rate during acute and chronic treatment of Parkinson's Disease. Circulation 45:97–106, 1972

165. Gould L, Gamprecht RF, Jaynal F: The effects of phentolamine on the duration of the phases of ventricular systole in man. Am J Med Sci 260: 29–33, 1970

166. Kennedy JW, Trenholme SE, Kasser I: Left ventricular volume and mass from single-plane cineangiocardiogram. A comparison of anteroposterior and right anterior oblique methods. Am Heart J 80:343–350, 1970

167. Wiggers CJ, Stimson B: Studies on the cardiodynamic actions of drugs. III. The mechanism of cardiac stimulation by digitalis and g-strophanthin. J Pharmacol Exp Ther 30:251–269, 1927

168. Weissler AM, Lewis RP, Leighton RF, et al: Comparative responses to the digitalis glycosides in man, in Marks BH, Weissler AM: Basic and Clinical Pharmacology of Digitalis. Fourt Lauderdale, Florida, Thomas, 1972, pp 260–280

169. Weissler AM, Snyder JR, Schoenfeld CD, et al: Assay of digitalis glycosides in man. Am J Cardiol 17:768–780, 1966

170. Lewis RP, Forester W, Willke TA, et al: A quantitative comparison of the onset and magnitude of inotropic action of commonly used digitalis glycosides in man. Circulation (Abstra) 45 and 46 (Suppl II):30, 1972

171. Wilson WS, Tolbert JH, Guilio W: Plasma digitoxin levels and serial left ventricular ejection times after a digitalizing dose of digitoxin. Am J Cardiol 26:162–164, 1970

172. Shapiro W, Narahara K, Neblett K: Relationship of plasma digitoxin and digoxin to cardiac response following intravenous digitalization in man. Circulation (Abstr) 42 (Suppl II):110, 1970

173. Doherty JE: The clinical pharmacology of digitalis glycosides: A review. Am J Med Sci 255:382–414, 1968

174. Bush CA, Caldwell JH, Lewis RP, et al: Relationship of digitoxin blood level to physiologic effect in man. Circulation (Abstr) 42 (Suppl III):111, 1970

175. Lewis RP, Yazel JJ, Weissler AM: Absorption patterns of digoxin tablets

and elixir in normal subjects. Circulation (Abstr) 45 and 46 (Suppl II): 182, 1972

176. Levy AM, Leaman DM, Hanson JS: Effects of digoxin on systolic time intervals of neonates and infants. Circulation 46:816–828, 1972

177. Cohen S, Weissler AM, Schoenfeld CD: Antagonism of the contractile effect of digitalis by EDTA in the normal human ventricle. Am Heart J 69:502–514, 1965

178. Kesteloot H, Brasseur L, Carlier J, et al: Effect of digitalis on the left ventricular ejection time: A multicenter double-blind comparative study of digitoxin and pentaformylgitoxin in normal subjects. Acta Cardiol 24:409–425, 1969

H. William Strauss
Bertram Pitt

7
Nuclear Cardiology

INTRODUCTION

Since the introduction of radioactive tracers to measure the circulation time by Blumgart et al in 1927,[1] tracer techniques have been applied to an increasing number of cardiovascular diagnostic problems. At present, total and regional blood volume, cardiac output, ejection fraction, shunt quantification, and detection of peripheral venous thrombosis can be performed with simple equipment requiring only analysis of time-dependent changes in activity concentration and a venous sample. Using a scintillation camera, the size, location, and filling sequence of cardiac chambers as well as a determination of regional ventricular wall motion and chamber volume can be obtained. In addition, the site and extent of myocardial ischemia can be evaluated by combining nuclear imaging procedures with pacing or exercise stress. All of these measurements can be performed without cardiac catherization, requiring only intravenous administration of tracer and an external radiation detector.

In this chapter the basic principles of nuclear medicine and their application to several diagnostic problems in cardiology are described.

PRINCIPLES

To obtain maximum use of nuclear medicine techniques in cardiovascular diagnosis, it is important to understand the types of radiation and the methods used to measure them.[2-5]

Radiation

The tracers used in nuclear cardiology are termed *radionuclides*.[2] Radionuclides are atoms of specific chemical elements which have an unstable configuration of the nucleus. The nucleus achieves a stable state by undergoing a nuclear rearrangement, usually accompanied by emission of excess energy in the form of particulate radiation; either alpha or beta particles; and/or packets of electromagnetic energy, gamma rays, or photons.

The quantity of radionuclide is measured by the number of atoms disintegrating per unit time. The unit of radioactive quantity is the Curie (3.7×10^{10} disintegrations/second). In nuclear cardiology, millicurie or microcurie amounts of radionuclide are most often used. Radionuclides can be characterized in several ways: (1) The chemical behavior of the element. The number of electrons, and hence, the chemical and physiological behavior of the atom is similar to non-radioactive atoms of the same element. (2) The time required for half the unstable atoms to emit their energy (disintegrate). This disintegration time is called the *half-life* and is important in selecting the quantity of tracer to be administered. (3) The type, number and energy of radiations emitted.

Tracers that emit gamma radiations are used to make most of the measurements in nuclear cardiology. These gamma photons have the greatest chance of penetrating tissues and are usually detectable externally. Alpha and beta radiation consist of charged particles which have a great likelihood of interacting in tissues a very short distance from their origin which makes external detection difficult or impossible. One special exception to this is the positron, which is a positively charged electron. When this particle interacts in tissues, the particle actually combines with an electron and annihilates itself. In keeping with the laws of conservation of matter and energy, in the place of this annihilated particle pair, two gamma photons are given off 180 degrees apart. These gamma rays can then be detected externally. Radionulclides undergoing this type of disintegration have been used to determine total myocardial blood flow and will probably be used for the determination of regional myocardial blood flow using tracers such as ammonia labelled with nitrogen—13.

Instrumentation

Gamma radiations are not perceptible by the ordinary senses. However, when these photons interact with matter, they cause heat, excitation, or ionization, which can be detected by devices sensitive to these parameters. The gamma radiation detector most commonly used in nuclear cardiology is the scintillation crystal. In the crystal, a photon interaction causes excitation of the electrons in the crystal lattice. These electrons give off energy in the form of light on returning to the ground state. When these flashes of light impinge on the photocathode of an optically coupled photomultiplier tube, a pulse of electrons is released. The height of the electrical pulse from the photomultiplier tube is proportional to the energy that the gamma photon deposited in the crystal. The scintillation crystal and phototube form a single unit called the *detector*.

The electrical pulse from the detector is then amplified and passed through a spectrometer. The spectrometer is an electronic device which can sort pulses of different heights (pulse-height analyzer), which permits separation of photons of different gamma energies. This is important when performing studies with two isotopes. One example is the combined use of [43]K for myocardial scanning to detect infarction or ischemia, and the determination of ventricular function with the gated cardiac blood pool scan using ^{99m}Tc-albumin. A more important reason for pulse-height analysis is elimination of scattered radiation. Photons may interact completely in matter giving up all their energy, or only partially giving off some of their energy and getting deflected (like a billiard ball striking a cushion). If counted, these lower energy photons would give a false impression of the quantity of radioactivity in a particular region. In an image, these scattered photons would cause distortion, particularly manifested by fuzziness at the border of the organ.

After pulses have passed through the spectrometer, the number of pulses are counted and expressed as the number of pulses per unit time. The information may be displayed on a digital scaler as the number of pulses for a given counting interval, or on an analog rate meter as a needle deflection on a calibrated meter. The information may be permanently recorded on a printer or strip chart recorder.

When images of the tracer distribution are obtained, the precise spatial origin of the photon must be determined. Two instruments are used to image the spatial distribution of a tracer in an organ or structure: The rectilinear scanner and the scintillation camera. The rectilinear scanner has a single scintillation crystal, usually viewed by a single photomultiplier tube. The region viewed by the detector is limited by a collimator so that only one small point in space is "seen" well. The collimator functions as a lens for these imaging devices. However, because gamma rays cannot be focused in the optical sense, the collimator permits only those radiations arising from the desired region to strike the crystal. Unfortunately, this is a very inefficient system. The detector perceives the quantity of radiation emitted from one point in space, and after suitable electronic processing activates a flashing light in the display. The brightness of the flashes in the display are proportional to the amount of radiation perceived. The flashes of light expose a piece of photographic film. The detector and display then move in tandem to an adjacent point along a horizontal line and repeat the process. On completion of a line, the detector and display move to the next line parallel to the first, but a small distance away, and the process is continued. The total image is built up point-by-point and line-by-line.

The scintillation camera produces an image of the entire distribution of tracer in a field of view without any movement of the detector. The camera is better suited to detect rapid changes in spatial distribution of tracer than the rectilinear scanner. There are four types of scintillation cameras, of which the Anger type is the most frequently used. The Anger scintillation camera has a single large crystal which is viewed by an array of photomultiplier tubes. When a scintillation occurs in the crystal, it produces a flash of light which is perceived by all tubes but the tube closest to the scintillation produces the largest signal; the others produce signals of lesser intensity. The electrical pulses produced by all tubes are subject to vector analysis to determine the location of the scintillation in the crystal. In addition, the sum of all pulses from one scintillation is subjected to pulse height analysis. A dot is then displayed on an oscilloscope screen in the same relative position as the scintillation which occurred in the crystal. Repetition of this process produces an image comprised of a large number of dots. A parallel hole collimator commonly used with the scintillation camera limits the field to view photons arising perpendicular to the detector. Because photons coming from an angle are eliminated, this collimator is essentially distortion free. There is, however, a limit to the spatial-resolving power of the scintillation camera which makes it difficult to image small objects. This can be partially overcome by enlarging the object on the surface of the detector using a pinhole collimator. The pinhole collimator is used to perform nuclear angiocardiograms in infants.

Radiopharmaceuticals

There are two components to the tracer substances administered: the radionuclide and the substance to be tagged (e.g., albumin).[4] The choice of nuclide and substance to be tagged will depend on the measurement to be made. If a determination of the total potassium space of the body is required, we can use a radionuclide of potassium.

No other substance need be tagged. On the other hand, if a determination of the blood volume is required, a tracer which remains in the blood stream is needed. This can be achieved by tagging a protein substance such as albumin with iodine or technetium. An alternative would be to tag red blood cells.

Technetium-99m is widely used in nuclear cardiology because it is readily available, has a suitable energy for the scintillation camera, no beta radiations, and has a 6-hr half-life. In the qualitative assessment of intracardiac shunting by nuclear angiocardiography, technetium (in the chemical form of pertechnitate) can be used without additional chemical compounding. The material remains in the blood stream for only a brief period of time, but this is sufficient to obtain images of the first pass of tracer through the heart. However, if detailed cardiac images are required over several minutes to hours, tracer technetium must be complexed with albumin. If measurements of the distribution of blood in the lungs (lung scan) are required, biodegradable particles of aggragated albumin labeled with technetium or iodine are suitable. The common radionuclides and their physical properties are listed in Table 7–1. The substrates which are usually labeled with these tracers and the measurements that can be made are listed in Table 7–2.

Dosimetry

The only theoretical deleterious effect attendant to the diagnostic use of tracer substances is possible radiation damage to the tissues. The chemical quantities of tracer are usually inconsequential. Radiation damage may occur when the photon or beta particle deposits all or part of its energy in tissues causing local excitation, ionization, or heat in the cell. The radiation dose is related to several factors:

1. The quantity of tracer administered;
2. The duration of exposure of the tissue to the nuclide;
3. The presence of beta radiation;
4. The energy and number of radiations emitted;
5. The distribution of tracer in the organ or throughout the patient's body.

Application of standard formulas to the above information permits determination of radiation dose to the patient or tissues.

We do not know at this time if a safe radiation dose exists (one in which no permanent damage to the tissues will occur). However, there are data to suggest that repair of radiation damage occurs if less

Table 7–1
Common Radionuclides and Their Physical Properties

Radionuclide[a]	Major Photon for Scanning	Physical Half-Life (hr)	Beta Emission	Remarks
1. Technetium-99m	140	6	No	Widely used for cardiac chamber visualization, dynamic studies either as $^{99m}TcO_4$ or chemically bound to a substrate
2. Iodine-131	364	192	Yes	Can label proteins and fatty acids in vitro
3. Indium-113m	393	1.7	No	Can label transferrin in vivo
4. Xenon-133	81	127	Yes	Low-photon yield and low energy; but it can be given in high doses because of short biological half-life due to excretion in breath
5. Iodine-123	159	13	No	Cyclotron produced, expensive (see ^{131}I)
6. Potassium-43	373	22	Yes	Exchanges with potassium; myocardial scanning for infarction and ischemia
7. Cesium-129	375	32	No	Exchanges with potassium; myocardial scanning—infarcts only
8. Rubidium-84	511	792	Yes	Exchanges with potassium; for measurement of total myocardial flow

[a] Radionuclides 1 through 5 are agents of proved usefulness; 6 through 8 are experimental.

Table 7–2
Substrates, Radionuclides, and Their Uses

Substrate*	Use	Radionuclide
1. Albumin	Visualization of blood pool, in vitro label, widely used	^{131}I or ^{99m}Tc
2. Transferrin	Visualization of blood pool, in vivo label	^{113m}In
3. Fibrinogen	Localization of blood clots, requires actively forming thrombi	^{131}I or ^{125}I
4. Streptokinase	Visualization of clots, rapidly localizes, even in old thrombi, labeled with iodine or technetium	^{131}I or ^{99m}Tc
5. Urokinase	See streptokinase	^{131}I or ^{99m}Tc
6. Oleic acid	Visualization of the myocardium	^{131}I or ^{99m}Tc

* Substrates 1 through 3, clinically proved; 4 through 6, research .

than a threshold amount is received. The radiation doses from studies of the cardiovascular system are no greater than those from a barium examination of the gastrointestinal tract. Since there are no other attendant risks, the use of tracers in patients with cardiac disease can be jusified.

CLINICAL APPLICATIONS

Nuclear Angiocardiography

Information regarding the size, configuration, and filling sequence of individual cardiac chambers can be achieved by following the course of a bolus of radionuclide with a scintillation camera as it traverses the heart and great vessels following intravenous injection.[6,7] This "nuclear angiocardiogram" is useful in the approach to the patient with congenital heart disease.[6,8,9] Although cardiac catheterization and contrast angiography remain the techniques of choice to obtain detailed anatomic evaluation, the nuclear angiocardiogram is of use as a screening technique to select patients for catheterization, and to provide preliminary anatomic information before catheterization. Knowledge of the major anatomic defects allows a more precise approach to the diagnostic questions and may shorten the time of catheterization. In addition, sequential studies can readily be performed.

An example of a normal nuclear angiocardiogram in the anterior and in the left anterior oblique projections is shown in Figs. 7–1 and 7–2. To perform this procedure the patient is placed beneath the detector of a scintillation camera in the appropriate position, and a dose of tracer (usually 10 to 20 mCi of ^{99m}Tc-pertechnetate) is administered intravenously. The passage of tracer through the circulation is recorded on film, videotape, or computer for analysis at a rate of at least 2 frames per sec for 1 min. After the tracer is distributed throughout the circulation, a cumulative image of 200,000 counts is recorded (Fig. 7–3). The cumulative image provides a more detailed outline of the cardiac blood pool. However, since chambers and vessels overlap, individual regions of the heart are best examined from the sequential images.

In viewing the nuclear angiocardiogram, it is useful to first evaluate the cumulative image to establish the relationship of the cardiac and pulmonary blood pools and the relationship of intracardiac blood pools. The sequential images should then be viewed to assess the temporal relationship of chamber filling. The vena cava is the first structure clearly delineated. The right atrium then appears as a bulge at the inferior aspect of the vena cava. Activity then courses medially and superiorly into the right ventricle and pulmonary outflow tract (Fig. 7–1A). There are two configurations of the right ventricle: vertical and horizontal. The pulmonary artery (PA) fills next, and courses superiorly to its bifurcation (Fig. 7–1B). In the left anterior oblique view, the PA angles posteriorly (Fig. 7–2B). A space between the PA and superior vena cava should be clearly seen in the anterior view (Fig. 7–1A, B), which is filled by the aorta in later frames. This observation is crucial to arrive at the diagnosis of transposition of the great vessels. The lungs sometimes appear asymmetrical, with the right somewhat better perfused than the left. The heart is then filled, occa-

---

Fig. 7–1. Normal nuclear angiocardiogram. Serial 0.3 sec frames in the anterior position. A. Activity filling SVC, RA, RV, pulmonary outflow tract and MPA. B. Activity no longer in SVC, but now extends to lungs. There is a space which is occupied by the LV which is not yet filled with activity. C. Activity in LA, LV, and Ao. D. Activity in LV and Ao. Note aortic activity definity extending below the diaphragm. Total time from A to D is 9 sec. (SC, superior vena cava; RA, right atrium; RV, right ventricle; LV, left ventricle; LA, left atrium; Ao, aorta; PA, pulmonary artery). (From Hurley PJ, Strauss HW, Wagner HN: Radionuclide angiography in cyanotic congenital heart disease, Johns Hopkins Med J 127:46, 1970, with permission.)

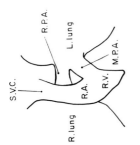

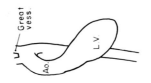

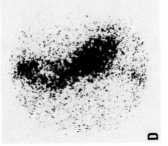

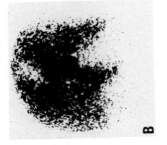

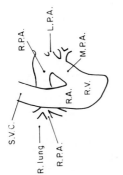

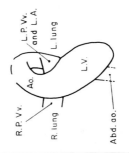

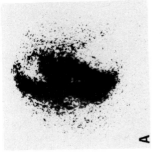

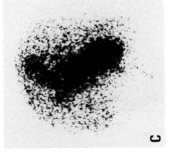

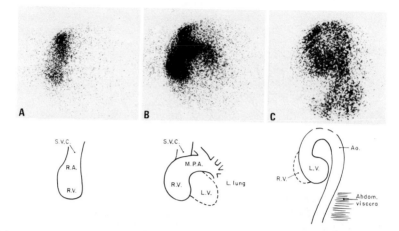

Fig. 7–2. Normal nuclear angiocardiogram. Serial 0.3 sec-images in the LAO position. A. Activity in SVC, RA and RV. B. Activity in SVC, RA, RV, MPA. Note PA arises anteriorly, curves posteriorly, and does not extend beneath the diaphragm. The space behind the RV will be filled by LV in later portions of the examination. C. Activity in LV, Ao extending into abdomen. Space where RV was earlier seen. (From Harley PJ, Strauss HW, Wagner HN: Radionuclide angiography in cyanotic congenital heart disease, Johns Hopkins Med J 129:46, 1970, with permission.)

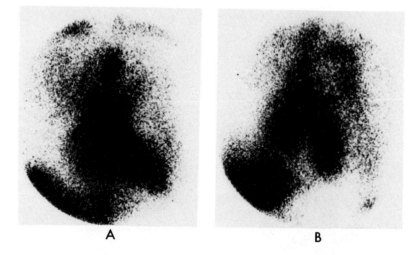

Fig. 7–3. Cardiac blood pool scan. A. Anterior view. B. LAO view. There is tracer in all chambers of the heart and great vessels. The liver is seen below the heart. The interventricular septum is clearly seen in the LAO view, separating RV from LV. This enlarges when ventricular hypertrophy occurs. (From Deland FH, Wagner HN: The lung and heart, in: Atlas of Nuclear Medicine, vol II, Philadelphia, Saunders, 1970, p 221, with permission.)

sionally without clear-cut delineation of the left atrium. If activity in the left atrium (LA) is persistent, the diagnosis of mitral stenosis or insufficiency should be suspected. In the pulmonary phase of the study, a definite clear region should be seen between the right ventricle and left lung which will fill during the left ventricular phase (Fig. 7–1B). In the left anterior oblique view, this region is located behind the right ventricle (Fig. 7–2B). The aorta arises from the superomedial aspect of the left ventricle and courses superiorly around the arch (the subclavian and carotid arteries may be seen) (Fig. 7–1C) and inferiorly (Fig. 7–1D). The abdominal aorta is usually well defined. If a pericardial effusion is present, there will be an abnormal separation of the heart and right lung blood pools. In pathologic states, either the sequence shape or size of the chambers may be altered.

Quantitative nuclear angiocardiology can be used to record the appearance of tracer and transit times through individual chambers[10],[11] (Fig. 7–4). This technique is particularly useful in the evaluation of intracardiac shunting.

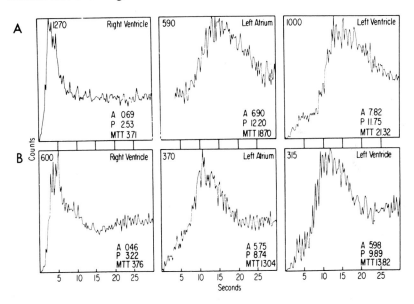

Fig. 7–4. Radiocardiogram in a patient with aortic stenosis (A) before and (B) after surgery. Counts are listed on the ordinate, time in seconds on the abscissa (A, arrival time after injection; P, peak time, MTT, mean transit time).[11] There is prolongation of the arrival, peak, and mean transit times which improves after surgery. (From Jones RH, Sabiston DC, Bates BB, Morris JJ, Anderson PAW, Goodrich JK: Quantitative radionuclide angiocardiography for determination of chamber cardiac transit times. Am J Cardiol 30:855, 1972, with permission.)

Acyanotic Congenital Heart Disease

The quantitative nuclear angiocardiogram can provide a noninvasive estimate of the magnitude of shunting in patients with atrial and ventricular septal defects. Since the magnitude of the shunt is often an important determinant in the selection of patients for surgery, the quantitative nuclear angiogram or radiocardiogram may be helpful in selecting patients for cardiac catheterization and surgery.[12] The most striking findings in these patients are persistence of activity in the lungs and refilling of a chamber or chambers which were previously emptied by the shunted activity.[13] It is frequently difficult to localize the precise site of shunting to an atrium or ventricle. Although criteria for the diagnosis of congenital pulmonary valvular stenosis, aortic stenosis, and coarctation of the aorta have been described, these diagnoses may be difficult to make from the nuclear angiocardiogram. Peripheral pulmonic stenosis, however, can be detected by nuclear angiocardiography, and by routine lung scanning as a unilateral decrease in perfusion (Fig. 7–5).

Cyanotic Congenital Heart Disease

Right-to-left shunting can be detected simply and quantified by the intravenous administration of a measured quantity of human serum albumin microspheres.[14] If a scintillation detector is placed over the patient's head, it will only detect activity caused by shunted patricles that were not trapped by the pulmonary capillary bed. If there are no intracardiac or transpulmonary shunts, no significant activity is recorded. No significant adverse effects have been seen in a large number of patients studied by this technique. Since the location of shunting is not determined with the microspheres, a nuclear angiocardiogram should also be performed if the study is abnormal. Right-to-left shunting is readily appreciated on the nuclear angiocardiogram by early visualization of the aorta.[6] In addition, there may be early left ventricular filling seen best in the left anterior oblique projection. Specific anatomic etiologies may often be difficult to define on the nuclear angiocardiogram.[15] However, it is possible to separate patients with ventricular septal defects from those with tetralogy of Fallot or truncus arteriosis. Patients with a hypoplastic left ventricle or hypoplastic right ventricle can be differentiated from those with normal or enlarged chambers.[8] In infants, a pinhole collimator is used to improve resolution. A normal pinhole nuclear angiocardiogram is shown in Figure 7–6, and a study

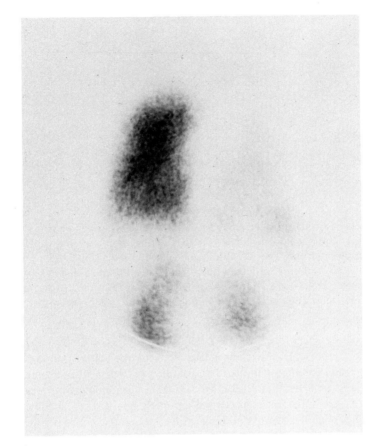

Fig. 7–5. Lung scan posterior view in a patient with tetralogy of Fallot. Activity is present in both kidneys indicating a right-to-left shunt. The left lung has a greater concentration of particles than the right which can be seen in a number of situations including peripheral pulmonic stenosis, or functioning Blalock Taussig anastomosis to left side, or massive pleural effusion. (From Deland FH, Wagner HN (Eds): The lung and heart, in Atlas of Nuclear Medicine, vol II, Philadelphia, Saunders, 1970, p 235, with permission.)

of a patient with truncus arteriosis and ventricular septal defect in Fig. 7–7.

The functional status of surgical shunts can also be evaluated by nuclear angiocardiography. A patient with tetralogy of Fallot who had an anastomosis of the superior vena cava to the left pulmonary artery is illustrated in Figure 7–8. Activity initially enters the right lung,

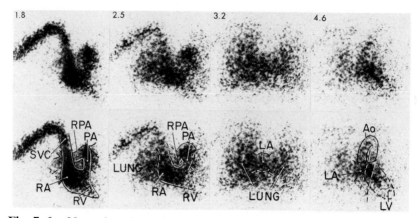

Fig. 7–6. Normal nuclear angiocardiogram in the anterior view done with pinhole collimator in a newborn. The circulation time is considerably faster than in an adult and the resolution somewhat poorer. The time after injection is listed at the upper left of each frame. (From Wesselhoeft H, Hurley PJ, Wagner HN, Rowe RD: Nuclear angiocardiography in the diagnosis of congenital heart disease in infants. Circulation 45:77, 1972, with permission.)

followed by entry into the left ventricle. In this example, the right ventricle represents the clear space seen in the early frames of the study. Shunt function can also be evaluated by the perfusion lung scan. In patients who have had a Blalock–Taussig anastomosis, the perfusion lung scan will demonstrate decreased perfusion to the shunted lung (Fig. 7–5). If the shunt is no longer functioning, there will be increased activity in the shunted lung.

Acquired Valvular Heart Disease

Severe isolated valvular lesions can be detected by nuclear angiocardiography (Fig. 7–9), but less severe lesions are easily missed.[13] In the presence of mixed valvular lesions, the diagnostic features are even more difficult to detect and may not permit a clear diagnosis. There have been several attempts to determine the magnitude of isolated valvular lesions by measuring the transit time from one chamber to another. For example, in a patient with aortic stenosis (Fig. 7–4), there is a delay in the appearance and transit of tracer in the left atrium and ventricle which is corrected after valve replacement.[11] The appearance and transit time, however, are dependent on many factors other than the magnitude of valvular lesions, such as cardiac output, which limits the usefulness of this method.

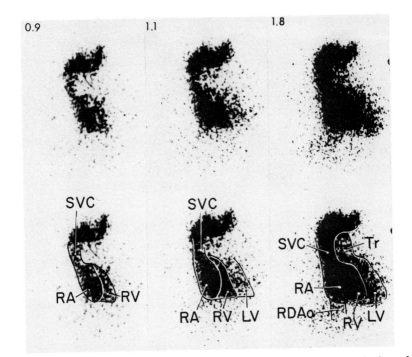

Fig. 7–7. Nuclear angiocardiogram in a patient with truncus arteriosis and ventricular septal defect. Tracer is injected into the left arm and the sub-clavian vein is seen emptying into the SVC, RA, and RV. In the next frame the LV fills, followed by the truncus and the right-sided aorta. (From Wessel-hoeft J, Hurley PJ, Wagner HN, Rowe RD: Nuclear angiocardiography in the diagnosis of congenital heart disease in infants, Circulation 45:77, 1972, with permission.)

Cardiomegaly

The nuclear angiocardiogram can be useful in differentiating cardiac dilatation from pericardial effusion[13] or tumor[16] in patients with car-diomegaly. Pericardial effusions of 150 ml or greater are easily diag-nosed by finding a relatively small cardiac blood pool in comparison to the cardiac silhouette on a nonmagnified x-ray (Fig. 7–10). An ab-normal separation of the superior portion of the hepatic from cardiac blood pool, separation of the pulmonary from the cardiac blood pool, and elevation of the hilar vessels are other findings characteristic of pericardial effusion.[15] Pericardial tumor may be differentiated from effusion or cardiac dilatation by the finding of a displacement of the cardiac blood pool to one side. In addition, intracardiac tumors and

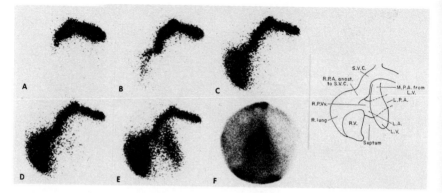

Fig. 7–8. Nuclear angiocardiogram in a patient with a SVC-RPA anastomosis. Tracer injected in the left arm. A. Subclavian vein and SVC are seen. B. Subclavian, SVC, RPA. C. Subclavian, SVC, RPA, right lung. D. and E. Progressive activity entering LV, clear area is filled in later by recirculating activity entering RV. F. Cumulative frame, with activity equilibrated through entire heart. (From Hurley PJ, Strauss HW, Wagner HN: Radionuclide angiography in cyanotic congenital heart disease, Johns Hopkins Med J 127:46, 1970, with permission.)

clots can be differentiated from cardiac dilatation on the blood pool scan[16] (Fig. 7–11).

Left Ventricular Dysfunction

The scintillation camera is useful in separating patients with diffuse cardiac dilatation from those with left ventricular aneurysms or lesser degrees of left ventricular dyskinesis by comparing detailed cardiac blood pool images of the heart at end-diastole and end-systole to determine the extent of left ventricular wall motion. These scans are obtained by triggering (gating) the scintillation camera so that images of the heart are collected only during a selected portion of the cardiac cycle (Fig. 7–12). Although sequential intervals during the cardiac cycle could be imaged, usually only end-systole and end-diastole are selected.[17] The end-systolic image is obtained by triggering the gate from the R wave of the patient's electrocardiogram and imaging only during the last 40 msecs of the T wave. The end-diastolic image is obtained by imaging only during the patient's P-R interval. A total of 200 to 300 cardiac cycles are summed to obtain a 200,000 count gated image. From these gated images at end-diastole or end-systole, the outline of the free left ventricular wall at these phases of the cardiac

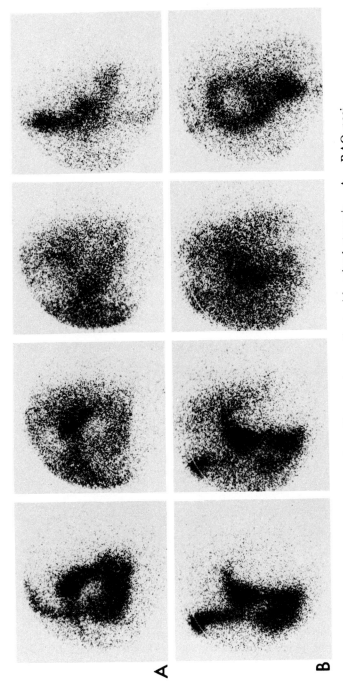

Fig. 7-9. Nuclear angiocardiogram in a patient with mitral stenosis. A. RAO position. B. LAO position. The apparent break in the SVC in the RAO view corresponds to the innominate vein emptying unlabeled blood into the SVC. The enlarged left atrium fills in the third frame on both RAO and LAO views and persists through the LV phase.

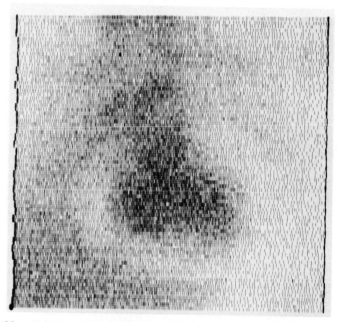

Fig. 7–10. Cardiac blood pool scan in anterior position in a patient with pericardial effusion. The scan was performed using the rectilinear instrument and reveals a zone of decreased activity between the cardiac and surrounding blood pools as well as elevation of the hilar vessels.

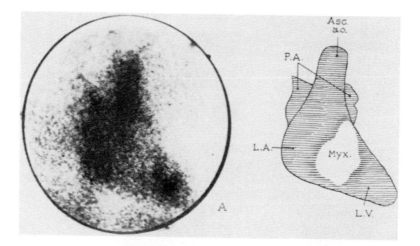

Fig. 7–11. Cardiac blood pool scan in the anterior position in a patient with myxoma of the left atrium. The mass appears as an area of decreased tracer concentration. (From Zaret BL, Hurley PJ, Pitt B: Noninvasive scintiphotographic diagnosis of left atrial myxoma, J Nucl Med 13:81, 1972, with permission.)

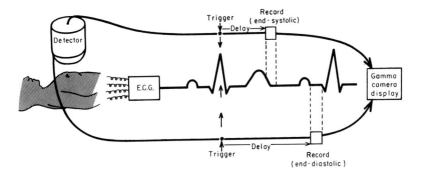

Fig. 7–12. Schematic representation of the gating unit which is triggered by the patient's ECG and permits signals to pass from the detector to the gamma camera display only during short portions of each cardiac cycle. The top line is the timing used at end-systole and the bottom line, for end-diastole. (From Strauss HW, Zaret BL, Hurley PJ, et al: A scintiphotographic method for measuring left ventricular ejection fraction in man without cardiac catheterization, Am J Cardiol 28:575, 1971, with permission.)

cycle can be obtained. The aortic and mitral valve planes, however, are poorly seen because of overlying activity in the great vessels and right ventricle. To localize the valve planes, a nuclear angiocardiogram is performed in the right anterior oblique projection when the tracer is first administered (Fig. 7–13). Sequential frames from the left ventricular phase of the study are examined to locate the filling and emptying of the left atrium to find the mitral valve plane. The aortic valve plane is determined by connecting the intersection of the left ventricular free wall and aorta to the mitral valve plane. Since the patient is not moved between the nuclear angiocardiogram and the gated portion of the study, the valve planes obtained from one portion may be transferred to the images obtained in a later portion of the examination (Fig. 7–14). The images are projected life-size for measurement.

In the gated right anterior oblique images, activity from the right ventricle falls within the borders of the left in most instances. In those cases with right ventricular dilatation in which a significant portion of the right ventricular activity lies outside the left ventricular border, a correction is made from the data obtained in the initial nuclear angiocardiogram. In patients with marked dilatation of the right ventricle, it may, however, be impossible to obtain the border of the left ventricular free wall in the right anterior oblique position (Fig. 7–15), and then only the left anterior oblique position is used.

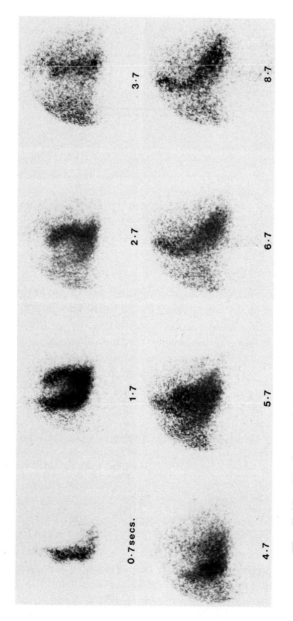

Fig. 7–13. Nuclear angiocardiogram in RAO position in a patient with coronary artery disease. The time of each frame in seconds is recorded at the bottom of each frame. The left atrium fills in frame 4.7, LV and Ao fill in 5.7, and the LA empties by 6.7. The plane of the mitral valve can be determined from examination of these sequential frames.

388

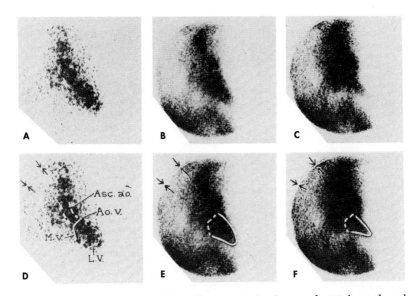

Fig. 7–14. The complete LV outline is obtained at end-systole and end-diastole by combining data from: A. LV phase of the nuclear angiocardiogram. B. End-diastolic gated image. C. End-systolic gated image. The mitral and aortic valve planes are determined from frame A and are superimposed on the scintiphoto. The recticule indicated by the arrow, is a constant reference. The valve planes are then superimposed on frame B and C. The outline of the LV at end-diastole and end-systole are traced and valve planes superimposed as shown. (From Strauss HW, Zaret BL, Hurley PJ, et al: A scintiphotographic method for measuring left ventricular ejection fraction in man without cardiac catheterization, Am J Cardiol 28:575, 1971, with permission.)

Ventricular Volume

To calculate left ventricular chamber volume from the right anterior oblique gated image, the long axis (L) of the ventricle from the midpoint of the aortic valve plane to the apex is drawn, and the area (A) is measured by planimetry. The volume (V) is then calculated using the formula for a prolate spheroid: $V = 0.848 \ A^2/L$; where L equals the length of the long axis of the ventricle. The ejection fraction (EF) is calculated using the formula

$$EF = \frac{EDV - ESV}{EDV}$$

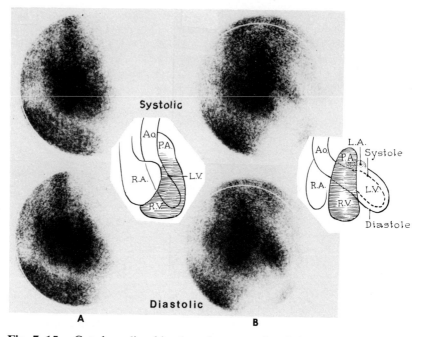

Fig. 7–15. Gated cardiac blood pool scans. A. RAO view. B. LAO view. The systolic frames are on top, diastolic below. Because of the unusual degree of RV enlargement, the LV is not seen in the RAO view, and an unusually low-ejection fraction is suspected. When the study is performed in the LAO view, excellent LV contraction is seen and the enlarged RV can be appreciated.

where EDV equals the end-diastolic volume and ESV equals the end-systolic volume. In those instances where the quality of the initial isotope angiogram is inadequate to allow accurate determination of the mitral valve plane, the long axis of the left ventricle from the junction of the free wall and aorta to the apex is drawn and then bisected to determine the short axis (M). Volume is then calculated using the formula

$$V = \frac{\pi}{6} LM^2$$

When biplane images are available, the formula is modified to include the short axis for both projections

$$V = \frac{\pi}{6} LM_{(RAO)}M_{(LAO)}$$

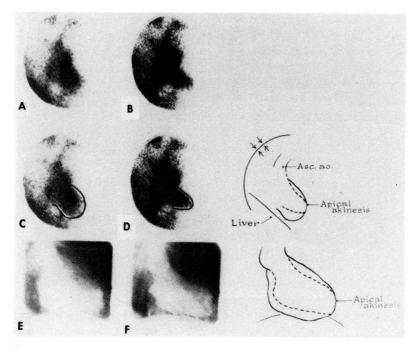

Fig. 7–16. Gated cardiac blood pool scans. A. End-diastolic image. B. End-systolic image. E. Contrast left ventriculogram in diastole. F. Contrast left ventriculogram in systole. The zone of akinesis can be appreciated by superimposing the traced ventricular outline from C to D. The site and extent of akinesis is similar on the gated blood pool scans and contrast angiograms.

where M(RAO) is the short axis in the right anterior oblique projection, and M (LAO) is the short axis in the left anterior oblique projection.* Using these techniques, a correlation coefficient of over 0.9 has been obtained when the scintiphotographs were compared with single-plane contrast angiocardiograms.[17]

Regional wall motion can be determined by superimposing the completed end-diastolic and end-systolic images (Fig. 7–16D). Regions of akinesis are quantitated by determining the percent change from end-systole to end-diastole in the long axis, anterior and inferior hemiaxis. These changes have also been correlated with single-plane contrast angiocardiograms (R = 0.9).[18]

The entire study takes approximately 30 min, and is easily

* An alternative method of defining short axis is $M = \dfrac{4A}{\pi L}$.

tolerated by most patients including those with severe orthopnea when the technique is modified by allowing the patient to sit upright in bed.

Several techniques have now been developed to determine left ventricular ejection fraction automatically using computers in conjunction with the scintillation camera.[19] One technique determines the counts in an area of interest in the left ventricle during systole and diastole. Ejection fraction is then determined by the formula

$$EF = \frac{\text{diastolic counts} - \text{systolic counts}}{\text{diastolic counts} - \text{background}}$$

This technique eliminates the assumption of an idealized ventricular geometry in the calculations. In addition to ejection fraction, regional akinesis, and chamber volume, other measurements can be made which include estimation of left ventricular circumferential fiber shortening, ventricular volume curves, and a measurement of dv/dt. These measurements require a means of recording data for later replay on a computer. Evaluation of the scintiphotographs alone, however, without additional equipment, can be used to assess the site and extent of regional wall motion in patients with a variety of heart diseases. In patients with congestive heart failure following myocardial infarction, the scintiphotographic studies are particularly useful in differentiating those with diffuse hypokinesis from those with aneurysms or localized akinesis (Fig. 7–16). Patients with diffuse hypokinesis can be treated medically without proceeding to contrast angiography, whereas those with suspected left ventricular aneurysm (Fig. 7–17) should undergo cardiac catheterization to evaluate them for surgery.

Radiocardiography

In 1948, Prinzmetal described the radiocardiogram which traces the passage of intravenously administered radionuclide through the right and left heart chambers using a detector placed over the precordium.[20] A curve with two peaks is recorded. The procedure has since been modified both in instrumentation and radiopharmaceuticals. The following calculations can be made from the radiocardiogram: cardiac output, regurgitant flow, and pulmonary blood volume.[21] The major advantage of this method is that it can be performed at the patient's bedside using portable equipment. A disadvantage of the method is that images are not obtained, making the differentition of

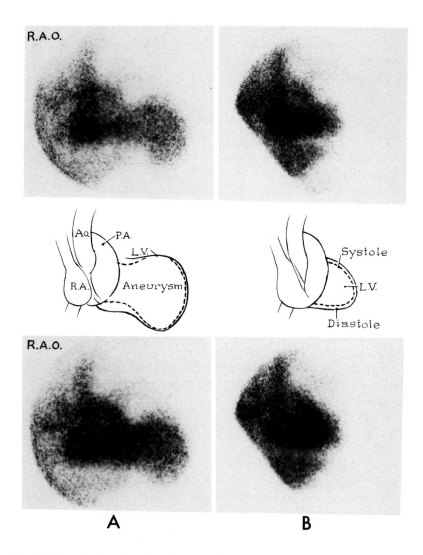

Fig. 7–17. Cardiac blood pool scans in the RAO position in a patient with anterior apical aneurysm. End-systolic images on top, end-diastolic images below. A. The preoperative studies reveal the aneurysm in the apex which hardly moves. B. The postoperative study shows a poorly contracting ventricle with no aneurysm.

multiple etiologies of left ventricular dysfunction difficult. Weber and associates have combined the scintillation camera and computer to obtain an image while recording information comparable to the radio-cardiogram on tape.[10] The method is complex, but the data provided are valuable and further application of this technique is awaited.

Myocardial Infarction and Ischemia

The site and extent of myocardial ischemia and infarction can be determined by myocardial scanning. Two approaches to the detection of infarction are possible: the infarct may be imaged either as a region of increased tracer concentration with little or no tracer in normal tissue (hot-spot scan) or as a region of little or no tracer accumulation with normal tissue having a high concentration (cold-spot scan).[22] Ideally, hot-spot scanning would be preferable for opti-mum imaging. Many tracers have been suggested for this purpose including tetracycline, chlormeridrin, and ^{67m}Ga.[23] However, because of the limited blood supply in the infarcted area, it is difficult to concen-trate enough tracer for adequate imaging. Although these agents may serve as prototypes, their use in patients has been disappointing. Cold-spot scanning has been shown to be practical for the detection of myocardial infarction.[24] The normal myocardial cell actively concen-trates potassium and its analogs cesium and rubidium. These tracers have been used to demonstrate myocardial infarcts as regions of de-creased tracer accumulation. The location and extent of infarction can be determined both acutely and long after the episode (Fig. 7–18). Other scanning agents which have been used intravenously include labeled fatty acids,[25] and ammonia.[26] A comparison of myocardial scanning for the detection of site and extent of infarction to gated cardiac blood pool imaging has suggested that there is correlation be-tween the site and extent of akinetic or hypokinetic regions to the areas of decreased activity on myocardial scan (Fig. 7–19). Therefore, the gated blood pool scan may also be of use in detecting the site and extent of infarction.

The site and extent of transient myocardial ischemia can be determined by scanning with ^{43}K.[27] If ^{43}K is given during angina pectoris induced by exercise or pacing, the ischemic area has a lower concen-tration of potassum than the normal region, and will appear as a "cold spot" compared to the normal region (Fig. 7–20). If a normal ^{43}K-scan is obtained on the same patient when injected during a pain-free interval, one can assume that the area of decreased uptake seen during ischemia is viable. Quantification of the ^{43}K-scan using computer tech-

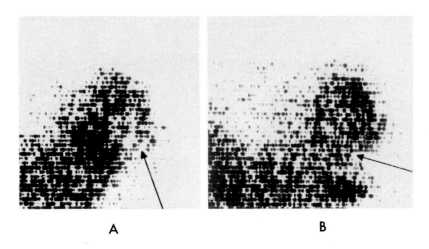

A   B

Fig. 7–18. Myocardial scan with ⁴³K in the anterior position performed on two patients with myocardial infarction. The regions of decreased tracer accumulation indicated by the arrows correspond to the electrocardiographic site of infarction. A. Anterior myocardial infarction. B. Inferior myocardial infarction. The tracer concentration in the liver may obscure lesions in the inferior wall of the heart. (From Strauss HW, Zaret BL, Martin ND, Wells HP, Flamm MD: Radiology 108:85–90, 1973, with permission.)

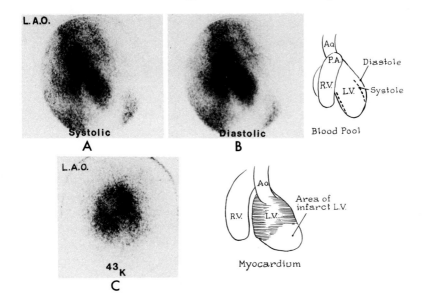

Fig. 7–19. Gated blood pool scan in the LAO position. A. In systole. B. In diastole. C. A ⁴³K myocardial scan on the same patient. The infarct appears as a dyskinetic region in the gated blood pool scan and corresponds to the region of decreased ⁴³K-uptake seen in the myocardial scan.

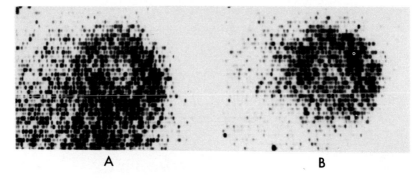

A   B

Fig. 7–20. Myocardial scans in a patient with angina pectoris using ^{43}K. A. Scan performed at rest. B. Scan performed after exercise to angina pectoris. The inferior wall has a decreased uptake of ^{43}K, and there is decreased tracer accumulation in the liver because of the decreased blood flow during exercise. (From Strauss HW, Zaret BL, Martin ND, Wells HP, Flamm MD: Radiology 108:85–90, 1973.)

niques may allow a noninvasive measurement of alterations in regional myocardial blood flow.

Pulmonary Embolism

Pulmonary embolism is frequently considered in the differential diagnosis of patients with dyspnea, chest discomfort, apprehension, or arrhythmia, particularly when some predisposing event such as recent surgery or congestive cardiac failure is also present. Since the manifestations of pulmonary embolism are so varied, clinical diagnosis is difficult. The lung scan provides information regarding the status of pulmonary perfusion. The specificity of the lung scan for diagnosing pulmonary embolism is greatly increased when ventilation scanning (by breathing a radioactive gas such as ^{33}Xe) is also performed.[28] Perfusion follows ventilation very closely. Thus, ventilation data is helpful in determining whether parenchymal lung disease, such as bronchitis, asthma, or emphysema are responsible for the perfusion abnormality. The perfusion scan is performed after the intravenous administration of particles of sufficient size to block a very small number of the pulmonary capillaries. The number of particles administered is very small compared to the size of the pulmonary capillary bed. The particles are usually made from albumin, either in the form of macroaggregates of albumin, or microspheres. Many tracers can be used, but technetium is most frequently used to label the particles. The lung scan must be interpreted

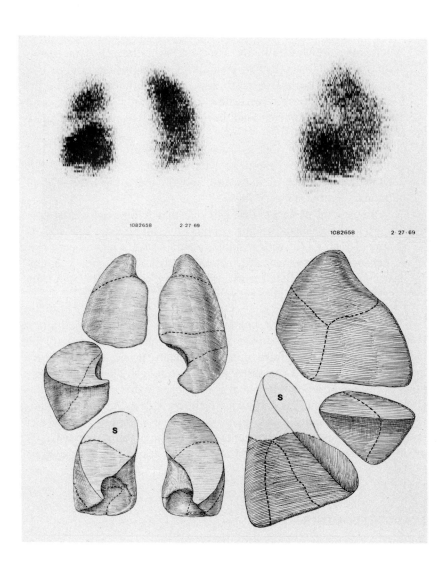

Fig. 7–21. Perfusion lung scan in the posterior and right lateral portions in a patient with pulmonary embolism. The superior segment of the lower lobe is not perfused. (From Deland FH, Wagner HN: The lung and heart, in Atlas of Nuclear Medicine, vol. II, Philadelphia, Saunders, 1970, pp 58–59, with permission.)

in conjunction with the chest radiograph. Abnormalities in the perfusion pattern can be divided into five categories:

1. Whole lung which is usually associated with bronchogenic carcinoma, congenital absence or stenosis of a pulmonary artery, or a large pleural effusion. It is rarely seen, with pulmonary embolus.
2. Lobar abnormalities in perfusion are commonly associated with infection such as pneumonia, but are also rare with pulmonary embolism.
3. Segmental perfusion defects, which are present with a normal ventilation scan, are frequent with pulmonary embolism (Fig. 7–21). The presence of these two findings make the likelihood of pulmonary embolism very high.
4. A subsegmental perfusion defect is one that follows segmental borders, but the segment is not completely obliterated. This too, is commonly associated with pulmonary embolism.
5. A nonsegmental perfusion defect is unusual in pulmonary embolism and when associated with a ventilatory abnormality, it is very suggestive of chronic obstructive pulmonary disease.

In congestive failure or pulmonary venous hypertension, there is increased perfusion to the upper zones of the lung compared to the bases. The fissures may also appear unusually prominent and there may be a patchiness to the distribution of traces in the lungs. These findings disappear when the patient is no longer in failure.

Although the nuclear cardiology techniques described in this chapter are already playing a role in cardiovascular diagnosis, we predict that further advances in instrumentation and radiopharmaceuticals will greatly improve the resolution and increase the use of these noninvasive studies.

ACKNOWLEDGMENTS

The authors wish to acknowledge the assistance of Pierre Rigo, M.D. and Malcolm Murray, M.D., Division of Cardiology, Johns Hopkins Hospital, for performing many of the gated cardiac blood pool studies; Buck A. Rhodes, Ph.D. and E. U. Buddemeyer, Ph.D., Department of Radiological Sciences, Johns Hopkins Medical Institutions, for their assistance in the section on principles, Barry L. Zaret, M.D., David Grant Hospital, Travis AFB, for providing the figures on myocardial ischemia with ^{43}K, and the Division of Nuclear Medicine,

Johns Hopkins Hospital, for the nuclear angiocardiograms and lung scans. We especially want to thank Dr. Henry N. Wagner Jr. and Dr. Richard S. Ross for their encouragement and guidance in applying many of the techniques of nuclear medicine to the cardiac patient.

REFERENCES

1. Blumgart HE, Weiss S: Studies on the velocity of blood flow III. The velocity of blood flow and its relation to other aspects of the circulation in patients with rheumatic and syphilitic heart disease. J Clin Invest 4:149, 1927
2. Maynard CD: Pharmaceuticals and instrumentation, in: Clinical Nuclear Medicine. Philadelphia, Lea and Feibeger, 1969, pp 3–23
3. Hine GJ: Sodium iodide scintillation detectors; Lorius, A: Systems for data accumulation and presentation, in, Hine GJ (ed): Instrumentation in Nuclear Medicine, vol 1. London, Academic Press, 1967, pp 95–116, 119–160
4. Wagner HN, Rhodes BA: The radiopharmaceutical, in Wagner HN (ed): Principles of Nuclear Medicine, Philadelphia, Saunders, 1968, pp 259–301
5. Smith EM, Brownell GL, Ellett WH: Radiation Dosemitry, in Wagner HN (ed): Principles of Nuclear Medicine, Philadelphia, Saunders, 1968, pp 742–784
6. Hurley PJ, Strauss HW, Wagner HN: Radionuclide angiography in cyanotic congenital heart disease. Johns Hopkins Med J 127:46, 1970
7. Mason DT, Ashburn WL, Harbert JC, Cohen LS, Braunwald E: Rapid sequential visualization of the heart and great vessels in man using the wide field anger scintillation camera. Circulation 39:19, 1969
8. Wesselhoeft H, Hurley PJ, Wagner HN, Rowe RD: Nuclear angiocardiography in the diagnosis of congenital heart disease in infants. Circulation 45:77, 1972
9. Graham TP, Goodrich JK, Robinson AE, Harris CC: Scintiangiocardiography in children: Rapid sequence visualization of the heart and great vessels after intravenous injection of radionuclide. Am J Cardiol 25:387, 1970
10. Weber PM, Dos Remedios LV, Jasko IA: Quantitative radioisotope angiocardiography. J Nucl Med 13:812, 1972
11. Jones RH, Sabiston DC, Bates BB, Morris JJ, Anderson PAW, Goodrich JK: Quantitative radionuclide angiocardiography for determination of chamber to chamber cardiac transit times. Am J Cardiol 30:855, 1972
12. Hagan AD, Friedman WF, Ashburn WL, Alazraki N: Further application of scintillation scanning techniques to the diagnosis and management of infants and children with congenital heart disease. Circulation 45:858, 1972
13. Kriss JP, Enright LP, Hayden WG, Wexler L, Shumway NE: Radioisotope angiocardiography: Wide scope of applicability in diagnosis and evaluation of the therapy in diseases of the heart and great vessels. Circulation 43:792, 1971
14. Strauss HW, Hurley PJ, Rhodes BA, Wagner HN: Quantification of right to left transpulmonary shunts in man. J Lab Clin Med 74:597, 1969
15. Donato L, Holmes RA, Wagner HN: The circulation, in Wagner HN (ed): Principles of Nuclear Medicine, Philadelphia, Saunders, 1968, pp 563–576

16. Zaret BL, Hurley PJ, Pitt B: Noninvasive scintiphotographic diagnosis of left atrial myxoma. J Nucl Med 13:81, 1972

17. Strauss HW, Zaret BL, Hurley PJ, Natarajan TK, Pitt B: A scintiphotographic method for measuring left ventricular ejection fraction in man without cardiac catheterization. Am J Cardiol 28:575, 1971

18. Zaret BL, Strauss HW, Hurley PJ, Natarajan TK, Pitt B: A noninvasive scintiphotographic method for detection of regional ventricular dysfunction in man. N Engl J Med 284:1165, 1971

19. Parker JA, Secker-Walker RH, Hill R, Siegel BA, Potchen EJ: Calculation of left ventricular ejection fraction. J Nucl Med 12:649, 1972

20. Prinzmetal M, Corday E, Spritzler RJ, Fleig W: Radiocardiography and its clinical applications. JAMA 139:617, 1949

21. Johnson DE, Liu CK, Akcay MM, Taplin GV: Radiopulmonary cardiography for measurement of central mean transit time and its arterial and venous subdivisions, in Knisely A, Tauxe WN (ed): Dynamic Clinical Studies with Radioisotopes. USAEC, June 1964, p 249

22. Zaret BL, Pitt B, Ross RS: Determination of the site, extent and significance of regional ventricular dysfunction during acute myocardial infarction. Circulation 45:441, 1972

23. Kramer RJ, Goldstein R, Hirshfeld IW, Johnston GS, Epstein SE: Visualization of acute myocardial infarction by radionuclide gallium 67. Circulation 45 (Suppl II):20, 1972

24. Carr EA, Gleason F, Shaw J, Krantz B: The direct diagnosis of myocardial infarction by photoscanning after administration of cesium 131. Am Heart J 68:627, 1964

25. Gunton RW, Evans JR, Baker RG, Spears JX, Beanlands DS: Demonstration of myocardial infarction by photoscans. Am J Cardiol 16:482, 1965

26. Harper PV, Schwartz J, Resnekov L, Hoffer PB, Krizek H, Stark VJ, Lathrop KA: Clinical myocardial imaging with ^{13}N-NH_3. J Nucl Med 13:782, 1972

27. Zaret BL, Strauss HW, Martin ND, Wells HP, Flamm MD: Noninvasive evaluation of regional myocardial perfusion with potassium 43. Study of patients at rest, exercise, and during angina pectoris. N Engl J Med 288:809, 1973

28. Wagner HN, Rhodes BA: Radioactive tracers in diagnosing of cardiovascular disease. Prog Cardiovasc Dis 15:1, 1972

Rashid A. Massumi, Robert Zelis,
Nayab Ali, and Dean T. Mason

8
External Venous and Arterial Pulses

INTRODUCTION

A thorough understanding of the physiologic events underlying venous and arterial pulses, their amplitude and the character of their individual components greatly enhances the value of the physical examination of the cardiovascular system. The important contribution of these pulsations to the teaching of clinical cardiology is matched by the useful information they provide concerning the dynamics of the heart, thereby permitting a physiologically based diagnosis of the nature and degree of cardiac dysfunction at the patient's bedside. Modern catheterization techniques have not displaced the art of examining the veins and the arteries, but actually have heightened its status by demonstrating good correlation between these pulses and intracardiac events.[1,2] Auscultation of the heart, in like manner, has benefited greatly from the knowledge gained in the cardiac catheterization laboratory. Moreover, it has become recognized that the careful study of venous and arterial pulses is indispensable in the proper evaluation of the cardiovascular system and, as demonstrated in this chapter, may provide valuable information not available by means other than invasive techniques. The suggestion for the first time of a specific cardiac abnor-

This investigation was supported in part by the American Heart Association (Grant #71-1072) and the National Heart and Lung Institute (Program Project Grant HL-14780).

mality by subtle alterations of the external pulses is familiar to the experienced cardiologist. For example, pulmonary embolic disease may be indicated initially by prominent, crisp *a* waves; early tricuspid valve endocarditis in heroin addicts by slightly larger than normal *v* waves in the jugular veins; and sharply rising, bifid carotid arterial pulses may suggest idiopathic hypertrophic subaortic stenosis. In the following sections, venous and arterial pulses are described in terms of their genesis and the method of detection and assessment of their abnormalities. Emphasis is placed on the less-appreciated aspects of these subjects rather than on the well-known features of the external pulses.

THE VENOUS PULSES

Pulsations of the veins are most commonly observed and recorded indirectly from the skin overlying the large veins of the neck. The jugular venous pulses may be of such great magnitude that they impart a rhythmic side-to-side "bobbing" to the head (Fig. 8–1).[3] Distant veins or venous reservoirs such as the veins of the upper arm and upper thorax (Fig. 8–2), the liver (Fig. 8–3), the femoral veins just below the inguinal ligament (Fig. 8–4), and even varicose veins of the calf (Fig. 8–5) may display detectable pulsations when venous pulses are of sufficiently high amplitude or are associated with retrograde displacement of large volumes of blood. We should emphasize that, although venous pulsations in these distant structures frequently result from tricuspid regurgitation, prominent *a* waves themselves can be transmitted readily to a congested liver and can be felt and recorded over this organ. These presystolic liver pulsations were recognized by MacKenzie in 1902[4,5] and have been described by a number of authors since.[6–11]

In normal individuals, only the veins of the neck have visible and recordable pulsations. In more peripheral veins, as the distance from the right atrium increases, the amplitude of the waves decreases, thus indicating clearly that the origin of the venous pulses is the right atrium itself. The energy of left ventricular contraction and the resultant arterial pressure pulse make no contribution to venous pulses, and are only important in moving blood centripetally in the veins. Arterial pressure transients become completely damped out in their passage through the capillaries; there remaining only an essentially nonpulsatile steady venous pressure to drive blood back toward the heart. The only exception is encountered in arteriovenous fistulas in which arterial pressure is transmitted directly to the veins for a variable distance from the

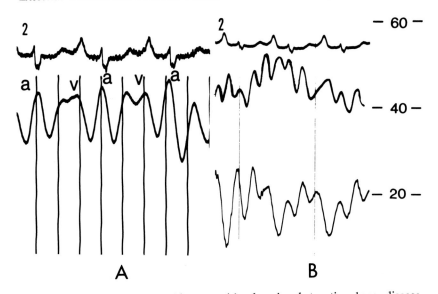

Fig. 8–1. In this 45-year-old man with chronic obstructive lung disease complicated by fibrosis and severe cor pulmonale, the head was found to vibrate visibly from side-to-side with two distinct components in each cardiac cycle. In A, one component corresponded to the *a* wave and the other to the *v* wave of the jugular venous pulses. These pulses were recorded using a peizoelectric crystal microphone applied to the side of the head and we noted that the pulsations were clearly venous in origin. The reason for the side-to-side motion of the head was thought to be the better transmission of right atrial pulse pressure to the right side of the head through the straight right internal jugular vein and diminished transmission to the left side of the head because of the angles present between the right atrium and the left internal jugular vein. In B, head pulses on top are recorded simultaneously with right atrial pressure pulse on bottom showing the components to be similar, the head pulse being slightly delayed. The right atrial pressure scale (mm Hg) is shown.

communication depending on the amplitude of the arterial pressure pulse, the cross-sectional area of the fistula, and the aggregate size of the recipient venous trunks. In one striking case of internal mammary arteriovenous fistula associated with occlusion of the right subclavian artery,[12] the fistula had grown so large and the recipient veins so heavily calcified that transmitted arterial pulsations could be seen and recorded in the veins of the dorsum of the right hand.

Visual inspection of the jugular veins permits a remarkably accurate estimation of the venous pressure. This is best executed by placing the patient in the supine position and then tilting the head of

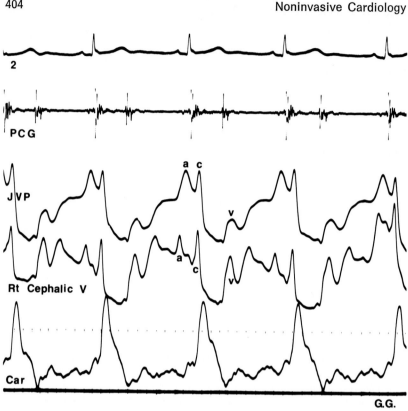

Fig. 8–2. Tracings from top to bottom are lead II of the electrocardiogram, phonocardiogram. (PCG), jugular venous pulse tracing (JVP), indirect pulse tracing from the right cephalic vein (rt cephalic v) and carotid pulse tracing (car). This 24-year-old man with history of heroin addiction had visible pulsations in the veins of the upper arms. Note that all three waves, *a*, *c*, and *v*, were visible and recordable. No tricuspid regurgitation could be documented. The explanation for transmission of the right atrial pulses to the arm veins was thought to be destruction of the venous valves as a result of chronic infection caused by self-administration of heroin in the veins of the arms.

the bed upward until the external jugular vein begins to empty and a pulsating meniscus, representing the summit of the column of blood, is clearly seen. The venous pressure is thereby equal in centimeters of water to the vertical height of this meniscus, measured in relation to the center of the right atrium which serves as the lowest point of the same column or the zero level. The spatial center of the right atrium is most easily localized 8 to 10 cm posterior from the sternal end of

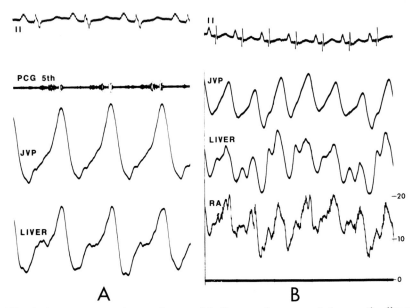

Fig. 8–3. Venous pulse tracings and indirect pulses recorded over the liver and direct right atrial pressure (RA). A. Gross tricuspid regurgitation with some congestive heart failure was present in this 34-year-old man with heroin addiction and destruction of the tricuspid valve by staphylococcal endocarditis. Note the identical monophasic waves, with slow rise and sharp descent recorded over the jugular vein and the liver. Both tracings display simultaneous peaks of the regurgitant wave and nadir of the *y* descent. B. Tracing from another patient with heroin addiction and tricuspid regurgitation. Here the similarity between the jugular venous pulse tracing, liver tracing, and direct right atrial pressure is noteworthy. Note that this patient's liver pulse peaked about 0.08 sec before the jugular venous pulse and was simultaneous with the right atrial pulse. Also, the *a* waves were more clearly visible in the liver pulse than in the jugular pulse. Again, note that the rate of rise of the V wave of the venous pulse and the liver pulse is less than the rate of *y* descent, and this highly important characteristic distinguished venous liver pulses from transmitted arterial pulse which rises more rapidly than it falls.

the fourth intercostal space. Elevation of jugular venous pressure without detectable pulsations is an indication of possible obstruction between the right atrium and the neck veins, most frequently in the superior vena cava, which is most commonly found in persons with lymphomatous mediastinal masses or direct invasion by bronchogenic carcinoma. On occasions, in severe right ventricular failure or constrictive pericarditis with the venous pressure greater than 25 cm of water,

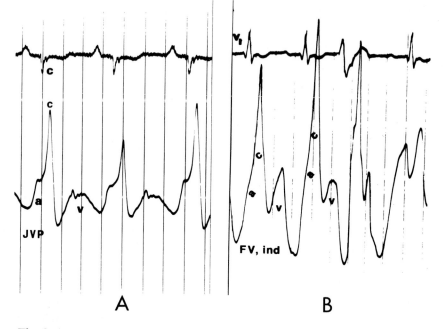
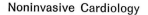

Fig. 8–4. A 68-year-old man with chronic obstructive lung disease and cor pulmonale. A. Jugular venous pulse tracings. B. Indirect femoral vein tracing (FV, ind). Note that the pulsations in the femoral vein are remarkably similar to those of jugular vein, and that there are giant *c* waves in both. The third beat in the femoral venous pulse tracing is a premature ventricular beat and is associated with a large *a* wave. This finding indicates that the venous pulses recorded over the femoral vein were not arterial in nature, for with a premature ventricular beat the arterial pulse would have been very small or imperceptible.

the neck veins remain full and nonpulsating even in the sitting position. In these circumstances, the scalp veins or the head itself may be found to pulsate, thus excluding the possibility of venous obstruction. Inferior vena caval obstruction is more difficult to recognize since pulsations of the leg veins are not readily appreciated. Simultaneous measurements of venous pressure in an arm and a leg vein may be necessary. One should keep in mind, however, that in the supine position, tense ascites can cause almost complete obstruction of the inferior vena cava and very high femoral venous pressures.

It is important to emphasize that venous pressure may be normal or even low in conditions that are expected to raise it. The reason is usually severe hypovolemia caused by vigorous diuretic therapy, gastro-

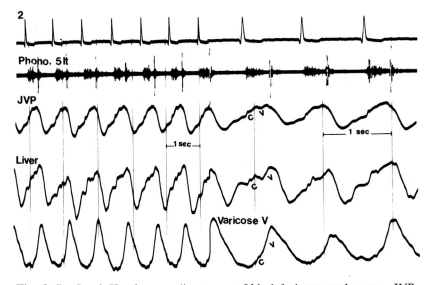

Fig. 8–5. Lead II, phonocardiogram at fifth left intercostal space, JVP, liver pulses and pulsations of varicose veins on the posterior aspect of the foreleg were recorded in this 72-year-old woman with chronic congestive heart failure and severe functional tricuspid regurgitation. Again the similarity of the tracings recorded from the jugular veins, the liver, and the varicose veins is quite impressive. The rate of rise in the JVP and the liver pulses appears slower than the rate of y descent. However, the pulsations of the varicose veins are so distant and damped that this particular characteristic is no longer recognizable.

intestinal loss, or inadequate fluid intake. We have observed cases of massive pulmonary embolism, pericardial tamponade, as well as severe heart failure of acute myocardial infarction in the presence of normal or subnormal venous pressures.

Normally, cervical venous pressure declines and the neck veins collapse during inspiration owing to the negative intrathoracic pressure and the suction applied to the extrathoracic veins. The inspiratory fall of venous pressure is diminished or obliterated when the right ventricle cannot accept this increment of blood because of severe heart failure, massive embolic obstruction of the pulmonary arteries, space-occupying lesions within the right ventricle, or constrictive pericarditis (Kussmaul's sign). In this respect, it is not universally appreciated that the inspiratory fall of venous pressure may be normal or only slightly reduced in pericardial tamponade. Thus the common practice of seeking Kussmaul's sign in patients suspected of tamponade is often unrewarding.

The morphology of the venous pulse is of great interest because it mirrors the dynamics which occur in the right atrium. A factor which may modify right atrial pressure events in their transmission to the extrathoracic veins is the pulsations of the proximal aortic root, since the aorta in this region is in immediate juxtaposition of the interatrial septum and the adjacent walls of both atria (Fig. 8–6). Also, to a lesser degree, the right ventricular outflow tract and supravalvular portion of the main pulmonary artery may transmit pulsations to the right atrium. In their retrograde propagation from the right atrium to the neck veins, venous pulses may be further modified by transmission of pulses from the innominate and carotid arteries. The strong arterial pulsations in patients with increased left ventricular stroke volume related to high cardiac output or to aortic run-off such as occurs with aortic regurgitation may make study of neck vein pulses practically impossible (Fig. 8–6A). Conversely, strong presytolic venous pulses can be transmitted to the arterial system and render recording of

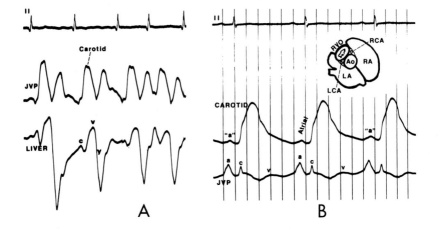

Fig. 8–6.   A.   JVP and liver pulses are recorded simultaneously in this patient with heart failure. It was impossible to record satisfactory jugular pulses because the carotid imprint could not be eliminated. The liver pulses, however, were completely free of arterial interference so that the *cv* waves and the sharp *y* descent could be clearly recognized.   B.   The carotid pulse tracing and JVP are recorded simultaneously, and it was impossible to eliminate the sharp venous *a* waves or the atrial imprint on the arterial pulses. The anatomic insert in B is intended to show the intimate relationship between the outflow tract of the right ventricle (RVO) and the aorta (Ao) on one hand, and the atria and interatrial septum on the other. Pulsations from the arterial trunks may easily be transmitted to the atria, and vice versa (LA, left atrium; LCA, left coronary artery; RCA, right coronary artery).

carotid pulses difficult (Fig. 8–6B). These arterial *a* waves are transmitted to the ascending aorta either by vigorous contractions of the right and left atria or result from contiguity of the pulsating veins with the arteries in the neck. Very large venous *a* and *v* waves in patients with low cardiac output, and therefore small arterial pulse pressure, make it impossible to record the carotid pulses.

In normal sinus rhythm, the *a* wave resulting from atrial systole reflects, through its amplitude, the strength of atrial contraction, and the ease with which blood can be driven into the right ventricle, i.e. right ventricular compliance. The *x* descent following the summit of the *a* wave is a manifestation of the fall in right atrial pressure caused by atrial relaxation. The terminal portion of this negative slope is caused by the downward movement of the tricuspid valve at the onset of right ventricular ejection. Between atrial relaxation and onset of right ventricular systole, the *x* descent is interrupted by a brief, positive deflection, called the *c* wave for the carotid pulsation, according to the originator of the term Sir James MacKenzie.[4] Today it is clear, however, that the *c* wave results from the upward bulge of the tricuspid valve during isovolumetric ventricular contraction. Although it is true that carotid pulsations are readily transmitted to the jugular veins, it is important to point out that *c* waves generally precede the onset of the carotid upstroke (Fig. 8–7). Moreover, *c* waves persist in patients in whom the carotid artery is congenitally atretic, occluded below the neck or surgically divided (Fig. 8–8). Another reason favoring a tricuspid origin for the *c* wave is that, in some cases, *c* waves can be clearly seen in liver pulse tracings (Fig. 8–9) as well as in right and left atrial pressure curves. Regardless of the mechanism involved, the diagnostic value of the *c* wave is negligible compared with that of the *a* wave.

After the nadir of the *x* descent, venous pressure rises slowly, corresponding to the gradual atrial filling from the venae cavae which occurs during ventricular contraction. The resultant *v* wave begins 0.06 to 0.08 sec before the second heart sound and ends 0.10 to 0.12 sec after it. Near the end of right ventricular isovolumetric relaxation, the tricuspid valve opens, the right atrium decompresses abruptly into the right ventricle (period of rapid or early ventricular filling) and the *v* wave collapses precipitously (*y* descent), unless there is obstruction to blood entering the right ventricle. The height of the *v* wave is determined by the volume of venous return into the atrium and the size and the compliance of the right atrium and the venae cavae. The slope of the *y* descent depends on the level of atrial pressure at the apex of the *v* wave, the speed with which the right atrium decompresses, and the

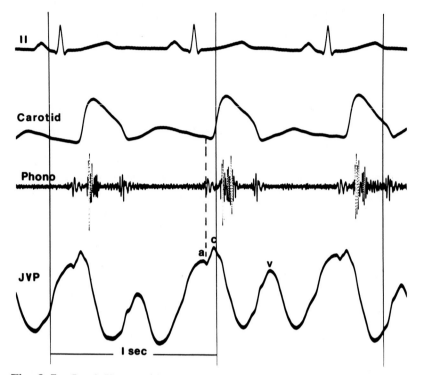

Fig. 8–7. Lead II, carotid pulse tracing, phonocardiogram at the apex, and JVP were recorded in this 17-year-old boy who had recovered completely 6 months after his surgery for subacute constrictive pericarditis. The *c* waves are clearly seen in JVP beginning before the carotid upstroke and simultaneously with the first heart sound. These *c* waves are undoubtedly related to the closure of the tricuspid valve and the hemodynamic phenomenon associated with it, and cannot be explained on the basis of transmission of arterial pulses from the carotid artery.

presence or absence of obstacles such as tricuspid stenosis (Fig. 8–10) or space-occupying masses or clots.

A new series of events take place at the nadir of the *y* descent. After the period of rapid ventricular filling ends, the period of slow filling and diastasis begins. At these times the tricuspid valve is widely open so that the right ventricle, atrium, and the venae cavae essentially form a single chamber. The gradual rise of the right ventricular pressure during its period of slow filling is transmitted to the veins, which can be seen as a late diastolic hump known as the *h* wave when the heart rate is slow (Fig. 8–11). This wave, much like the *c* wave, is of little diagnostic significance. For practical purposes, the *a* wave, the *x* descent, the *v* wave, and the *y* descent are the only venous transients

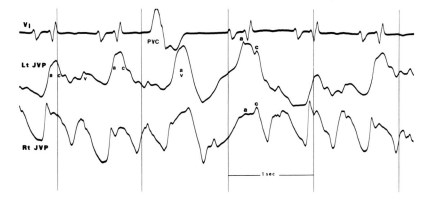

Fig. 8–8. This 54-year-old man with tetralogy of Fallot had a Blalock-Taussig operation in 1946 at the age of 28. Because of technical difficulties, the right carotid artery was used for the shunt. Examination of his neck at the present time showed no arterial pulses on the right, but the left carotid artery was quite forceful. Tracings of the jugular venous pulses simultaneously on the right and on the left clearly showed *c* waves on both sides, thus indicating a tricuspid origin for these waves.

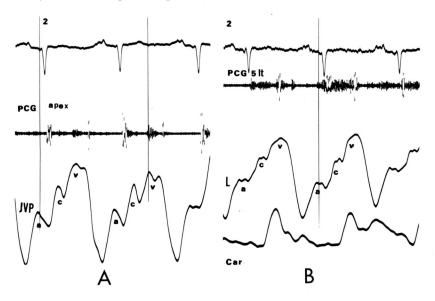

Fig. 8–9. In this patient with congestive heart failure and tricuspid regurgitation, *a-c-v* waves were recorded from the jugular vein and also from the liver (L). In both areas the *c* waves began a considerable interval before the upstroke of the carotid pulse tracing. The slow rise of the venous pulse and the sharp *y* descent contrast with the rapid rise and slow fall of the carotid arterial pulse (Cap) shown in B.

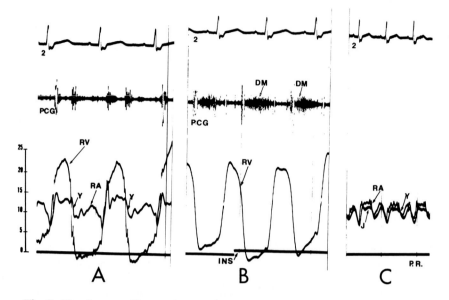

Fig. 8–10. Intracardiac tracings of sounds and pressures in this patient with severe tricuspid stenosis resulting from formation of clots on the tricuspid prosthesis which was inserted 5 months earlier because his tricuspid valve was completely destroyed by staphylococcal endocarditis resulting from heroin addiction.   A.   The surface phonocardiogram from the fifth left intercostal space and lead II of the electrocardiogram are recorded simultaneously with right ventricular (RV) and right atrial (RA) pressures.   B. The intracavitary phonocardiogram shows a loud diastolic murmur (DM) of tricuspid stenosis.   C.   Jugular venous pulse (J) and right atrial pressure are recorded simultaneously showing persistently elevated RA pressure and short y descent with slow rate of fall. The RA and RV pressure scale (mm Hg) is shown. INS = inspiration.

which provide useful clinical information. We must emphasize that changes in the temporal relationship between atrial and ventricular systoles (changing P-R relationship) profoundly affect the venous wave form by superimposing or separating the component waves. Even a simple sinus tachycardia can cause superimposition of the *a,v,* and *h* waves. The ideal heart rate for the study of the venous pulses is between 40 and 60 beats/min.

It is not always easy or even possible to examine neck vein pulsations. The most common problems are the short neck in infants, heavy breathing causing large fluctuations in the level of the venous pressure, large bounding arterial pulses imparting motion to the veins and the overlying skin, and finally tense muscles at the thoracic inlet

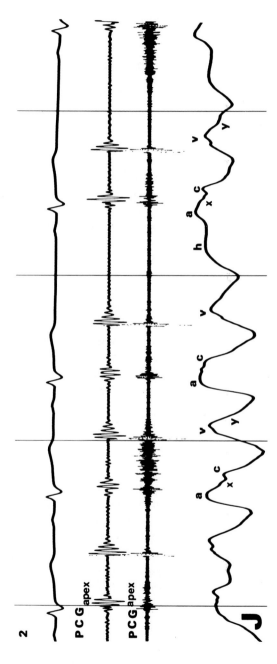

Fig. 8–11. Lead II, apex phonocardiograms at low and high frequencies, and jugular venous pulse tracing in a patient with sinus arrhythmia. During the first two cycles *a*, *c*, and *v* waves can be recognized. The last two cycles are considerably slower and show a third rise in venous pulse marked *h*. This corresponds to the late, slow period of right ventricular filling at a time when the right ventricle, the right atrium, and the jugular veins form almost a single communicating chamber.

preventing free transmission of right atrial waves to the neck veins. In these circumstances, an attempt should be made to study the internal jugular vein instead of the external and to evaluate both sides of the neck because the left jugular vein pulsates more visibly than the right in approximately 10 percent of persons. Occasionally, the small veins coursing over the thyroid area are suitable for examination. In the lower and midneck regions, pulsations of the internal jugular vein are not seen directly but are clearly transmitted to the sternocleido-mastiod muscle provided the vein is fully distended. In the upper regions of the neck, this vein separates from the muscle and emerges between it and the external ear. Its pulsations at this level are readily detected by focusing on the groove between the mastoid process and the posterior edge of the mandibular bone just behind the ear lobe.

Transmission of arterial pulses, both to the veins and to the over-lying structures in the neck, is a frequent source of difficulty in the analysis of venous wave forms. Differentiation usually becomes quite simple if one keeps certain principles in mind. (1) Arterial pulse rises more rapidly than it falls, whereas venous pulses behave in the opposite manner. (2) Venous pulses are readily affected by body position and changes in intrathoracic pressure, so that assumption of erect posture may empty the veins and cause their pulsations to disappear. Further, mild straining may bring about overfilling of veins or, conversely, forceful performance of this maneuver reduces venous return to the right atrium, thereby making the pulses invisible. Inspection of the veins during the early phase of a gentle Valsalva maneuver demonstrates gradual distention and clearly identifies their pulsations. (3) In severe congestive heart failure, arterial pulses are generally small, unless aortic regurgitation is present, whereas venous *a* waves in pulmonary valvular stenosis and pulmonary hypertension may be very forceful, rapidly rising, and easily palpable. The rapid fall from the summit in these large *a* waves is generally sufficient to distinguish them from arterial pulses (Fig. 8–12). (4) With premature beats, particularly those of junctional or ventricular origin which are likely to cause simultaneous contractions of the right ventricle and atrium, venous *a* waves are considerably amplified (cannon *a* waves), whereas arterial pulses are invaribly smaller. This difference serves as a valuable clue to distinguishing venous from arterial pulses in the neck, and also in separating pulmonary artery from pulmonary capillary wedge pressure during catheterization (Fig. 8–12, 8–13). (5) The pulsating structure in the neck may be compressed with the examining finger and venous waves disappear above the finger. In contrast, arterial pulses are not easily obliterated by finger pressure; if they are sufficiently weak to be

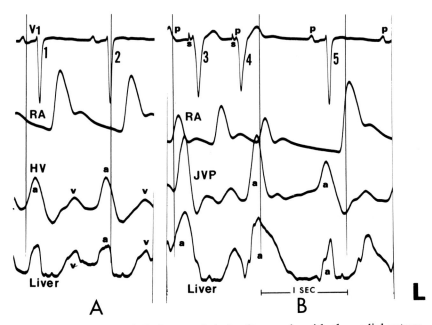

Fig. 8–12. A. Lead V_1 is recorded simultaneously with the radial artery pressure (RA), hepatic vein pressure (HV) and indirect liver pulses. B. Lead V_1 is recorded with radial artery pressure, JVP, and liver pulses. The sharp, peaked *a* waves in the venous and hepatic pulses occur earlier than the arterial upstroke. However, the shape of these *a* waves, especially their rate of rise and fall, is not sufficiently distinctive in this particular case for differentiation from arterial pulses. The reason is that the *a* waves were markedly enhanced because of severe pulmonary hypertension and right ventricular hypertrophy in this patient with severe mitral regurgitation and chronic heart failure. Also note that the first two beats B are electrically induced premature ventricular beats from the right ventricle so that the P waves have variable relationships with the QRS complexes. The large *a* waves in JVP and liver pulses appear after the P waves irrespective of their location in relation to the cardiac cycle, where as the arterial pulses always follow the QRS. Moreover, the *a* waves appear larger with premature ventricular beats, whereas the arterial pulses are smaller.

obliterated, they should not be visible. Therefore, prominently visible and palpable pulses that are easily compressed by finger pressure are venous in origin.

In a sizable proportion of patients, venous pulses cannot be satisfactorily examined because of one or more of the circumstances enumerated earlier. Here, study of liver pulses assumes great importance. Noncongested livers do not have detectable pulses. Venous

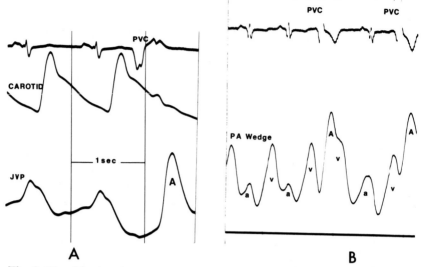

Fig. 8–13. The jugular venous pulse in A and the pulmonary artery wedge pressure in B are intended to show that the *a* waves are generally larger following premature ventricular beats (PVC) when the next P is situated in the ST segment of the QRS of the extrasystole. The arterial pressure pulse associated with premature ventricular beats is frequently quite weak or imperceptible. This is shown in the carotid artery pulse tracing below the ECG in A, showing only a gentle wave representing the pulse in the carotid artery following the PVC, whereas the JVP at this time shows a giant *a* wave. During cardiac catheterization, it is sometimes difficult to differentiate pulmonary arterial pressure from wedge pressure. However, the behavior of the pulmonary artery wedge pressure (PA) in the manner of a venous pressure (i.e., greater amplitude of the *a* wave following premature ventricular beats) distinguished venous pressure, and therefore indicates a proper wedging of the catheter.

congestion of a modest degree is generally required, probably because it renders the edge of the liver accessible for examination. Gentle liver pulses are best appreciated if the palm of the hand is rested on the lower ribs and the fingers are curved and extended over the right hypochondrium. Large liver pulses in tricuspid regurgitation are felt with great ease and even seen as expansile *v* waves (Fig. 8–3, 8–5, 8–9). Prominent *a* waves in pulmonic stenosis and in severe pulmonary hypertension can readily be detected only when there is moderate liver congestion (Fig. 8–14). Pulsations transmitted from a dilated or aneurysmal abdominal aorta are recognized simply by attention to their rapid rise and slow fall. Both the *a* and the *v* waves and on occasion the *c* waves may be recorded (Fig. 8–5, 8–9). Liver pulses are par-

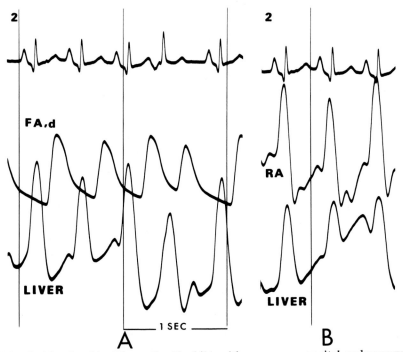

Fig. 8–14. In this 15-month-old child with severe congenital pulmonary valve stenosis with a peak systolic gradient of 120 mm Hg across the valve, complicated by severe anemia and congestive heart failure, very large, peaked *a* waves were recorded both in the liver and in the right atrium (RA). There were numerous premature atrial beats present, one of which is represented by the fourth beat in panel A. A negative P is clearly visible before the QRS, and a sharp *a* wave is present in the liver pulse. The simultaneously recorded intraarterial pressure from the femoral artery (FA,d) demonstrates a smaller amplitude for the premature beat. This patient exemplifies the ease with which atrial systolic waves can be felt and recorded over a congested liver. In this child, like in most infants and small children, it was impossible to record jugular venous pulses because of the short neck and the child's inability to cooperate. In such situations, the liver pulse becomes truly the only accessible venous pulse to be studied. The precipitous fall of the venous *a* waves contrasts with the gradual, slow fall of the arterial pressure.

ticularly suitable for study of the *y* descent. This parameter can be appreciated both visually and through palpation. A steep *y* descent becomes the only detectable negative wave in the venous system when the *x* descent is obliterated by the regurgitant jet in tricuspid insufficiency, or by loss of atrial contraction in atrial fibrillation (Fig. 8–3, 8–5, 8–9). Occasionally in patients with normal sinus rhythm, atrial contractions are so weakened by myocardial disease that no significant *a* wave, and therefore no detectable *x* descent, are present. In such cases, the term *electromechanical dissociation* may be applied to the atrium. Usually, both atria are involved in the same pathologic process and thereby their contractions produce weak or imperceptible pulsations; neither an atrial gallop nor presystolic accentuation nor a diastolic murmur of atrioventricular valvular stenosis would be expected.

In supraventricular and ventricular tachycardias, superimposition of antegrade or retrograde P waves on the QRS, ST, and T deflections make identification of the P wave difficult and frequently impossible. Contrariwise, careful analysis of the jugular venous pulse shows augmentation of *a* waves when atrial and ventricular contractions are approximated or superimposed. We have found the study of venous waveforms to be an important adjunct to a thorough analysis of arrhythmias, first with respect to the existence of atrial contractions, and second, in terms of the temporal relationship between atrial to ventricular depolarizations. Figure 8–15 demonstrates the ease with which inspection of the jugular veins serves to indicate the presence of P waves after ectopic beats by showing very large *a* waves in the neck. In Figure 8–16 unexplained pauses in the routine electrocardiogram were thought to be caused by blocked premature atrial beats because on inspection of the neck veins, large *a* waves could be identified within those pauses. This was subsequently documented by direct right atrial leads.

Atrial flutter and fibrillation may not be easily differentiated from each other by electrocardiography. However, in flutter, examination of the neck veins frequently shows small *a* waves corresponding to regular atrial contractions, and larger *a* waves when atrial systole occurs during ventricular systole (Fig. 8–17). Prominent flutter waves may be associated with audible sounds.[13] A clinical problem which occurs with

---

Fig. 8–15. A. A direct right atrial (RA) lead is recorded with lead V₁, phonocardiogram at the apex and JVP which shows the expected *a*, *c*, and *v* waves. B. One normal sinus beat (3) is followed by an escape beat (4), most probably from the ventricle, and another escape beat with narrow QRS complex (5), is presumed to be junctional in origin. A third ectopic beat from the ventricle which is probably premature (6) is also present. All three ectopic beats are followed by retrograde P waves as seen in the right atrial lead on top, and giant *a* waves (A) in the jugular tracing. It matters little whether the ectopic beats arise from the ventricle or the junction. What determines the extreme height of the *a* waves is the temporal relationship causing contraction of the right atrium against a closed tricuspid valve.

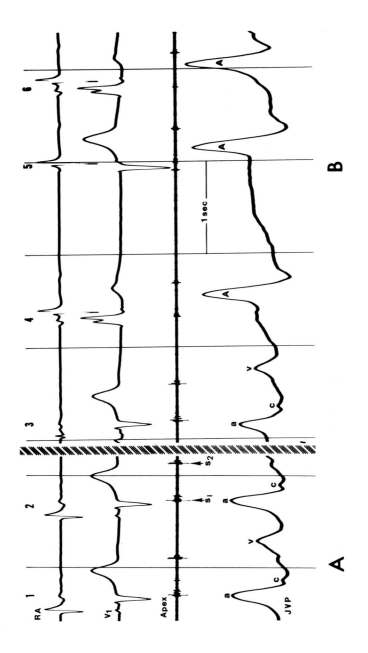

419

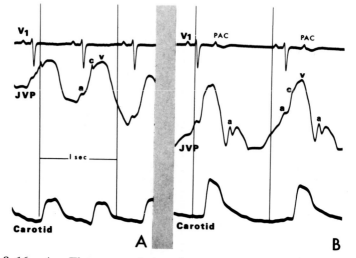

Fig. 8–16. A. Three normal sinus beats are recorded. The JVP tracing shows *a*, *c*, and *v* waves with loss of the *x* descent because of tricuspid regurgitation in this 62-year-old woman with congestive heart failure. The carotid pulse tracing shown at the bottom of panel A is unremarkable.   B. This tracing represents a sudden slowing of the heart rate. A higher than usual V_1 was taken and this allowed the recognition of premature atrial beats marked PAC after each normal sinus beat causing the pause and the apparent slowing of the heart rate. Inspection of the JVP clearly demonstrated the presence of a second *a* wave corresponding to the premature atrial contraction. The pulse from the carotid artery lacks a dicrotic wave and thus the origin of the *a* wave in the JVP was purely venous.

considerable frequency is the differentiation between sinus rhythm and atrial tachycardia or flutter with fixed 2:1 AV conduction, the blocked P generally being hidden in the QRS complexes. Figure 8–18 is from a 17-year-old boy with severe mitral regurgitation and heart failure in whom flutter was present intermittently (Fig. 8–18A). On this occasion, his ventricular rate was regular at 66/min. However, because of large *a* waves during ventricular systole and also changing intensity of the first heart sound, atrial tachycardia with variable block caused by digitalis intoxication was suspected and documented by an atrial augmented lead 2. Two days later (Fig. 8–18B), the pulse rate was still slow but the absence of large venous *a* waves immediately after the QRS complex proved that, at this time, there were no hidden P waves within the QRS, and that the rhythm was truly sinus bradycardia associated with first-degree AV block.

Large atrial contractions or cannon waves resulting from super-

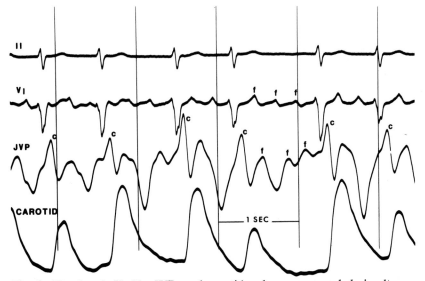

Fig. 8–17. Leads II, V_1, JVP, and carotid pulses are recorded simultaneously in this 58-year-old patient with severe long-standing congestive heart failure secondary to myocardial infarctions in the past. The atrial rhythm is predominantly one of flutter and the f waves can be clearly recognized in lead V_1. Corresponding to these f waves are undulations also marked f in JVP. Recognition of these venous waves at the patient's bedside is generally sufficient for making the diagnosis of atrial flutter or atrial tachycardia. Of course, these atrial systolic waves cannot be recognized if ventricular rate is rapid (see left-hand portion of this figure).

imposition or close proximity of P and QRS deflections can be impressive even in the absence of heart failure and pulmonary hypertension. Furthermore, it does not matter whether the atrial contraction is in response to a normal sinus P wave, an ectopic atrial P wave, or a retrograde P wave coming after an AV junctional or ventricular beat. In Figure 8-19, taken 3 months postoperatively from a patient who developed complete heart block after aortic valve surgery, sinus P waves are seen throughout the tracing. Giant a waves (A) can be seen after beats 3,4 and 5 where P waves occur within or shortly after the QRS complexes. That the mere superimposition of the c wave on the a wave is not responsible for the extreme height of the a wave is shown beneath beat 5 where the separation of the c and a waves has not altered the high amplitude of the a wave. Our studies on the hemodynamic significance of the giant a waves produced by retrograde 1:1 VA conduction during electrical pacing of the right ventricle both in man and in animals suggest that the greatly increased amplitude of

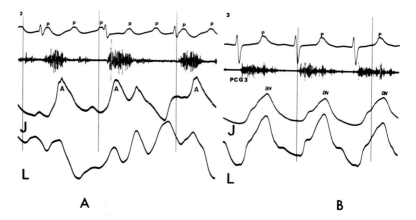

Fig. 8–18.   Recordings from a 17-year-old boy with mitral regurgitation and chronic recurrent atrial flutter.   A.   Lead II, phonocardiogram from the apex, JVP (J), and liver pulses (L) were recorded simultaneously. The atrial rhythm is clearly one of atrial tachycardia with varying AV conduction. Corresponding to each P wave, there is a hump in the JVP, the amplitude of which depends on the relationship between the P and the QRS. The three humps marked A occur during ventricular systole. The liver pulse at the bottom could not be recorded satisfactorily at this time.   B.   Recording taken three days later because the cardiac rhythm had suddenly changed. The effective ventricular rate was about the same as in A, in the vicinity of 72–75 beats/min. However, only one P wave for each cycle could be clearly recognized. Whether the rhythm was one of sinus or one of atrial tachycardia with 2:1 block could not be easily decided from the electrocardiogram. Inspection of the JVP and liver pulses recorded below the electrocardiogram clearly showed the presence of only one *a* wave for each cardiac cycle, indicating the disappearance of the atrial tachycardia and return of normal sinus rhythm with long PR interval.

these waves is generated not only by atrial contraction against a closed tricuspid valve but also by retrograde flow of blood into the venae cavae which can be visualized by selective injection of contrast medium into the superior vena cava. Further, this unfavorable movement of blood together with loss of atrial contribution to ventricular filling substantially diminishes venous return to the ventricles resulting in a 10 to 15 percent fall in cardiac output and associated decline in arterial pressure (Fig. 8–20).

Figure 8–21 depicts arterial pressure in a patient with coronary artery disease who developed junctional rhythm with 1:1 retrograde conduction during periods of myocardial ischemia and angina pectoris. Simultaneously, venous pulses displayed giant *a* waves indicating 1:1

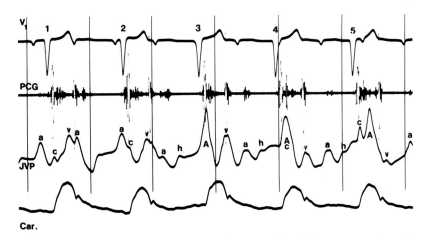

Fig. 8–19. In this 54-year-old man with coarctation of the aorta and aortic valve stenosis, complete heart block occurred after prosthetic valve surgery for the aortic valve. The basic atrial rhythm is normal sinus at the rate of approximately 100 beats/min, and there is complete heart block with wide QRS complexes at the rate of 47 beats/min. The resultant variations in the PR relationship causes marked changes in the *a* waves. In beats 1 and 2 the P waves occur before the QRS and the *a* waves are small in amplitude. The *a* wave of the blocked P between beats 1 and 2 is also small. The P waves occurring within or shortly after the QRS complexes 3, 4, and 5 are associated with giant *a* waves (A). The P wave occurring after the QRS in beat 5 is not within the QRS complex, and it occurs in the ST segment of that beat. The *c* wave of this beat, therefore, is separated from the *a* wave so that both can be clearly recognized. In spite of the separation, the *a* wave (A) is still large. This indicates that the large peaked *a* waves in beats 3 and 4 were not related entirely to the superimposition of the *a* and *c* waves, and that contraction of the right atrium against the closed triscuspid valve played a major role in generating the large *a* waves.

retrograde conduction while the arterial pressure fell precipitously and contributed to the prolongation of the anginal episode. In order to discriminate between the effect of the simple rise in heart rate and that of retrograde flow of blood from the atria into the cavae and pulmonary veins in the production of arterial hypotension, the right atrium was paced at a rate very close to that of the spontaneous junctional tachycardia. In this fashion, two rhythms at nearly equal rates and normal QRS complexes, differing only in their P-R relationship, could be compared. We can see that arterial pressure was markedly lowered when junctional rhythm was present (end of top strip and middle of bottom strip). The retrograde flow of blood in the veins coincident

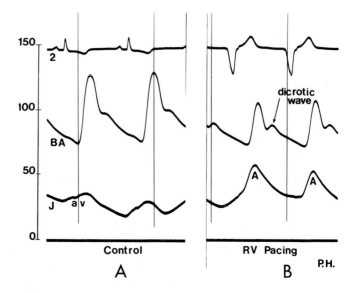

Fig. 8–20. A. Two normal beats in patient P. H. The arterial pressure shows the rapid rate of rise and the JVP shown below that displays *a* and *v* waves with a gentle rate of *y* descent. B. Two beats resulting from stimulation of the right ventricle. The arterial pressure is lower and the dicrotic wave is more prominent. This is related to the lower stroke volume during right ventricular pacing. Each QRS is associated with retrograde conduction to the atrium marked by a distinct notch at the end of the QRS complexes. Together with the retrograde conduction the right jugular venous pulse shows considerably increased amplitude of the *a* waves (A). Because of the time relationship between the QRS and the P, the *a* waves which occur after the QRS merge with the *v* and form single monophasic waves. During these *a* waves (A), blood was forced back from the atrium into both superior and inferior venae cavae, and this was visualized by injection of contrast medium through a catheter with side holes into these veins at the time of right ventricular pacing. The diminished cardiac output at this time could be explained at least in part on the basis of the unfavorable flow of some blood from the atrium retrogradely into the veins and thereby reduced filling of the right ventricle during subsequent diastole.

with the cannon *a* waves was thought to be in great part responsible for the fall in blood pressure. The loss of atrial contribution to ventricular filling is the other important factor. However, the relative contribution of each to the reduction of cardiac output and arterial pressure is not known at this time.

Simultaneous with giant *a* waves, loud sounds are often heard over the jugular veins (Fig. 8–22), their intensity being proportional to the amplitude of the *a* waves. These prominent pulsations occur with sudden, marked distention of the neck veins. Patients may interpret these pulsations as "throbbing" or "beating" in the neck. In taking history from patients suspected of having paroxysmal tachycardias, it is useful to ask if abnormal throbbing of the neck occurs during the paroxysms. Its presence favors ventricular or junctional tachycardia with retrograde conduction. Otherwise, during paroxysms of tachycardia, arterial pulses are diminished or normal in amplitude and, therefore, are unlikely to be interpreted by the subject as forceful throbbing. The large *a* waves associated with retrograde conduction may be preceded by *c* waves if retrograde first-degree AV block is present. Under such circumstances, the *a* wave appears to be bifid (Fig. 8–23).

The study of venous pulses is often of considerable help in differentiating pericardial from myocardial causes of systemic venous hypertension. In pericardial tamponade, the inspiratory augmentation of venous return to the right ventricle is usually preserved and the normal inspiratory fall in cervical venous pressure can be detected. In constrictive pericarditis, on the other hand, jugular venous pressure may paradoxically rise during inspiration (the venous Kussmaul's sign). This is perhaps caused by downward pull of the pericardium which is adherent to the diaphragm, with resultant decrease in the capacity of the right ventricle. The phenomenon of inspiratory rise of cervical venous pressure is also found in severe right ventricular failure and in massive pulmonary embolization, in both of which the right ventricle cannot accept a normal increment of blood during inspiration.

In practice, assessment of respiratory changes of venous pressure is best achieved by inspection of the neck veins, normally showing filling or ascent of the summit of the column of blood as the venous pressure rises during expiration. In pericardial tamponade, it is thought that the limited increase in venous return which is allowed on inspiration results in augmentation in the volume of the right heart chambers within the tense, maximally stretched pericardium. It is postulated that the left heart chambers are thereby compressed which prevents them from accepting venous return from the lungs.[14,15] This differential behavior of the venous return to the right ventricle during inspiration

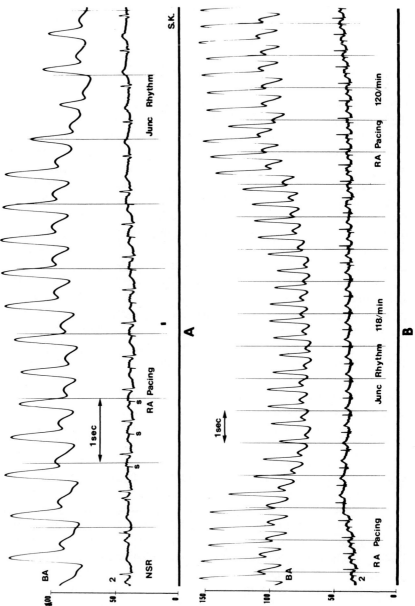

appears to be the reason for the universal existence of marked pulsus paradoxus in pericardial tamponade, as compared with a more modest or even absent paradoxus in chronic constructive pericarditis.

In patients with congestive heart failure and systemic venous engorgement, examination of the jugular venous waveform offers substantial help in distinguishing constrictive pericarditis from heart failure associated with dilation of the right ventricle. Thus, tricuspid regurgitation is usually absent in constrictive pericarditis but present in cardiomyopathies. Further, obliteration of the x descent is characteristic of tricuspid regurgitation, whereas it is present and sometimes exaggerated in constrictive pericarditis (Fig. 8–24). Further, in restrictive cardiomyopathy which is capable of closely mimicking constrictive

---

Fig. 8–21. These tracings of brachial arterial pressure (BA) together with leads II were taken from a 61-year-old man with ischemic heart disease. Attacks of coronary insufficiency were associated with emergence of a junctional rhythm at the rate of 118 per min. During the junctional rhythm, there was 1:1 retrograde conduction to the atrium so that the P waves were situated behind the QRS complexes. A. Rhythm begins with normal sinus and the arterial pressure is about 140/75. The pressure pulse displays a sharp rate of rise. Right atrial pacing began with the third beat and captured the atrium with the fourth beat in which the electrical artifact is marked with an S. The rate of stimulation at this time is slightly faster than the normal sinus rhythm and this is associated with minimal fall in blood pressure. Toward the end of the top strip, atrial stimulation is stopped, following which a self-sustaining junctional rhythm begins. This is best seen in the last four beats of the top strip (Junc Rhythm). Note the precipitous fall in the arterial blood pressure. B. The same phenomenon at a slower rate of paper speed so that larger number of beats can be studied. This strip begins with right atrial pacing for the first four beats with the blood pressure in excess of 150/80. A self-sustaining junctional tachycardia of 118/min begins after cessation of pacing. Now the arterial pressure has fallen to nearly 80 mm Hg systolic pressure. Toward the right-hand portion of the lower strip, atrial pacing is resumed in order to capture the atrium and bring the P waves once again in front of the QRS. Once this is achieved, the blood pressure begins to rise and reaches the previous level of 150 mm Hg systolic. This case, therefore, demonstrates the importance of the position of the P waves in relation to the QRS. The patient is unique in that the QRS complexes remain unchanged during the three different rhythms so that asynchronous intraventricular activation does not play a role. In this patient, giant a waves were visible in the neck during the junctional rhythm. Also note the presence of atrial imprints on the arterial pressure pulse best seen in the first three beats of strip A. It is important to note that atrial impulses can reach as far distally as the brachial artery.

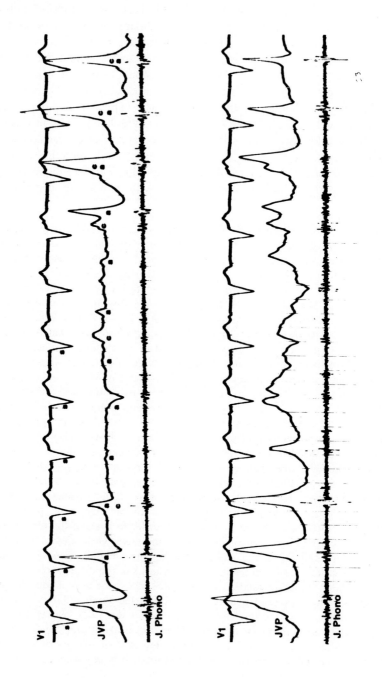

pericarditis, the venous pulses generally show absent or diminished slope of the x descent (Fig. 8–25). Note that the presence of atrial fibrillation in constrictive pericarditis tends to render the x descent shallow and thus detract from its diagnostic value. This may be partly related to the considerable extension of pericardial fibrosis into the myocardium in many of these patients with atrial fibrillation and, therefore, they do not remain relatively pure cases of pericardial involvement. The y descent is brief in constrictive pericarditis because of the restricted volume of the right ventricle, but is usually quite deep and sharp in congestive failure associated with tricuspid regurgitation.

ARTERIAL PULSES

In general, assessment of the arterial waveform may be of less specific value than the venous pulses because the former is more complex and influenced by several factors including the performance of the left ventricle, the caliber of the outflow tract, the nature of any outflow obstruction, the presence of aortic regurgitation, the characteristics of the wall of the large arteries, the systemic arteriolar resistance, and the volume of circulating blood. However, recording of the carotid arterial pulses is indispensable for timing of the cardiac events; the onset of the upstroke indicates aortic valve opening and the incisura on the descending limb coincides with the closure of the semilunar valve (Fig. 8–7). Differentiation between A_2 and P_2 becomes particu-

---

Fig. 8–22. Two strips, each displaying lead V_1, JVP and a phonocardiogram obtained over the right internal jugular vein, are recorded in this patient with complete heart block. The P waves are clearly dissociated from the QRS complexes with constantly changing P-R relationship. The QRS complexes are produced by right ventricular pacing, pacemaker impulses marked by S. When the P waves move into the QRS or appear immediately thereafter in the ST segment, giant a waves are seen and simultaneously prominent sounds are recorded over the jugular veins. This can be seen at the beginning and the end of both strips. In the middle of the top strip, P waves are in front of the QRS and consequently a waves and jugular sounds occurring simultaneously with the a waves are very small. The audible sounds of jugular a waves are usually associated with very large, visible and recordable a waves and retrograde flow of blood with distention of the jugular veins. It is possible that the venous valves play a role in the genesis of these sounds. However, observation of contrast medium moving up the jugular veins has not suggested to us that these valves stop the retrograde flow of blood and contribute to the genesis of venous sounds.

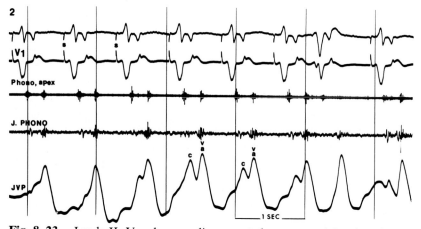

Fig. 8–23. Leads II, V$_1$, phonocardiogram at the apex, and jugular phonocardiogram are recorded with JVP in this patient who had an implanted pacemaker because of persistent sinus bradycardia. Retrograde conduction to the atria is present at 1 : 1 ratio so that the retrograde P waves are seen in the ST segments in lead V$_1$. The result is that the c waves near the end of the QRS complexes occur before the a waves of retrograde P waves. Moreover, the retrograde P waves and the resultant large a waves coincide with ventricular systole and therefore the v waves of the JVP. This reverse temporal relationship makes interpretation of the jugular venous pulse at the patient's bedside difficult. The beat before the last is a premature ventricular beat which is, in turn, followed by a retrograde P wave. Because of prematurity, right ventricular contraction was weak and closure of the triscupid valve was thereby executed with diminished force, the result of which caused the first heart sound and the c wave to be considerably reduced in amplitude, whereas the a wave in the jugular venous pulse and the consequent jugular sound remained unchanged as compared with other beats.

larly certain if simultaneous recordings can be obtained of external pulsations of the main pulmonary artery, from which P$_2$ can be identified. Thus, using the same piezoelectric crystal microphone used for carotid pulses, we have been able to record pulmonary arterial pulses in the second left intercostal space in patients with pulmonary hypertension, especially when large left-to-right shunts are present (Fig. 8–26).

　　Relatively few clinical entities alter the configuration of the arterial pulses in a characteristic and specific manner. Of these, valvular aortic stenosis and idiopathic hypertrophic subaortic stenosis are the best examples (Fig. 8–27, 8–28). The rapidly rising pulse and even its bisferiens quality in aortic regurgitation (Fig. 8–29) can be simulated

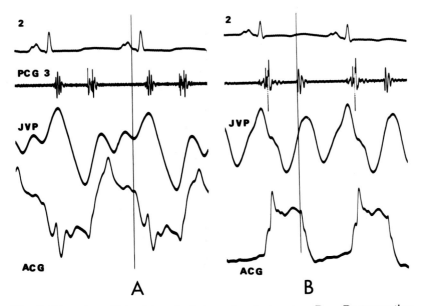

Fig. 8–24. A. Strip taken before pericardectomy. B. Postoperative strip in a 16-year-old boy with subacute constructive pericarditis. The phonocardiogram from the third intercostal space, lead II, and JVP are taken simultaneously with apexcardiogram (ACG). The notable feature here is the sharp and deep x descent which is present preoperatively but becomes normal in appearance postoperatively. The v wave in the preoperative tracing follows a steep rise from the nadir of the x descent, but the y descent is aborted because of the inability of the right ventricle to expand and accept the incoming blood. In the postoperative tracing the y descent has also returned to normal in this patient who derived considerable benefit and became asymptomatic after surgery. The apexcardiogram show an inverted systolic component in the preoperative tracing related to the inward motion of the apex because of adhesions between the heart and the chest wall. In the postoperative tracing, the systolic component has regained its outward displacement.

by high-output cardiac states regardless of the basic mechanism, and also by conditions associated with increased left ventricular preload such as mitral regurgitation and ventricular septal defect. Although the rate of rise of the arterial pressure pulse as recorded indirectly from the carotid arteries may be markedly increased in these conditions, with shortened t time, i.e., the interval from the onset of carotid upstroke to a point midway on its ascending limb, the diastolic pressure is seldom below 60 mm Hg in the absence of aortic regurgitation. Patent ductus

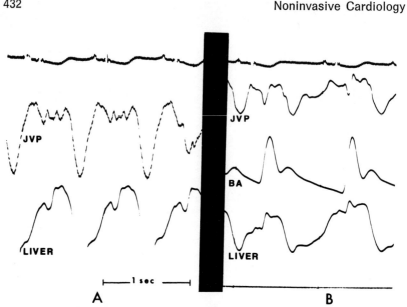

Fig. 8–25. A 54-year-old man suspected of having constrictive pericarditis for a period of 2 years. A. JVP and liver pulses. B. JVP, brachial arterial pulses (BA), and liver pulses. The clinical features were those of marked venous hypertension, a small heart, congested and pulsatile liver, and ascites. Although the steep *y* descent present in the tracing in A did not strongly indicate constrictive pericarditis, the patient underwent exploratory thoracotomy. No pericarditis was found and a myocardial biopsy revealed extensive myocardial fibrosis with the final diagnosis of restrictive cardiomyopathy. In retrospect, the absence of a steep *x* descent and the presence of the deep *y* descent were more compatible with cardiomyopathy than with constrictive pericarditis.

arteriosus and large arteriovenous fistulas exhibit rapidly rising arterial pulses with diastolic arterial pressures which are intermediate between aortic regurgitation and the high-output states.

An exceptional case of high pulse pressure and low arterial diastolic pressure occurred in a 21-year-old girl with advanced obliterative giant cell aortitis occluding all of the major brachiocephalic trunks, leaving the right vertebral artery as the only supply to the brain, and otherwise sparing only the right femoral artery. The arterial pulses in the right leg were strikingly sharp, the pulse pressure wide, and the diastolic pressures very low in the vicinity of 25 mm Hg. There was no diastolic murmur of aortic regurgitation and aortic regurgitation was not present on retrograde aortography (Fig. 8–30). The skin tempera-

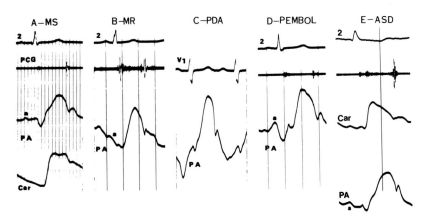

Fig. 8–26. An electrocardiographic lead and phonocardiogram from the third intercostal space are recorded together with impulses from the second left intercostal space in five patients with documented severe pulmonary hypertension. Diagnoses included mitral stenosis (MS), mitral regurgitation (MR), patent ductus arteriosus (PDA), pulmonary emboli (PEmbol) and atrial septal defect (ASD). Note that all the characteristic features of an arterial pulse tracing are present in these records. The incisural notch in the pulmonary artery tracing (PA) corresponds with the pulmonary second sound and, in fact, serves as an excellent indicator of temporal events because, unlike the carotid pulse, little delay related to transmission time is present. We have been able to record pulmonary artery impulses in a variety of situations associated with pulmonary hypertension, especially in patients who have relatively thin chest walls. Such tracings have been useful in identifying the two components of the second sound in complex cases. Generally, pulmonary artery pressure in these patients has been near the systemic level.

ture in the right lower extremity was elevated and the capillaries appeared engorged. The dorsalis pedis artery on the right was dilated on palpation and was as large as a normal brachial artery. The explanation appeared to be that a large portion of left ventricular output entered the right leg in which vascular resistance became minimal and its arterial trunks served as wide-open conduits.

Determination of the arterial diastolic pressure in aortic regurgitation may present a problem when Korotkoff sounds remain audible even when cuff pressure is completely eliminated. The diastolic pressure in such patients is often incorrectly recorded as zero, a value which is physiologically untenable, for even with total destruction of the aortic valve, the arterial diastolic pressure cannot be lower than left

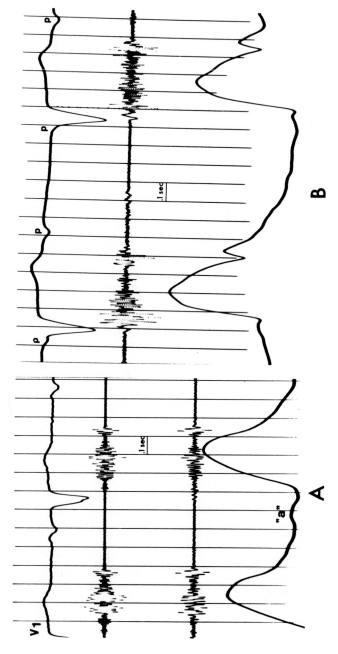

Fig. 8–27. Preoperative (A) and postoperative (B) tracings of lead V_1, phonocardiograms, and carotid artery pulses in a patient with coarctation of the aorta and aortic valve stenosis (same patient as in Fig. 8–19). The postoperative tracing shows very loud clicks of the aortic prosthetic valve. The complete heart block was produced at the time of surgery. Note the characteristic configuration of the carotid artery pulse tracing in the preoperative period: the slow rate of rise, the subtle incisura, and the atrial imprint marked "a." In the postoperative tracing the rate of rise is clearly much higher and the dicrotic notch is better defined.

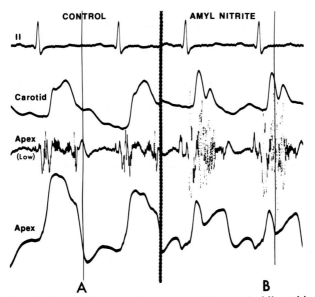

Fig. 8–28. A 52-year-old woman with occult idiopathic hypertrophic subaortic stenosis (IHSS). A. Control tracings at rest show only an unimpressive notch in the carotid artery pulse tracing and an indistinct ejection murmur at the apex of the heart. B. Inhalation of amyl nitrite clearly brought out the midsystolic notch and late-systolic rise in the carotid pulse tracing, very loud systolic ejection murmur at the apex, and midsystolic trough in the apex cardiogram all of which are characteristic of this condition. Patients with IHSS with little or no obstruction at rest have normal carotid pulse and apex tracings before provocative tests such as amyl nitrite inhalation, Valsalva maneuver and isoproterenol infusion which augment stenosis.

ventricular diastolic pressure, which would certainly be markedly elevated under such circumstances (Fig. 8–31). When Korotkoff sounds are audible to the zero level, the diastolic pressure may be determined either by direct manometric recording of the intraarterial pressure, or by the use of the palpation technique. In this technique, the cuff is inflated to above systolic blood pressure and the examiner's index finger is used on the brachial artery instead of the stethoscope. The cuff pressure is then lowered slowly and gradually. At the point of systolic pressure, a brief, sharp tap corresponding to the passage of the summit of the arterial pressure pulse under the cuff is felt. With

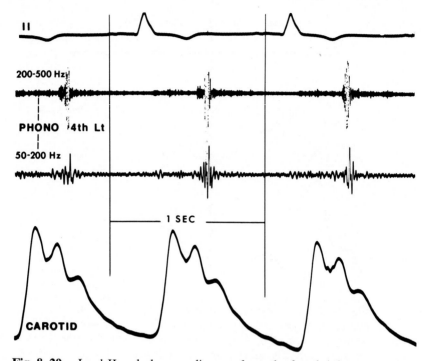

Fig. 8–29. Lead II and phonocardiogram from the fourth left space at two different frequency settings are recorded simultaneously with the carotid artery pulses in a patient with marked aortic regurgitation. The extremely sharp rate of rise in the carotid artery pulse and the midsystolic trough (pulsus bisferiens) are clearly recorded. Note that a similar pulse with a rapid upstroke and bifid configuration can be obtained in patients with high-output states and in IHSS. Differentiation depends upon hearing a decrescendo diastolic murmur of aortic regurgitation.

further lowering of the cuff pressure, greater portions of the arterial pressure pulse make their way through the compressed segment of the brachial artery, imparting the sensation of increasingly full pulse to the examining finger. Finally, at the point of true diastolic pressure the pulse loses its brisk quality and becomes soft and maximally full.

As pointed out earlier, pulsus paradoxus is of great diagnostic significance. We must stress, however, that an elevated central venous pressure is inseparably associated with the mechanism of paradoxus caused by pericardial disease or severe right ventricular failure. When pulsus paradoxus of 10 mm Hg or greater is associated with normal or decreased central venous pressure, subtle arrhythmias (Fig. 8–32) and hypovolemia should be suspected (Fig. 8–33).

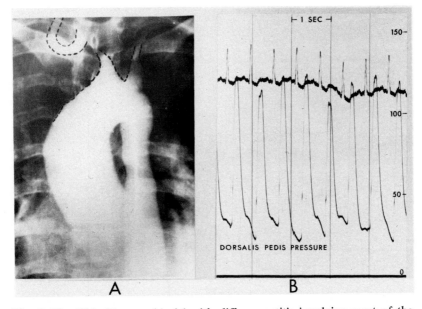

Fig. 8–30. This 21-year-old girl with diffuse aortitis involving most of the major arteries had a retrograde aortagram (A) which documented absence of aortic regurgitation. There was nearly complete occlusion of all of the brachiocephalic trunks, the vertebral artery remaining as the dominant supply to the brain. Further studies in this young woman showed that the left femoral artery was almost completely occluded. The right femoral artery, on the other hand, was wide open and the peripheral arteries in this leg appeared extremely dilated and very pulsatile. The dorsalis pedis on the right was markedly enlarged and pulsated with great vigor. A needle was easily placed in this vessel for the pressure tracings shown in B. The arterial pressure was found to average 120/25. This extremely low diastolic pressure was interpreted as a manifestation of extreme dilation of the arterial channels in the right leg attempting to accommodate a substantial portion of the cardiac output.

In patients with severe left ventricular dysfunction, relatively evenly spaced alterations of strong and weak peripheral pulses may occur with each beat (Fig. 8–34). This phenomenon, known as *pulsus alternans*, is observed most commonly in aortic stenosis, systemic hypertension, cardiomyopathies and coronary artery disease. The precise mechanism leading to the development and perpetuation of pulsus alternans is not firmly established. However, it is generally regarded that there is alteration of the force of ventricular contraction and that variations in contractility, preload, electrical excitability and refrac-

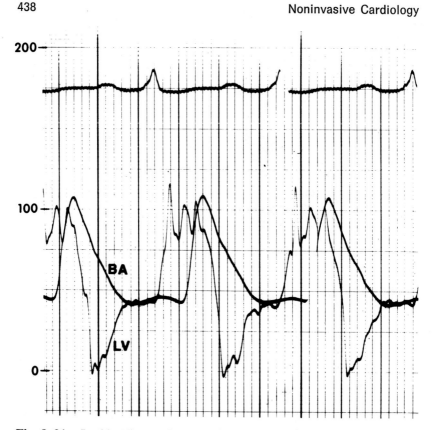

Fig. 8–31. In this 25-year-old man with heroin addiction and bacterial endocarditis, destruction of the aortic valve with a large perforation in one of the cusps was associated with extreme aortic regurgitation and very severe left ventricular failure. Simultaneous left ventricular (LV) and brachial artery (BA) pressures showed equalization of diastolic pressures at the level of 40 mm Hg because the aortic valve no longer served as an obstable between these two chambers. Even complete destruction of the aortic valve cannot lower the arterial diastolic pressure to a level below about 25 mm Hg which would be a reflection of the left ventricular end-diastolic pressure under such circumstances.

toriness, and the number of contracting myocardial fibers might be important.[16] In some patients, pulsus alternans may persist for several days, whereas in other individuals it may be initiated by a premature ventricular contraction and last for only a few beats. In general, the discrepancy between the amplitude of the strong and weak beats and the duration of the phenomenon are directly related to the depression of left ventricular contractile state.

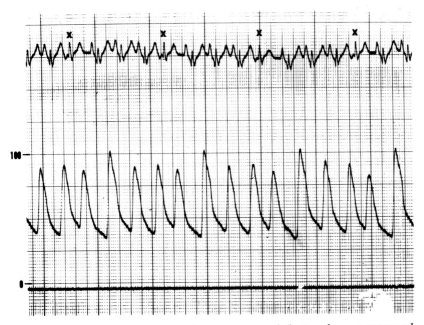

Fig. 8–32. Arterial pressure tracings were recorded at a slow paper speed in this patient with congenital pulmonic stenosis. An apparent pulsus paradoxus was noted for which no explanation could be found. Careful analysis of the electrocardiogram showed that every fourth beat was, in fact, a premature atrial beat (marked *x*). These beats were associated with relatively small arterial pressure pulses. This was, in turn, followed by an amplified pressure pulse and then a return to the normal level in the subsequent two beats. This combination gave the arterial pressure the typical configuration of paradoxus.

SUMMARY

Pulsations of the neck veins, the liver, and more distant venous channels mirror the hemodynamic events taking place in the right atrium and, therefore, are of considerable assistance in the assessment of right ventricular disease and cardiac performance. Some of these useful observations include prominent *a* waves in pulmonary embolism, pulmonic and tricuspid stenosis, reduced right ventricular compliance and certain disorders of cardiac rhythm; large *v* waves with rapid *y* descent in tricuspid regurgitation; inspiratory augmentation of venous pressure in constrictive pericarditis; and steep *x* descent and short *y* segment in differentiating constrictive pericarditis from cardiomyopathy.

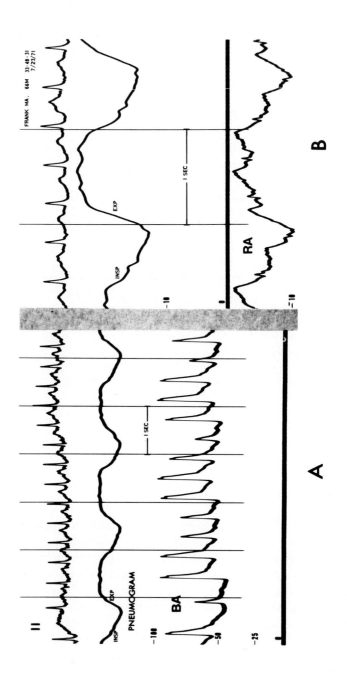

440

Fig. 8–33. A. Marked pulsus paradoxus recorded together with a pneumogram and lead II of the electrocardiogram in a patient with pulmonary embolism of moderate size and congestive heart failure who had been vigorously diuresed. There was no indication of pericardial disease. B. The pneumogram is again recorded together with the right atrial (RA) pressure through a catheter showing the central venous pressure to be below zero and diminishing further with inspiration (Insp). Excessive diuresis in this patient resulted in low blood volume and strong inspiratory efforts produced considerable negative pressure on the pulmonary capillaries, thus holding substantial quantities of blood in the pulmonary bed and markedly reducing left ventricular preload during inspiration. Pulsus paradoxus caused by hypovolemia may be related to low left ventricular preload with this chamber operating on the steep portion of the ascending limb of its function curve. Restoration of blood volume in this patient resulted in disappearance of the pulsus paradoxus.

Transmission of the adjacent arterial channels frequently renders interpretation of the venous waveforms difficult. However, analysis is possible by evaluation of the differential rates of rise and fall of the venous and arterial pulses and the characteristic behavior of these pulses during premature beats and arrhythmias. Study of the configuration of the carotid arterial pulse provides important information concerning specific disorders of the left heart chambers, usually those owing to abnor-

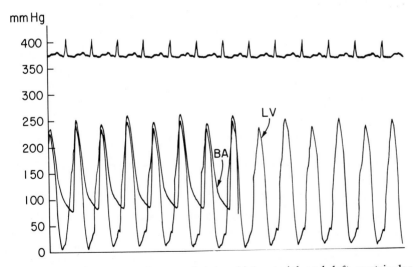

Fig. 8–34. Simultaneously recorded brachial arterial and left ventricular pressures in a patient with severe aortic regurgitation. Pulsus alterans of approximately 15 mm Hg is demonstrated.

malities of the aortic valve and outflow tract. In addition, severe disturbances of left ventricular filling and function may be revealed by peripheral arterial pulsus paradoxus or alterans. Finally, careful inspection of the venous and arterial pulses together with satisfactory recordings often prove to be of great assistance in the analysis of complex arrhythmias.

REFERENCES

1. Colman AL: Clinical Examinations of the Venous Pulse. Springfield, Thomas, 1966, p 15
2. Tavel ME: Clinical Phonocardiography and External Pulse Recording. Chicago, Year Book, 1967, pp 56–58
3. Rios JC, Massumi RA, and Ewy GA: Presytolic displacement of the head: A sign of decreased right ventricular compliance. Circulation 47 (Suppl III):32, 1970
4. MacKenzie J: The Study of the Pulse, Arterial, Venous and Hepatic, and of the Movements of the Heart. New York, Macmillan, 1902
5. Gelfand D: Jugular tracings, in Luisada AA (ed): Cardiology, vol 2. New York, McGraw-Hill, 1959, p 247
6. Turnbull HH: The circular form of liver pulsation and its relation to tricuspid stenosis. Heart 3:243, 1911–1912
7. Colman AL: Demonstration of the jugular venous pulse. N Engl J Med 268: 548, 1963
8. Kerr WJ, Warren SL: Peripheral pulsations in the veins in congestive failure of the heart associated with pulsations of the liver and tricuspid regurgitation. Arch Intern Med 36, 593, 1925
9. Grishman A, Kroop IG, Steinberg MF, Dack S: Presystolic pulsations of the liver in the absence of tricuspid disease. Am Heart J 40:739, 1950
10. Hartman H: Simultaneous recordings of the phonocardiograms, venous and arterial pulses. Arch Inst Cardiol (Mexico) 31:39, 1961
11. Calleja HB, Rosenow OF, Clark TE: Pulsations of the liver in heart disease. Am J Med 202, 1961
12. Massumi RA: Internal mammary arterio-venous fistula. Med Ann Dist Columbia 36:163, 1967
13. Massumi RA: The audible-sounds of atrial tachyarrhythmia (flutter). Circulation, 33:65, 1966
14. Massumi RA: The mechanism of pulsus paradoxus in pericardial effusion. Circulation 39: (Suppl III):142, 1969
15. Gabe IT, Mason DT, Gault HJ, et al: Effect of respiration on venous return and stroke volume in cardiac tamponade. Br Heart J 32:592, 1970
16. Zelis R, Amsterdam EA, Mason DT: Spontaneous pulsus alternans in man: Beat to beat alterations in contractile state. Circulation 43 (Suppl II):242, 1971

Index

        b
  5   c
  6   d
  7   e
  8   f
  9   g
  0   h
  1   i
8 2   j